Clinical Ethics in Pediatrics

A Case-Based Textbook

Clinical Ethics in Pediatrics

A Case-Based Textbook

Edited by

Douglas S. Diekema MD, MPH

Professor of Pediatrics and Adjunct Professor of Bioethics & Humanities, University of Washington School of Medicine; Director of Education, Treuman Katz Center for Pediatric Bioethics, Seattle Children's Hospital, Seattle, WA, USA

Mark R. Mercurio MD, MA

Director, Program for Biomedical Ethics and Professor of Pediatrics, Yale University School of Medicine, New Haven, CT, USA

Mary B. Adam MD, MA, PhD

Clinical Lecturer in Pediatrics, University of Arizona College of Medicine; Research Fellow in Evaluation, Research, and Development Unit, Department of Psychology, University of Arizona, Tucson, AZ, USA

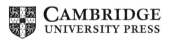

CAMBRIDGE
UNIVERSITY PRESS

CAMBRIDGE
UNIVERSITY PRESS

University Printing House, Cambridge CB2 8BS, United Kingdom

One Liberty Plaza, 20th Floor, New York, NY 10006, USA

477 Williamstown Road, Port Melbourne, VIC 3207, Australia

4843/24, 2nd Floor, Ansari Road, Daryaganj, Delhi - 110002, India

79 Anson Road, #06-04/06, Singapore 079906

Cambridge University Press is part of the University of Cambridge.

It furthers the University's mission by disseminating knowledge in the pursuit of
education, learning and research at the highest international levels of excellence.

www.cambridge.org
Information on this title: www.cambridge.org/9780521173612

First published 2011

A catalogue record for this publication is available from the British Library

Library of Congress Cataloging in Publication data
  Clinical ethics in pediatrics : a case-based textbook / [edited by]
  Douglas S. Diekema, Mark R. Mercurio, Mary B. Adam.
      p. ; cm.
  Includes bibliographical references and index.
  ISBN 978-0-521-17361-2 (pbk.)
  1. Pediatrics–Moral and ethical aspects–Case studies.   2. Professional ethics.
  I. Diekema, Douglas S.   II. Mercurio, Mark R.   III. Adam,
  Mary B.   IV. Title.
  [DNLM: 1. Pediatrics–ethics–Case Reports.   2. Ethics, Medical–Case Reports.
  3. Ethics, Professional–Case Reports. WS 21]
  RJ47.8.C55 2011
  174.2′9892–dc23
  2011017978

ISBN 978-0-521-17361-2 Paperback

Contents

Contents

Contributors

Armand H. Matheny Antommaria, MD, PhD
Associate Professor, Division of Pediatric Inpatient
Medicine
Adjunct Associate Professor, Division of Medical
Ethics and Humanities
University of Utah School of Medicine
Salt Lake City, Utah, USA

Andrew C. Beckstrom, MD
Fellow, Department of Pediatrics, Division of
Neonatology
University of Washington School of Medicine
Seattle, Washington, USA

Jessica Wilen Berg, JD, MPH
Professor of Law, Bioethics & Public Health
Case Western Reserve University
Cleveland, Ohio, USA

Valarie Blake, JD, MA
Fellow, Cleveland Fellowship in Advanced Bioethics
Department of Bioethics, Cleveland Clinic
Cleveland, Ohio, USA

Ellen L. Blank, MD, MA
Associate Professor of Pediatrics and Bioethics
Medical College of Wisconsin
Pediatric Gastroenterologist, Children's Hospital of
Wisconsin
Milwaukee, Wisconsin, USA

Jeffrey R. Botkin, MD, MPH
Professor of Pediatrics
Chief, Division of Medical Ethics and Humanities
Associate Vice President for Research Integrity
University of Utah
Salt Lake City, Utah, USA

Donald Brunnquell, PhD, MA, LP
Director, Office of Ethics
Children's Hospitals and Clinics of Minnesota
Minneapolis and St. Paul, Minnesota, USA

Jeffrey P. Burns, MD, MPH
Chief, Division of Critical Care Medicine
Children's Hospital Boston
Edward & Barbara Shapiro Chair of Critical Care
Medicine
Associate Professor of Anesthesia and Pediatrics
Harvard Medical School
Boston, Massachusetts, USA

E. Charlisse Caga-anan, JD
Fellow, Cleveland Fellowship in Advanced
Bioethics
Department of Bioethics, Cleveland Clinic
Cleveland, Ohio, USA

John C. Carey, MD, MPH
Professor and Vice Chair, Academic Affairs
Department of Pediatrics, University of Utah
Editor-in-Chief, *American Journal of Medical
Genetics*
Salt Lake City, Utah, USA

Christy L. Cummings, MD
Department of Pediatrics, Division of Neonatal-
Perinatal Medicine
Yale Pediatric Ethics Program
Yale University School of Medicine
New Haven, Connecticut, USA

Douglas S. Diekema, MD, MPH
Professor of Pediatrics, University of Washington
School of Medicine
Director of Education, Treuman Katz Center for
Pediatric Bioethics
Seattle Children's Hospital
Seattle, Washington, USA

Denise M. Dudzinski, PhD, MTS
Associate Professor & Director of Graduate Studies
Department of Bioethics and Humanities
University of Washington School of Medicine
Seattle, Washington, USA

Jeffrey Ecker, MD
Associate Professor
Massachusetts General Hospital
Harvard Medical School
Boston, Massachusetts, USA

Norman Fost, MD, MPH
Professor, Departments of Pediatrics and Medical
History & Bioethics
University of Wisconsin School of Medicine and
Public Health
Madison, Wisconsin, USA

Joel Frader, MD, MA
A Todd Davis Professor of General Academic
Pediatrics
Professor of Medical Humanities and Bioethics
Feinberg School of Medicine, Northwestern
University and Children's Memorial Hospital
Chicago, Illinois, USA

Thomas H. Gallagher, MD
Associate Professor of Medicine, Bioethics &
Humanities
University of Washington School of Medicine
Seattle, Washington, USA

Aviva M. Goldberg, MD, MA
Assistant Professor, Section of Pediatrics and Child
Health
Faculty of Medicine, University of Manitoba
Winnipeg, Manitoba, Canada

Emily C. Goodlander, JD
Baltimore, Maryland, USA

Jennifer Guon, JD, MA
Fellow, Treuman Katz Center for Pediatric Bioethics
Seattle Children's Hospital
Seattle, Washington, USA

Rebecca M. Harris
Medical Scientist Training Program Candidate
Medical Humanities and Bioethics Candidate
Feinberg School of Medicine, Northwestern University
Chicago, Illinois, USA

Christine Harrison, PhD
Associate Professor, Department of Paediatrics and
The Joint Centre for Bioethics
University of Toronto
Toronto, Ontario, Canada

D. Micah Hester, PhD
Chief, Division of Medical Humanities
Associate Professor of Medical Humanities and
Pediatrics
University of Arkansas for Medical Sciences, College
of Medicine
Clinical Ethicist, Arkansas Children's Hospital
Little Rock, Arkansas, USA

Ian R. Holzman, MD
Professor of Pediatrics, Obstetrics, Gynecology and
Reproductive Sciences
Chief, Division of Newborn Medicine
Vice Chair for Clinical Affairs
Department of Pediatrics, Mount Sinai School of
Medicine
New York, New York, USA

Annie Janvier, MD, PhD, FRCPC
Associate Professor of Pediatrics, University of
Montreal
Neonatologist and Clinical Ethicist, Sainte-Justine
Hospital
Montreal, Quebec, Canada

Maureen Kelley, PhD
Assistant Professor of Pediatrics, Division of Bioethics
University of Washington School of Medicine
Scholar, Treuman Katz Center for Pediatric Bioethics
Seattle Children's Hospital
Seattle, Washington, USA

Jennifer C. Kesselheim, MD, MBE, M.Ed.
Instructor in Pediatrics, Harvard Medical School
Division of Pediatric Hematology-Oncology
Dana-Farber/Children's Hospital Cancer Center
Boston, Massachusetts, USA

Eric Kodish, MD
Center for Ethics, Humanities and Spiritual Care
F.J. O'Neill Professor and Chair, Department of
Bioethics
Professor of Pediatrics, Lerner College of Medicine
Cleveland Clinic
Cleveland, Ohio, USA

Alexander A. Kon, MD, FAAP, FCCM
Chief, Pediatric Critical Care Medicine
Medical Director, Pediatric Intensive Care Unit
Naval Medical Center San Diego
San Diego, California, USA

Carolyn Korfiatis, BA
Research Associate, Treuman Katz Center for
Pediatric Bioethics
Seattle Children's Hospital
Seattle, Washington, USA

John D. Lantos, MD
Director, Children's Mercy Bioethics Center
Children's Mercy Hospital
Professor of Pediatrics, University of Missouri –
Kansas City
Kansas City, Missouri, USA

Steven Leuthner, MD, MA
Professor of Bioethics and Medical Humanities
Medical College of Wisconsin
Director of the Fetal Concerns Program
Children's Hospital of Wisconsin
Milwaukee, Wisconsin, USA

Marcia Levetown, MD
Principal, Health Care Communication Associates
Houston, Texas, USA

David J. Loren, MD
Assistant Professor of Pediatrics, Division of
Neonatology
University of Washington School of Medicine
Seattle Children's Hospital
Seattle, Washington, USA

Mark R. Mercurio, MD, MA
Professor of Pediatrics
Director, Program for Biomedical Ethics
Yale School of Medicine
Director, Pediatric Ethics Program
Yale-New Haven Children's Hospital
New Haven, Connecticut, USA

Kelly Michelson, MD, MPH
Assistant Professor of Pediatrics
Division of Critical Care Medicine, Children's
Memorial Hospital
Northwestern University Feinberg School of Medicine
Associate Physician, Buehler Center on Aging, Health
& Society
Chicago, Illinois, USA

Geoffrey Miller, MA, MB, MPhil, MD, FRCP, FRACP
Professor of Pediatrics and Neurology
Yale University
New Haven, Connecticut, USA

Howard Minkoff, MD
Distinguished Professor Obstetrics and Gynecology
State University of New York Downstate
Chair, Department of Obstetrics and Gynecology
Maimonides Medical Center
Brooklyn, New York, USA

Christine Mitchell, RN, MS, MTS
Director, Office of Ethics
Children's Hospital Boston
Associate Director, Clinical Ethics
Harvard Medical School
Division of Medical Ethics
Boston, MA, USA

Douglas J. Opel, MD, MPH
Acting Assistant Professor of Pediatrics
University of Washington School of Medicine
Scholar, Treuman Katz Center for Pediatric Bioethics
Seattle Children's Hospital
Seattle, Washington, USA

Malcolm Parker, MB BS, MLitt, LLM
Associate Professor of Medical Ethics
School of Medicine, University of Queensland
Brisbane, Australia

Lainie Friedman Ross, MD, PhD
Carolyn and Matthew Bucksbaum Professor of
Clinical Ethics
Professor in the Departments of Pediatrics, Medicine,
Surgery and the College
Associate Director of the MacLean Center for Clinical
Medical Ethics
University of Chicago
Chicago, Illinois, USA

Stephanya B. Shear, MD
Rochester, New York, USA

Halle Showalter Salas, MPhil
Research and Family Liaison, Seattle Children's
Research Institute
Seattle, Washington, USA

Anthony J. Thomas, Jr., MD, MA, FACS
Professor of Surgery
Department of Bioethics
Center for Bioethics, Humanities and
Spiritual Care
Cleveland Clinic
Cleveland, Ohio, USA

Yoram Unguru, MD, MS, MA
Attending Physician
Division of Pediatric Hematology/Oncology
The Herman and Walter Samuelson Children's
Hospital at Sinai
Berman Institute of Bioethics, Johns Hopkins
University
Baltimore, Maryland, USA

A.A. Eduard Verhagen, MD, PhD, JD
Head of Section General Pediatrics, Dept of Pediatrics
University Medical Center Groningen,
Groningen, the Netherlands

Benjamin S. Wilfond, MD
Professor and Chair, Division of Bioethics,
Department of Pediatrics
University of Washington School of Medicine
Director, Treuman Katz Center for Pediatric Bioethics
Seattle Children's Hospital
Seattle, Washington, USA

David E. Woodrum, MD
Professor of Pediatrics, Division of Neonatology
University of Washington School of Medicine
Scholar, Treuman Katz Center for Pediatric Bioethics
Seattle Children's Hospital
Seattle, Washington, USA

Roger Worthington, PhD
Lecturer and Law and Ethics Lead
Keele University School of Medicine
City General Hospital, Stoke-on-Trent, UK
Assistant (Adjunct) Professor of Medicine
Department of General Internal Medicine
Yale University
New Haven, Connecticut, USA

John Wyatt, MBBS, FRCP
Professor of Ethics & Perinatology
Institute for Women's Health
University College London
London, UK

Preface

Douglas S. Diekema, Mark R. Mercurio, and Mary B. Adam

This is a book for individuals who struggle with the ethical issues that inevitably arise when providing medical care to children. The contributing authors possess expertise in clinical ethics and experience in the clinical world. Most of the authors are clinicians, intimately familiar with the issues they discuss in their chapters. Those who are not clinicians serve as ethics consultants in clinical settings. All of the authors have struggled with difficult ethical situations involving children.

The three of us have been teaching clinical ethics to undergraduates, medical students, and residents for a combined total of over 50 years. Because our clinical practice is pediatrics, most of our teaching involves clinical ethics as it relates to the care of children and their families. Twenty years ago, one of us (DSD) developed a structured curriculum for teaching clinical ethics to the pediatric residents at Seattle Children's Hospital. A description of that curriculum was published in *Archives of Pediatrics and Adolescent Medicine* in 1997 (Diekema & Shugerman, 1997). That article generated significant interest, including pleas from residency programs around the country for resources to help teach the topics outlined in that paper. At the same time physicians and trainees frequently ask whether we can recommend a book that provides a good overview of pediatric ethics. But while there are some terrific books that deal with specific areas within the field (research ethics, neonatal ethics, decision-making on behalf of children), we find ourselves at a loss in identifying a volume that provides a comprehensive overview of the rich array of issues faced by those who care for children in the medical context. This volume is an attempt to provide such a resource.

The aim of this book is to provide a comprehensive overview of the ethical issues faced in pediatric practice. Each chapter begins with a case that illustrates the topic. The discussion that follows in each chapter is grounded by the specific case. We wanted this text to be accessible to readers who did not necessarily have an extensive background in ethics or philosophy, but who wanted to deepen their understanding of the ethical issues faced in pediatrics. Our hope is that this volume will be a useful resource for health care providers who take care of children – an introductory text for those who want to learn about and better understand ethical issues in pediatrics as well as a teaching resource for those who might teach these topics in a residency program, medical school, or undergraduate setting.

Why a case-based textbook of clinical pediatric ethics?

Cases involving children have always been central to discussions of ethics in medicine. In *The Birth of Bioethics*, Albert Jonsen (1998) identifies the 1960s and 1970s as the beginning of the modern era of bioethics. While the Tuskegee Syphilis Studies and the case of Karen Ann Quinlan, among others, are representative of the case studies that initiated some of those early discussions, the truth is that many of the earliest cases discussed by philosophers and theologians in those years involved children. Saul Krugman's *Willowbrook Hepatitis studies* elicited intense discussion in the early 1960s. In 1970, Paul Ramsey published *The Patient as Person*, one of the first texts on medical ethics. A key chapter in that book centers on the question of whether children should serve as research subjects. One of the earliest clinical cases to engender public discourse on ethical issues was the Johns Hopkins Baby Doe story. The year was 1970, and the story involves the birth of a baby with trisomy 21 and multiple anomalies, including duodenal atresia. The parents chose not to allow surgery and the physicians agreed, with the baby dying after two weeks. Several members of the pediatric team, however, questioned the decision. A year later the Joseph P. Kennedy Foundation produced a film titled *Who Should Survive?* that re-enacted the events surrounding the baby's short life and death. That film was shown to thousands of medical students in the decades that followed and became a staple of medical ethics education in a time before clinical ethicists were a common sight in medical centers and medical schools. As an interesting side note, two of the physicians involved in the events surrounding the Hopkins baby, Norman Fost and William Bartholome, went on to become prominent academic bioethicists who helped maintain the focus on issues related to children.

It should be noted that cases remain central to the recognition and discussion of ethical issues in medicine. The early philosophical and theological explorations of ethical issues in the 1960s and 1970s were prompted by events like those that occurred at Willowbrook and Johns Hopkins. The events comprising those cases caused someone to raise an eyebrow, and then ask a question to which nobody could provide a satisfactory answer. Those questions became the source of ethical discourse that over time has changed the way we think about certain issues faced in the care of patients. As new cases arise, they continue to raise new questions that challenge our assumptions and existing standards. Clinical ethics is a living, breathing discipline that continues to evolve as a result of cases. And each of those cases represents a real person with real interests at stake.

Ethical issues faced by pediatricians certainly share features in common with those faced by providers in other specialties. Yet they can also be distinguished. Most decisions in pediatric medicine involve three parties – the clinician, the child/patient, and the parent. Infants and children cannot make decisions for themselves and have not yet developed the kind of narrative that allows a surrogate decision-maker to discern the patient's preferences regarding medical intervention. While we generally assume parents seek the best interests of their children, we may not always be convinced that a specific parental decision accomplishes that goal. A recurring theme through many of the chapters in this book is the struggle to identify the limits of parental decision-making authority, and determine when a parental decision should be challenged. Older children and adolescent patients add another dimension. These individuals may have the ability and desire to be involved in decision-making, but their capacity for "adult-like" decision-making may not yet be fully developed. Determining the right balance between respecting the preferences of an adolescent patient and protecting their future interests represents another common theme in pediatric bioethics. Even the so-called boundary issues may manifest themselves differently in pediatrics, since the boundary being delimited usually involves that between the clinician and the patient's parent or relative rather than between the clinician and the child/patient.

In addition to the clinical realm, health care professionals can be found on hospital ethics committees, institutional review boards, national committees that set policy related to ethics and law, national organ procurement agencies, local, state, and federal committees evaluating triage and scare resource allocation strategies, and state and federal committees concerned with vaccine allocation strategies (i.e., for pandemic influenza) or vaccination requirements for children. These responsibilities involve the application of ethical analysis to issues that affect policy, public health, and populations. Health care professionals who serve these roles will benefit from some understanding of ethical analysis.

The purpose of this book

This book is intended for a broad audience. Its intent is to serve as a primer on pediatric clinical ethics for health care professionals, undergraduates, graduate students, medical students, and residents who seek to better understand the issues that arise in pediatric practice. At the same time, we have written this book to provide a useful resource for those who teach pediatric clinical ethics. Each case-based chapter could easily form the basis of a course lecture, classroom or seminar discussion, small group discussion, or residency ethics conference. Cases represent the soul of each chapter and provide an anchor around which the discussion of each topic can take place. They also remind the reader that ethics is not simply about opinions and theories, but ultimately about coming to a reasoned solution to a difficult problem that involves a very real patient. Taken as a whole, the chapters not only provide an overview of the broad range of issues that comprise pediatric ethics, but also give the reader a sense for the common themes shared by seemingly different ethical issues.

Clinical practice inevitably poses difficult ethical questions. Caring for patients will inevitably lead to situations in which there are disagreements over what is "best" for a patient, over which values should prevail in a given situation, about who ultimately should be able to decide what to do. Clinical practice is driven by the ethical principle of beneficence – the obligation to apply the tools of the health care professions for the good of the patient. This ideally involves the application of medical science. But it also inevitably requires value judgments; for every medical decision is premised on the assumption that what is being proposed medically is good or best for the patient. Disagreements will arise in those situations, and it is important for clinicians to recognize that those disagreements are, at their core, disagreements about values. Recognizing, understanding, and learning how to approach, mediate, and even solve ethical dilemmas requires applying the appropriate tools – the tools of ethical reasoning. Ethics is not ultimately about forming an opinion about a difficult issue, but about being able to give reasons and arguments that have the potential to convince others about the best approach in a difficult situation. These are serious questions that have significant impacts on patients. They deserve serious, thoughtful, well-considered, and reasoned solutions. We have given the chapter authors the freedom to approach their chapter topic as they see fit. This is intentional. Our hope is that it provides the reader with a sampling of different approaches to ethical issues. What is important, however, is that the authors have approached each topic thoughtfully – outlining the issues, making an argument to support a specific approach, and ultimately offering a resolution to the problem.

We do not expect the reader to agree with everything in these chapters. We have asked our expert contributors to provide an overview of each issue, but the issues are by nature controversial. We don't necessarily agree with everything written on these pages, and we don't expect that our readers will. Our hope, however, is that if nothing else the chapters will engender discussion, debate, and further reflection. If we can hope more grandly, our desire is that this book will provide a means for readers to enhance their ability to recognize ethical issues and improve their skills in seeking a reasonable resolution to difficult ethical dilemmas. In many cases, one will come to the conclusion that more than one approach is acceptable. Many ethical issues are difficult precisely because they offer no clearly good way to navigate the conflict. They represent conflicts between important values or commitments. They are frequently infused with uncertainty. In many cases, they are truly tragic in the sense that one must choose between two or more good options, but choosing for one good will forgo the other – as when one must choose between potential recipients in allocating a single kidney, liver, or heart for transplant. Alternatively, tragic ethical dilemmas in medicine take the other form – we must choose between options that can only be described as bad – as when those gathered around the bed of a child who has suffered a severe anoxic brain injury after a prolonged submersion event face the decision of whether to allow the child to die or continue to

use medical technology that may maintain life, but life accompanied by a vegetative existence.

The structure and organization of this book

This volume provides a practical overview of the ethical issues arising in pediatric practice. The case-based approach grounds the bioethical concepts in real-life situations, covering a broad range of important and controversial topics encountered by those who provide health care to children, including informed consent, confidentiality, truthfulness and fidelity, ethical issues relating to perinatology and neonatology, end-of-life issues, new technologies, and problems of justice and public health in pediatrics. A dedicated section also addresses the topics of professionalism, including boundary issues, conflicts of interests and relationships with industry, ethical issues arising during training, and dealing with the impaired or unethical colleague. Each chapter contains a summary of the key issues covered and recommendations for approaching similar situations in other contexts.

We have organized this textbook around six sections. Section 1 addresses core issues in pediatric clinical ethics. These include the topics of parental permission and refusal, the assent of children, adolescent involvement in decision-making, confidentiality, disclosure and keeping diagnostic secrets from children and adolescents, truth-telling, disclosure of errors, parental refusals of certain treatments on the basis of religious or cultural beliefs, and requests for treatments that the physician may be uncomfortable providing.

Many difficult ethical issues face prospective parents and clinicians during pregnancy and at the time of birth. Section 2 encompasses a broad range of ethical issues that arise during the perinatal and neonatal period. These include maternal–fetal conflicts, fetal therapy, the responsible use of assisted reproductive technology, preimplantation and prenatal genetic testing for inherited disorders, dispositions, or traits, and the ethical issues that arise in making decisions in the delivery room and in the newborn period regarding the initiation or continuation of life-sustaining interventions. We have included two chapters related to the latter topic that address quality of life assessment and international variations in the way these decisions get made.

Death is tragic when it occurs in children, and decisions surrounding the death of a child can be difficult for all involved. Section 3 addresses the ethical issues that arise at the end of a child's life, including resolving disputes that occur in making decisions about continuation or initiation of life-sustaining interventions, futility, advanced directives and do-not-resuscitate orders in children, the definition of death, physician-assisted death, and palliative care.

New technologies are frequently accompanied by ethical issues, in some cases ethical issues that have not previously been considered. Section 4 addresses several of the issues that new technologies in pediatrics pose for parents and providers. This section includes discussions of transplantation, enhancement technologies (growth hormone treatment, cognitive enhancement), genetic screening and testing, the introduction of innovative technology in practice, and ethical aspects of human subjects research. Three of the chapters in this section explore the impact of medical innovation or new technologies on groups that may or may not perceive the interventions as beneficial, either because they carry social implications for the group in question (cochlear implants and the Deaf community) or because of disagreement about whether the intervention provides net benefit to the child (sterilizing procedures in children with profound developmental delay and the surgical management of children with disorders of sex development).

Section 5 addresses issues of policy that directly impact the medical care of children. These include allocation decisions (related to resources during a pandemic or disaster) and policy related to school vaccine mandates. We have also included here a chapter that addresses the interesting question of whether health care providers should provide medical support at events that may pose significant risks to the participants (in this case youth boxing).

Finally, we have included a section to address the professional responsibilities of providers. These are topics frequently left unaddressed in other texts. While most of these issues are not directly related to clinical care, they do have implications for the care patients receive. Included in Section 6 are discussions about the impaired health care provider, ethical issues that arise in training (practicing procedures, disclosure of level of experience), physician relationships with industry, and boundary issues in pediatrics (gifts from patients, romantic relationships with patients/family members, caring for the children of friends/relatives). We have also included a final chapter in this section about ethics consultation and ethics committees, since these

mechanisms provide an important resource for clinicians and families struggling with the issues raised in many of the other chapters in this book.

Acknowledgments

This text was truly a collaborative effort. We owe a debt of gratitude to the contributing authors for their stimulating and thoughtful chapters. It is truly remarkable that we could find 50 talented individuals to participate in this endeavor. Almost nobody we asked refused to write a chapter. For your willingness to work with us and for your wonderful contributions, we are deeply grateful.

We are also truly grateful to the wonderful editors at Cambridge University Press. In particular, Nick Dunton helped launch this project. It has been completed only because of his encouragement, patience, and persistence during the early phases of writing this book. Likewise, thanks to Richard Marley for taking over mid-stream and providing us with the support we needed to complete this project. Finally, we couldn't have asked for a better editor than Nisha Doshi. She gently kept us on task, provided superb organizational support, and offered us timely and helpful advice whenever we needed it. We are also grateful to Carolyn Korfiatis, research associate at the Treuman Katz Center for Pediatric Bioethics, whose organizational and editing skills helped make this a better book.

Mark would like to thank his wife, Anna, for her support, patience, and encouragement that made this and so many other professional projects possible. Mary would like to thank her husband, Rod, for his support and encouragement that allowed her the flexibility to pursue this project in the midst of transitioning their lives and work to Africa. Doug would like to thank his wife, Susan, for her support and encouragement, and his children, Nathan and Katie, for their inspiration and patience. All three displayed more patience and understanding as he labored to finish this book than he had a right to expect.

References

Diekema, D.S. & Shugerman, R.P. (1997). An ethics curriculum for the pediatric residency program: confronting barriers to implementation. *Archives of Pediatrics and Adolescent Medicine*, **151**, 609–614.

Jonsen, A.R. (1998). *The Birth of Bioethics*. New York: Oxford University Press.

Ramsey, P. (1970). *The Patient as Person*. New Haven, CT: Yale University Press.

Chapter

Pediatric decision-making: informed consent, parental permission, and child assent

Yoram Unguru

Case narrative

Osteosarcoma is a highly malignant bone cancer with a predilection for spreading to the lungs that primarily affects adolescents. Non-metastatic osteosarcoma has an approximate cure rate of 70%. Patients with osteosarcoma *and* metastases at the time of diagnosis are cured less than 20% of the time. Treatment consists of surgery and chemotherapy. Many children with cancer are treated according to clinical research trials.

Michael, a 15-year-old with metastatic osteosarcoma, has not responded to conventional therapy. For almost one year, he was treated on a therapeutic randomized clinical trial, which consisted of standard therapy (up-front chemotherapy, limb salvage surgery, and postsurgical chemotherapy). When his cancer responded poorly to up-front therapy he was randomized to receive additional "experimental" chemotherapy.

Michael has a very close relationship with his mother, and he has been an active participant in every treatment conference. For the most part, Michael tolerated the treatment; however, he struggled both physically and emotionally with the last 3 months of treatment. Michael's end-of-therapy scans confirmed that tumor was still present in both the bone and the lungs.

Michael's mother wants to proceed with an (unproven) experimental therapy in an effort to prolong his life. Michael, on the other hand, does not desire this intervention. Michael asks the physician not to administer the drug and to allow him to die on his "own terms." Michael's mother (emphatically) states that this is her decision to make and not his. She adds that if the physician is not willing to treat him, she will take him to a doctor who will.

Introduction to ethical issues

Decision-making in pediatrics presents numerous challenges for children, parents, and physicians alike. The related, yet distinct concepts of assent and consent are central to pediatric decision-making. While informed consent is largely accepted as an important ethical and legal principle in adult medicine, the limits of parental permission and the concept of assent continue to be mired in debate. This chapter will examine the issues of parental permission and assent, explore how to resolve disputes between children and their parents, consider the relationship between assent and consent, and offer an effective, practical, and realistically applicable decision-making model.

Ethical principles and discussion

Parental permission and surrogate decision-making

Parents have the legal and moral authority to make medical and other decisions on behalf of their children for several reasons (Diekema, 2004). First, unless proven otherwise, parents are assumed to care about their children, know the unique needs of their children better than others, and are invested in promoting their child's well-being. Second, the interests of family members may conflict, and parents are presumably more able than outsiders to balance the competing interests of family members in making a final decision. Finally, as caretakers, parents will have to contend with the consequences of the choices they make on behalf of their children.

Parenthood alone, however, does not qualify one as an adequate surrogate decision-maker. A parent or guardian must meet four preconditions in order

Clinical Ethics in Pediatrics: A Case-Based Textbook, ed. Douglas S. Diekema, Mark R. Mercurio and Mary B. Adam. Published by Cambridge University Press. © Cambridge University Press 2011.

to make decisions for someone else (Beauchamp & Childress, 2001, p. 154). Surrogate decision-makers must: (1) be competent to make reasoned judgments; (2) possess adequate knowledge and information; (3) be emotionally stable; and (4) be committed to the incompetent patient's interests.

The second and fourth preconditions seem particularly relevant for pediatricians. Specifically, physicians have a duty to make sure that parents have enough information to make a thoughtful decision. How much information is truly "adequate?" While this question is frequently discussed, it should minimally include the information that a reasonable person would consider relevant to the decision-making task. Physicians also have an independent duty to guard the welfare of those patients, like children, who cannot protect their own interests. While most parents seek to act in their child's best interest, there are times where a parental decision might place a child at risk of serious harm. In those situations, the physician has a duty to identify when a parent or surrogate's decision jeopardizes a child's well-being.

Assent is not consent

Informed consent is a process grounded in the notion of respect for persons. Autonomy is the right of a rational person to make his or her own decisions and provides a moral justification for the doctrine of informed consent. Capacity to consent requires the legal ability to enter into a valid contract and the psychological or developmental ability to make sound decisions. Hence, minors cannot give valid consent, but they may give assent. Consent for adults is based on the principle of autonomy, which in turn focuses on competence, a legal term. Assent on the other hand is better viewed as focusing on capacity, a developmental term.

Participation of children in non-therapeutic research notwithstanding, assent refers to the active agreement of a minor to participate in a diagnostic or treatment regimen. The ethical principle of pediatric assent recognizes that children (especially adolescents) are capable of participating at some level in decision-making related to their care. The assent requirement seeks to respect children as individuals with emerging autonomy (National Commission, 1978). Above all else, assent is about respecting children's "developing capacity" (Bartholome, 1996), assisting them in understanding their condition and treatment at a developmentally appropriate level, and involving them in appropriate decision-making tasks.

In contrast to informed consent, a less exacting capacity for decision-making is necessary for a child to meaningfully assent. Assent empowers children to the extent that they are capable. Meaningful assent requires an appreciation of the child's developmental stage *and* recognition of his or her basic preferences. Children should be included in medical decisions to the extent they are able to and want to be involved (Unguru et al., 2008). Children need to be encouraged by parents and physicians to communicate openly so that they may be active participants in the assent process. Shared decision-making empowers children to the extent of their capacity (Geller et al., 2003).

Assent differs from consent to the extent that, while the willingness of a minor to accept treatment is an important goal, the minor is not the ultimate decision-maker. Treatment (based on a child's best interest) often may proceed against the minor's wishes if his or her parents consent. Thus, parental permission may trump assent and is legally binding.

Assent and decision-making capacity

Beyond a child's desire to make decisions, understanding or capacity is a critical component of assent. Capacity for decision-making is not a fixed phenomenon, but rather a process that matures with time and experience. Not all children experience life, health, or disease in exactly the same way, and each child's personal experiences with decision-making are unique. These experiences contribute to the child's unique capacity for decision-making. Children of varying ages possess varying abilities to synthesize information and to make decisions accordingly. In general, children 14 years and older appear to be as competent as adults in making informed treatment decisions (Weithorn & Campbell, 1982). Age alone, however, does not indicate a child's ability to understand. Knowledge, health status, anxiety, experience with decision-making, and each child's unique cultural, familial, religious background, and values all play a role in children's understanding of their situation and impact their ability to make decisions. Children with poor health (often resulting in more experiences and a greater role in decision-making) or whose parents have allowed them to make "life decisions," seem better equipped to appreciate that their choices carry certain consequences and thus, they may have a greater understanding of what is required to assent to participate in medical (and research) decisions than healthy children or children whose parents have insulated them from making decisions.

Barriers influencing a child's ability to participate in decisions

For assent to be valid, it must be voluntary. A child's freedom to choose may be influenced by many competing interests that call into question if a child is ever truly a voluntary decision-maker. Each decision or choice a person makes is ultimately influenced by and affects others, and children are no exception. It is useful to consider how children, especially sick children, see themselves and view their place within their larger social networks and how that may affect their ability to participate in decision-making. In their seminal work on informed consent, Faden and Beauchamp (1986) identified the concept of "role constraints," which serve to limit a person's ability for autonomous expression. They assert that the expectations associated with the role of a patient are constraining, and a unique feature of this role is to place the (child) patient in a passive position with authority figures, i.e., physicians and parents, who assume a more powerful and controlling position. Therefore, the ability of a child to voluntarily make a decision is limited by the child's role as a hospitalized or an ill patient. Children are particularly vulnerable to influences in medical consent/assent situations because of their physical, emotional, and financial dependency upon adults (Grodin & Alpert, 1983) and because of their relative inexperience with health care-related decisions. Subsequently, minors may regress to dependency on significant others (Weithorn & Scherer, 1994) rather than achieving their potential as developing decision-makers. Although adolescents may possess the skills to make informed treatment decisions, they often lack perspective and life experience. As such, they are more likely to act impulsively and to focus on their current situation rather than the future.

Parents present another barrier to children's involvement in medical decision-making. Many parents feel that decisions about a child's health care belong to them alone, regardless of the child's awareness or capacity (Bluebond-Langer et al., 2005). Some parents are not aware that it is acceptable to include their child in the decision-making process (Angst & Deatrick, 1996). Thus, it may become the *physician's* responsibility to broach the topic of children participating in decisions about their care. Ideally, physicians need to do this relatively early in discussions with families and should revisit the point periodically to assure that a child's increased decision-making parallels their developmental growth. For assent to be more than a mere symbolic gesture, it needs to be viewed as a *process*, rather than as a one-time event. This necessitates that assent be periodically revisited. As a child matures, gaining both life- and health-related experience, physicians must ensure that the information provided and issues discussed are commensurate with the child's increased level of maturity and experience. Physicians need to continually remind themselves that a meaningful application of assent requires the involvement of the child, physician, *and* parents.

Determining the validity of a child's decision

For a decision to be valid, it must be voluntary and informed. No universally accepted standard defines decisional capacity. Whether a person possesses decisional capacity depends on the *type* of decision and the *risks and benefits* involved. Capacity is linked both to developing cognition and to prior life experiences.

Decision-making capacity by children requires that the child possess the freedom to make a choice. The choice must be both reasonable and rational, and the child must understand information that is relevant to that choice. Thus, prior to soliciting assent from a child, it is crucial that the physician assess the child's level of understanding of the details of the proposed diagnostic and treatment plan (including potential risks and benefits). This is one way to assure that assent is significant and meaningful. However, assessing understanding alone is not sufficient. The process of obtaining a child's assent requires several steps (American Academy of Pediatrics, 1995): the physician must (1) help the patient achieve awareness of their condition; (2) tell the patient what they can expect regarding diagnosis and treatment; (3) assess the patient's understanding; (4) assess factors influencing patient responses (i.e., undue pressure); and (5) solicit the patient's willingness to accept care.

Balancing children's, parents', and caregivers' goals

Children typically want to be involved in decisions that concern their bodies and health. They also generally recognize their role in decision-making as intertwined with that of their parents and appreciate and respect their parents' input (Rossi et al., 2003; Unguru et al., 2010), particularly when they perceive a situation to be more risky (Geller et al., 2003). Most children do not expect to make decisions on their own, but wish to be involved in the process and have their opinions respected. Shared decision-making helps children to clarify values and preferences (Geller et al., 2003). Although most children prefer joint decision-making with their parents, many do not believe that decisions made by parents or physicians should be absolute (Levenson et al., 1982; Dunsmore & Quine, 1995; Snethen et al., 2006; Unguru et al., 2010). This emphasizes the importance of parents helping children to recognize their abilities and responsibilities as part of the process that constitutes meaningful assent.

The AAP encourages pediatricians to evaluate each child's capacity for assent on an individual basis. Based on their development, children are encouraged to "provide assent to care whenever possible" (American Academy of Pediatrics, 1995). The AAP views assent as a process that ideally incorporates *joint decision-making* by all parties. The Academy endorses the view that discussion leads to the development of a meaningful relationship between a child and physician and it is this aspect of assent that is paramount in the process.

Clinicians should make every effort to provide parents with the tools to allow their children to think independently. Doing so enables children to make reasoned and valid, age-appropriate decisions knowing that they can rely on their parents to support these decisions. Children learn to make good, sound decisions with practice and by relying on those they trust. Parents and children may not be in a position to fully recognize the extent to which their relationship may serve to limit a child's ability to make free or voluntary decisions. Thus, it is the physician's responsibility, as the child's advocate, to serve as a facilitator and to assure that this process occurs.

Suggestions for a practical decision-making model with appropriate roles for children, parents, and physicians

A strategy that accounts for a child's developmental level as well as his or her unique medical background and history of decision-making combined with familial preferences is most appropriate. A tangible model of assent gives children of all ages choices (King & Cross, 1989). As children age and gain experience with decision-making they ought to be involved to a greater extent in decisions. Parents and physicians should

evaluate a child's decision-making prowess and then designate a role that not only allows the child to make appropriate decisions but which concurrently challenges his or her abilities.

This strategy results in one of three decision-making roles determined by the child's capacity and the gravity of the decision to be made. Some decisions will be made exclusively by the child with minimal to no parental input; some decisions will place the parents in a more central role while children will be "consulted" for their preferences; and finally, some decisions will be made exclusively by parents and children will be asked only to ratify the decision. For example, (1) a child might have decisional priority for choosing how blood is to be drawn (i.e., right or left arm; with or without a local anesthetic); (2) the child could decide at what time of day a medication is taken, but not refuse to take it; (3) the child could approve of a life-saving intervention, but not be permitted to refuse it. Allowing children a developmentally appropriate role in decision-making respects them as persons with developing autonomy, it allows them to learn from the decisions they make and to improve upon future decisions, and it provides them with a sense of control and ownership that comes with making decisions related to one's health.

Children, parents, and physicians need not be equal in status when it comes to medical decision-making, but it is vital that each party have the opportunity to voice his or her desires and concerns (Bluebond-Langer et al., 2005). Parents need to understand the importance of listening to their child's voice and consider what the child says as meaningful. Children need to appreciate that decision-making is a joint endeavor and while their input will be factored into the final decision, it is not theirs alone to make, nor will it necessarily be binding. Thus, by establishing ground rules and intervening where appropriate, the physician is able to shoulder some of the burden and ease what is a potentially contentious and stressful time for both children and parents.

Conclusions and practical suggestions

Since children do not, in general, have the ability to protect their own interests, they must rely on others to do so. Parents provide that function as the legal decision-makers for their children. The process of assent serves a different function. Assent gives children a voice in decisions, showing respect for their developing autonomy. Physicians are in a unique position to educate parents and the child about the child's condition and options, and to help parents and children understand each other's role and responsibilities. Parents need to know that their authority will be honored, but that they must consider their child's opinions. Children must be given a range of choices. This will enable them to be involved in the assent process and provide them with a sense of control and empowerment. Children also need to know that while they will be allowed to participate in the process, their decisions may be overridden and the reasons for this should be revealed to them. Effective communication is a prerequisite for shared decision-making and shared decision-making is a strong foundation on which to base assent.

Case resolution

As a 15-year-old, Michael is sufficiently mature to understand the issues related to his treatment and to participate in decision-making. His experience with his disease and past treatment regimens has also resulted in a level of maturity that exceeds his age. Michael understands the nature of the proposed treatment, including its risks and expected benefits. He has voiced the opinion that he does not wish to proceed with an experimental regimen, an opinion not shared by his mother. Given his level of maturity, failure to respect his wishes, especially regarding an experimental treatment regimen that is unlikely to significantly alter the course of his illness, would be profoundly disrespectful and potentially harmful, leading to feelings of isolation and distress (American Academy of Pediatrics, 2000). Situations like this one do not lend themselves to easy solutions. By helping to facilitate, clarify, and resolve areas of contention, pediatricians can be extremely helpful. The challenge for pediatricians is to do so in a way that is both sensitive and respectful of the child's, parents', and providers' needs, needs that are often in conflict with one another. In many cases, simply by providing a space where Michael and his mother can speak freely about their choices and the reasons for those choices will lead to a solution that is acceptable to both. Michael needs his mother to hear what he is saying, and the physician's role in this case is not simply to override his desires, but to facilitate the opportunity for his mother to understand what he needs in this difficult situation.

References

American Academy of Pediatrics, Committee on Bioethics (1995). Informed consent, parental permission, and assent in pediatric practice. *Pediatrics*, **95**, 314–317.

American Academy of Pediatrics, Committee on Bioethics and Committee on Hospital Care (2000). Policy Statement: Palliative Care for Children. *Pediatrics*, **106**, 351–357.

Angst, D.B. & Deatrick, J.A. (1996). Involvement in health care decisions: Parents and children with chronic illness. *Journal of Family Nursing*, **2**, 174–194.

Bartholome, W.G. (1996). Ethical issues in pediatric research. In *The Ethics of Research Involving Human Subjects*, ed. H.Y. Vanderpool. Frederick, MD: University Publishing Group, 339–370.

Beauchamp, T.L. & Childress, J.F. (2001). *Principles of Biomedical Ethics*, 5th edn. New York: Oxford University Press.

Bluebond-Langer, M., DeCicco, A., & Belsco, J. (2005). Involving children with life-shortening illnesses in decisions about participation in clinical research: A proposal for shuttle diplomacy and negotiation. In *Ethics and Research with Children: A Case-Based Approach*, ed. E. Kodish. New York: Oxford University Press, 336.

Diekema, D. (2004). Parental refusals of medical treatment: the harm principle as threshold for state intervention. *Theoretical Medicine*, **25**, 243–264.

Dunsmore, J. & Quine, S. (1995). Information, support, and decision-making needs and preferences of adolescents with cancer: implications for health professionals. *Journal of Psychosocial Oncology*, **13**(4), 39–56.

Faden, R.R. & Beauchamp, T.L. (1986). *A History and Theory of Informed Consent*. New York: Oxford University Press, 368–373.

Geller, G., Tambor, E.S., Bcrhardt, B.A., Fraser, G., & Wissow, L.S. (2003). Informed consent for enrolling minors in genetic susceptibility research: a qualitative study of at-risk children's and parent's views about children's role in decision-making. *Journal of Adolescent Health*, **32**, 260–271.

Grodin, M.A. & Alpert, J.J. (1983). Informed consent and pediatric care. In *Children's Competence to Consent*, ed. G.B. Melton, G.P. Koocher, & M.J. Saks. New York: Plenum Press, 93–110.

King, N. & Cross, A. (1989). Children as decision makers: Guidelines for pediatricians. *Journal of Pediatrics*, **115**, 10–16.

Levenson, P.M., Pfefferbaum, B.J., Copeland, D.R., & Silberberg, Y. (1982). Information preferences of cancer patients ages 11–20 years. *Journal of Adolescent Health Care*, **3**(1), 9–13.

National Commission for the Protection of Human Subjects of Biomedical and Behavioral Research (1978). Research involving children: Report and Recommendations of the National Commission for Human Subjects of Biomedical and Behavioral Research. *Federal Register*, **43**(9), 2084–2114.

Rossi, W.C., Reynolds, W., & Nelson, R.M. (2003). Child assent and parental permission in pediatric research. *Theoretical Medicine*, **24**, 131–148.

Snethen, J.A., Broome, M.E., Knafl, K., Deatrick, J.A., & Angst, D.B. (2006). Family patterns of decision-making in pediatric clinical trials. *Research in Nursing and Health*, **29**(3), 223–232.

Unguru, Y., Coppes, M.J., & Kamani, N. (2008). Rethinking pediatric assent: from requirement to ideal. *Pediatric Clinics of North America*, **55**, 211–222.

Unguru, Y., Sill, A., & Kamani, N. (2010). The experiences of children enrolled in pediatric oncology research: implications for assent. *Pediatrics*, **125**, e876–e883.

Weithorn, L.A. & Campbell, S.R. (1982). The competency of children and adolescents to make informed treatment decisions. *Child Development*, **53**, 1589–1598.

Weithorn, L.A. & Scherer, D.G. (1994). Children's involvement in research participation decisions: psychological consideration. In *Children as Research Subjects: Science, Ethics, and Law*, ed. M.A. Grodin & L.H. Glanz. New York: Oxford University Press, 133–179.

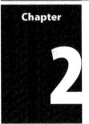

Pediatric decision-making: adolescent patients

Emily C. Goodlander and Jessica Wilen Berg

Case narrative

Daniel Hauser was a 13-year-old boy from Sleepy Eye, Minnesota who, in early 2009, was diagnosed with stage IIB nodular sclerosing Hodgkin disease. Doctors determined that the cancer was readily treatable with chemotherapy, predicting an 80–95% chance of complete remission after 5 years. Daniel was prescribed six cycles of chemotherapy followed by radiation to treat the cancer. Daniel's parents initially consented to the course of treatment, but abruptly refused to continue treatment after only one round of chemotherapy because of side effects (e.g., fatigue and nausea). The Hausers sought opinions from five other physicians, including three pediatric oncologists, who all strongly recommended continued chemotherapy.

Despite a bleak chance of survival without chemotherapy and radiation, Daniel and his parents refused to continue the prescribed treatment and decided to use alternative therapies. Specifically, Colleen Hauser sought to treat her son with dietary changes and ionized water that would "starve the cancer" from his body (*In the Matter of Hauser*, 2009, p. 28). The Hausers justified their refusal of further chemotherapy by claiming it would violate the family's and Daniel's religious beliefs. Although the Hauser family was not of Native American descent, the family subscribed to the beliefs of Nemenhah, a Native American religious organization. Nemenhah doctrine advocates the use of Native American holistic medical practices, and a central tenet is the principle of "do no harm." Colleen Hauser, in particular, believed that "God intends for the body to be healed in a natural way." (*In the Matter of Hauser*, 2009, p. 29). As such, the Hausers viewed chemotherapy as self-destructive and poisonous. Daniel, himself, asserted that he was a Medicine Man in the Nemenhah

tradition, and that use of chemotherapy would violate his religious beliefs and status.

General ethical and legal issues in decision-making for adolescents

This chapter will discuss the ethical and legal issues involved in adolescent medical decision-making. It focuses on treatment decision-making and does not address the specific requirements for adolescent participation in research protocols. We start below with a general discussion of the issues, including adolescent autonomy, capacity, and the scope of parental authority. We then outline the situations in which adolescents are legally authorized to make medical decisions without parental involvement. The final section applies the key points to the case study described above.

Adolescent autonomy and decision-making capacity

Autonomy

The principle of respect for autonomy remains a fundamental hallmark of modern bioethics. Autonomy has been defined as "at a minimum, self-rule free from both controlling interference by others and from limitations, such as inadequate understanding, that prevent meaningful choice" (Beauchamp & Childress, 2001, p. 58). This conception of autonomy requires two elements: liberty (freedom from controlling influences) and agency (capacity for self-rule) (Beauchamp & Childress, 2001, p. 58). Decision-making capacity develops during the adolescent years, raising questions about how to deal with minors' emerging autonomy. During this time, parents wield enormous control over their minor children both directly and indirectly

Clinical Ethics in Pediatrics: A Case-Based Textbook, ed. Douglas S. Diekema, Mark R. Mercurio and Mary B. Adam. Published by Cambridge University Press. © Cambridge University Press 2011.

through the values and beliefs they instill. Adolescents are usually socially and economically dependent on their parents, both of which challenge the notion of freedom from controlling influences. This raises a particularly difficult conflict in the pediatric setting – we must simultaneously recognize the limits parental influences place on adolescent autonomy, and also that in some cases the minor may be making certain choices as a way of rejecting parental influence. Autonomy in the adolescent context is thus a fluid concept. As a result, adolescents fall into an ethical and legal gray area, where the contours of decision-making capacity and autonomy are imprecise and frequently determined on a case-by-case basis.

Capacity

As noted above, autonomy requires both liberty and agency, or capacity. Key elements of capacity include the "degree to which an individual has the ability to understand a proposed therapy or procedure, including its risks and benefits, and alternatives; to communicate relevant questions; and to arrive at a decision consistent with his or her values" (Cummings & Mercurio, 2010). The fields of law and medicine have struggled with identifying a particular age or uniform standards to determine when adolescents develop sufficient decision-making abilities. The result has traditionally been a blanket legal presumption that patients who have not yet attained the age of majority (which may vary between 16 and 18 years old, depending on the state in question) lack capacity, with a few exceptions discussed below.

A more nuanced approach, but one that still relies on generalities, is the "Rule of Sevens." Minors under the age of 7 years are presumed to be lacking the relevant capacities, minors aged 7–13 years old are presumed to be developing capacity and decisions may be made on a case-by-case basis, and minors 14 years and older are presumed to have capacity to make medical decisions, unless evidence is provided to the contrary (*Cardwell v. Bechtol*, 1987). The Rule of Sevens is supported by growing medical evidence. For instance, several sources (Weithorn & Scherer, 1994; Hartman, 2000) have identified the age of 14 as a developmentally relevant watermark for decision-making capacity. Based on their research, Weithorn and Scherer have noted that "the cognitive functioning of a fourteen year-old clearly appears sophisticated enough and sufficiently grounded in reason to meet legal criteria of competency to consent to most types of treatment" (1994,

p. 152). This view is not without its drawbacks. It still groups minors by age, and may not accommodate vast individual differences based on actual development or experience. The approach also fails to take into account the maturity required for different types of decisions (e.g., simple versus complex, life-sustaining versus routine treatment). Furthermore, although minors 14 years and older may have greater decision-making capacity than younger minors, "competent children are not similarly situated to their adult counterparts" due to a shortage of life experience (Ross, 1997, p. 166). Finally, the most recent data on brain development suggest that some abilities crucial to medical decision-making (such as the capacity to appreciate long-term risks) may not fully develop until the mid-twenties – far beyond even the legal age of majority.

Parental authority – source and limits

Parents are legally authorized to consent to (or refuse) medical treatment for their minor children. We assume that parents are best able to ascertain their children's interests and act in accordance. This parental right is deeply rooted in ethical and legal traditions. The Supreme Court of the United States has long recognized the right of parents to the care, custody, and nurture of their children as a protected liberty interest under the Fourteenth Amendment (*Meyer* v. *Nebraska*; *Pierce* v. *Society of Sisters*; *Wisconsin* v. *Yoder*). Parents have wide latitude to direct their children's upbringing, from schooling to religious training to reasonable corporal punishment. This right has been expressly extended to include the right to make medical decisions for their children. Parents' status as decision-makers has a practical component as well. When a patient makes an informed decision, he or she must be prepared to live with the attendant consequences. Parents are responsible for caring for their minor children, including any corresponding financial obligations. Thus, a parental role in decision-making seems necessary and appropriate.

A parent's right to make medical treatment decisions for a minor is limited. Under certain circumstances, the state and courts will intervene in the decision-making process. Laws pertaining to child abuse and medical neglect may restrain parents from refusing beneficial medical treatment for their children. The propriety of state intervention often depends on balancing the potential harm of refusal (including whether the harm is life-threatening or irreversible) against the strength of the preferences and values of the minor and the parents. The vast majority of refusals of medical care, made by parents and/or minors, are based on religious objections. Although religious freedom is a highly protected constitutional right, religiously motivated treatment decisions are not immune to being overridden when a child's welfare is at stake. Religious objections to medical treatment are frequently upheld on legal grounds, but some professional associations have called for an end to such exemptions when children are denied therapeutic treatment (Committee on Bioethics, 1997). As the Supreme Court famously stated in limiting religious freedom, "Parents are free to become martyrs themselves. However, it does not follow that they are free, in identical circumstances, to make martyrs of their children before they have reached the age of full and legal discretion when they can make that choice for themselves" (*Prince* v. *Massachusetts*, 1944, p. 170).

Legal authority of minors to make decisions

The law recognizes certain situations in which the balance between a minor's autonomy and parental authority has been resolved in favor of allowing adolescent decision-making. Every state has laws identifying circumstances in which an adolescent's consent alone is legally sufficient to obtain medical care. In addition to the exceptions described below, there are specific legal rules in two other areas, which we will not discuss in this chapter. The first, adolescent decision-making for abortion, varies from state to state and may require judicial involvement. The second is the general emergency exception to informed consent, which functions for both adults and minors, allowing treatment in the absence of any decision-making by either the patient or the patient's family. The exception applies only in the case of true emergencies, when there is no time to elicit consent.

Public health exceptions

The majority of minor consent laws are rooted in public health policy. The laws primarily address: (1) access to contraception and family planning services (not including sterilization or abortion); (2) diagnosis and treatment of sexually transmitted infections (STIs); (3) mental health treatment; and (4) substance abuse treatment. All states have enacted minor consent laws in some or all of these areas, but there remains little uniformity regarding the prerequisites

to consent. Age and status requirements, types of treatment permitted, and other limitations on consent vary considerably. The public health exceptions to the parental consent requirement were enacted for two reasons. The primary reason is based on community public health needs rather than on the recognition of adolescent autonomy or capacity. Minors will be encouraged to seek certain treatments if they know it can be done confidentially, thereby reducing the spread of STIs, the incidence of unplanned teenage pregnancies, substance abuse, and teenage suicide. Legislators acknowledge that minors will not seek access to these treatments if parental consent is required (Jones & Boonstra, 2004). This reasoning is especially apparent in the case of STIs. Every state has a law allowing minors to consent to STI diagnosis and treatment. Forty-one of these states permit all minors to consent at any age, highlighting the public health imperative to reduce community infections regardless of minors' capacity to make informed decisions. States have made this policy determination not because they believe adolescents are more capable of making these decisions, as opposed to general medical treatment decisions, but because minors would not seek treatment at all if parental consent or involvement was required (Rosato, 1996). The second reason for minor consent laws in the particular treatment areas noted above is the recognition that adolescents have a limited constitutional right to privacy. This right has been most robustly developed in the area of reproductive health care decision-making, with a limited focus on public health consequences.[1] Thus, laws allowing adolescent consent to contraception may be a product of both public health reasoning and legal recognition of autonomy in the reproductive context.

Emancipated minor exception

The emancipated minor exception authorizes adolescents who have reached specific life milestones to make their own medical treatment decisions. There is little uniformity across the states, but typical laws designate marriage, joining the armed forces, bearing a child, graduating from secondary school, living apart from one's parents, or managing one's own finances as relevant life experiences. Essentially, these life experiences serve as proxies for determining decision-making capacity and maturity. Emancipated minor laws grant broader decision-making authority to adolescents than public health exceptions or mature minor determinations (discussed below). If an adolescent is found to be sufficiently emancipated, he or she can usually consent to any health care procedure. In contrast, the public health exceptions apply only to specific services, and mature minor status is often limited to a particular illness or treatment decision. In addition, emancipated minors are not subject to parental notification statutes, which still may be required under the public health laws. One problem with the emancipated minor exception is that the legal or social status of an adolescent is not always an adequate representation of decision-making capacity. For instance, a 14-year-old may well lack the ability to weigh the risks and benefits of treatment, even though she has borne a child. Similarly, a 10-year-old "genius" who has already graduated from high school likely has not had adequate life experience to inform his/her medical decision-making. For this reason, the emancipated minor determination is sometimes made on a case-by-case basis by a judge rather than automatically springing from the minor's "emancipated" circumstances.

Mature minor exception

Mature minors are minors by virtue of their chronological age. However, because of their ability to understand the risks and benefits of a proposed medical treatment, they are granted limited decision-making power. Under this exception, a court may extend the right to consent to or refuse medical treatment if the minor demonstrates that he/she can "appreciate the consequences of her actions, and [...] is mature enough to exercise the judgment of an adult." (*In re E.G.*, 1989, pp. 327–328). One court stated that the consent of a minor will be effective if the minor is capable of appreciating the "extent and probable consequences of the conduct consented to, although the consent of a parent, guardian or other person responsible is not obtained or is expressly refused" (*Cardwell* v. *Bechtol*, 1987, p. 746). Relevant factors to be weighed include the age, ability, life experience, education, and degree of maturity of the minor (*Cardwell* v. *Bechtol*, 1987). In comparison with the emancipated minor exception, mature minor determinations focus on actual decision-making capacity rather than attainment of specific life experiences. The mature minor exception has garnered support from the medical and academic communities (Committee on Bioethics, 1995). The Institute of Medicine has even promoted using the mature minor standard in obtaining adolescents' informed consent to research (Institute of Medicine, 2004).

A primary benefit of the mature minor exception is that it acknowledges emerging adolescent autonomy and is based on a fact-specific review of the minor's decision-making abilities. Despite its utility, the mature minor exception has several disadvantages. As an initial matter, the maturity determination must be conducted on a case-by-case basis because there is no uniform objective scale to evaluate a minor's maturity. Although judges may have general criteria to guide them, some determinations may come down to mere instinct. The case-by-case nature of the determination can also prove problematic when time is of the essence. Judicial rulings take time for deliberation, during which the health of a minor refusing treatment could significantly deteriorate. A final disadvantage is that a court may simply be reluctant to find a minor "mature" if the result would be the adolescent making a decision that poses a substantial risk to his or her health. For example, a judge may otherwise find a minor mature, but believe that the minor's refusal of life-sustaining treatment is evidence itself of impaired decision-making. Thus, the court may be willing to grant a mature minor petition more readily when the adolescent's proposed decision comports with some external perception of what is in the minor's best interests. The problem lies in the potential assumption that an "unwise" decision is the product of faulty or impaired decision-making, focusing on the choice we think the minor should make rather than the minor's capacity to make the decision at all. This highlights a disadvantage shared by all of the minor consent exceptions: they are tailored mainly to an adolescent's right to consent to treatment, not the corollary right to refuse.

Conflicts between adolescents, parents, and clinicians

In all situations adolescents should be involved in decision-making to the extent they are capable. This both recognizes their developing autonomy and has the practical effect of involving them in their care. Similar to the reasons proffered for encouraging informed consent from adult patients, adolescents need to be prepared for the consequences of treatment choices and to sometimes actively engage in their own treatment. Involving adolescents in medical decision-making can facilitate this. Even where parents retain ultimate legal authority for consenting to or refusing treatment, adolescent patients will likely play some role in the decision-making process. While a formal concept of "assent" has only been articulated in the research setting, it may play a useful role in the treatment setting as well. Adolescent assent may provide the ethically required permission to proceed with treatment, but may not rise to the same legal level as "consent." Moreover, although the failure of an adolescent to assent may not be equivalent to a legal refusal of treatment, it should be given weight in the decision-making process. The exact balance between adolescent assent and parental consent depends both on the level of capacity demonstrated by the minor and on the type of decision at hand.

There are four basic categories of adolescent–parent agreement or disagreement over treatment decisions. The simplest scenario occurs when both the adolescent and parent consent to medical treatment. The adolescent's wishes are respected, the parent's consent is legally operative, and no conflict ensues. The remaining three scenarios (adolescent consents but parent refuses; adolescent refuses but parent consents; both adolescent and parent refuse) create ethical and legal complications. For example, when a parent consents to medical intervention, but the adolescent adamantly refuses, a clinician is faced with the unenviable choice of potentially treating a patient against his or her will. Resolving this sort of conflict will often hinge on a determination of whether the adolescent possesses requisite decision-making capacity. When the minor lacks capacity, the scale will tip in favor of the parent's choice unless it is clear that the parent is not acting in the child's best interest by consenting to or refusing treatment. In those extremely rare situations, the treatment team (or treating institution) is obligated to seek judicial involvement and possible appointment of a separate decision-maker. If, on the other hand, the adolescent has exhibited the necessary decision-making abilities, his or her preferences will be entitled to greater weight and the conflict will be more acute.

The allocation of decision-making power between an adolescent and the parent invariably depends upon the type of treatment decision contemplated. Medical interventions exist along a continuum where the consequences of consent or refusal progressively become more significant. At the one end, minor and routine treatment decisions require a lesser degree of decision-making capacity, often carry fewer serious consequences, and present ripe opportunities to solicit adolescent participation. At the other end of the spectrum lie decisions regarding life-sustaining treatment where a higher magnitude of potential harm requires the adolescent patient to demonstrate a greater level of capacity.

End-of-life treatment decisions are particularly problematic when there is a refusal of treatment by the adolescent, the parent, or both. When parents consent to life-preserving measures against the wishes of the minor, the parents' decision almost always prevails. In the reverse scenario, when only the adolescent consents, the parents' refusal will generally be overridden to protect the life of the minor, at least in cases where the potential for benefit is substantial.[2] When both the adolescent and the parent refuse, the irreversible consequences of forgoing treatment must be weighed against the basis for refusal, including the minor's maturity, and the probability of the intervention's success. A paradigmatic case is *In re E.G.* (1989), where a Jehovah's Witness teenager and her mother both refused consent to life-saving blood transfusions. The adolescent patient sincerely believed that consenting to treatment would violate her religious beliefs and bar her from eternal salvation. E.G. was found mature enough to refuse treatment, and the court gave great deference to her religious objections as a highly protected ground for refusal. Granting E.G. the authority to refuse life-sustaining treatment ultimately hinged on a positive assessment of her decision-making capacity.

While most of this chapter has focused on whether adolescents are permitted to exercise decision-making authority in the therapeutic treatment context, it should be noted that similar issues are raised by elective treatments. Elective procedures can range from purely cosmetic (e.g., rhinoplasty, dental veneers) to quasi-therapeutic or corrective (e.g., lap-band or weight-loss surgery, breast reduction surgery). Treatments such as the use of human growth hormone can have both therapeutic and cosmetic elements. Many of these procedures have life-altering consequences that implicate an adolescent's decision-making capacity. Moreover, some elective treatments are only effective during narrow windows of adolescent growth, and requiring patients to wait until they are adults may deny them any benefits of treatment. In almost no situation would a purely elective procedure be performed without the minor's assent. For those situations in which waiting until the minor reaches the age of majority is possible, either the minor's or the parent's refusal is usually sufficient to prevent treatment against the wishes of the other party. In situations where waiting until the age of majority would result in the loss of a significant benefit, clinicians will need to evaluate the minor's capacity, and judicial involvement may be necessary to accord the minor legal authority to make decisions.

Case resolution

The Daniel Hauser case described at the beginning of this chapter provides a mechanism for better understanding how the ethical and legal framework can be applied. After Daniel Hauser refused to submit to further chemotherapy, the State of Minnesota charged his parents with medical neglect for failing to provide their son with necessary medical care as required by state law. In the court hearing that followed, the judge found that the state's interest in Daniel's life and welfare was compelling enough to override the preferences and even religious beliefs of both Daniel and his parents. While the court made no comment on the validity of the Nemenhah religion, it found that Daniel's parents could not base their refusal of life-sustaining medical care for their son on their own religious beliefs. In particular, the judge focused on the necessity of the chemotherapy and the risk of death without intervention. Here, as in *Prince v. Massachusetts*, the parents were not free to martyr their child by refusing life-sustaining care. Furthermore, the consensus among all of the physicians who were consulted regarding an appropriate course of treatment, and the understanding that chemotherapy is the standard of care for Daniel's condition with a high likelihood of success, weighed in favor of overriding the parents' choice.

In addition to the evaluation of parental decision-making authority, the judge specifically held that Daniel lacked the ability to give or refuse consent due to his age and limited capacity to comprehend the nature of his cancer or treatment alternatives. The judge also determined that Daniel's religious beliefs, although sincerely held, were insufficient justification for refusing life-preserving treatment. In part, the judge rested this determination on the fact that Daniel was unable to describe the precepts of the Nemenhah tradition or his responsibilities as a Medicine Man. Daniel and his mother were ordered to report for a chest X-ray to evaluate the growth of his tumor and to ascertain whether chemotherapy was still an effective treatment option. Unless the tumor had progressed to a point where treatment would be futile, Daniel was ordered to undergo chemotherapy. Refusal of treatment by Daniel or his parents would result in Daniel being placed in protective custody by the state. Daniel and his mother remained so resistant to chemotherapy treatment that they fled the state shortly after the hearing to avoid complying with the court's order, although they eventually returned.

The decision in the Daniel Hauser case stands in contrast to *In re E.G.*, where the adolescent's religious objections were considered sufficient grounds for refusing life-saving treatment. The fundamental distinction between the two cases is that unlike E.G., Daniel Hauser failed to demonstrate the decision-making capacity needed to make an end-of-life decision. He was not an emancipated minor and did not meet the requirements for a mature minor determination. As the court noted, Daniel was only 13 years old, still in the fifth grade, and could neither read nor write. Perhaps most importantly, Daniel did not believe that he had life-threatening cancer because he did not feel sick without chemotherapy. His inability to comprehend the nature of his disease, coupled with a failure to appreciate the risks of forgoing treatment, weighed heavily against a finding of decision-making capacity. The legal authority to consent therefore remained with his parents, who continued to refuse consent to treatment. Daniel's case illustrates one of the rare occasions when parents' medical decision-making for their child can be overridden because the decision is not in the child's best interests. The Hauser family's preferences were ultimately outweighed by the highly probable success of chemotherapy and the near certainty of Daniel's death without treatment.

These situations, like others involving adolescent decision-makers, are evaluated on a case-by-case basis by focusing on certain key elements: the nature and seriousness of the decision, the parental interest in making decisions for one's children, and the child's maturity and ability to exercise autonomy in making his or her own decisions. In the Daniel Hauser case, the determination came out in favor of requiring treatment even against both the parents' and the adolescent's wishes. Not all cases will be resolved this way. Nonetheless, clinicians may use the discussion of the Hauser case and the relevant factors to guide their understanding of other cases involving adolescent patients.

Notes

1. For instance, the Supreme Court held that minors should be accorded a constitutional right to privacy in limited circumstances, stating that "constitutional rights do not mature and come into being magically only when one attains the state-defined age of majority" (*Planned Parenthood of Central Missouri v. Danforth*, 1976, p. 74).

2. A court may find the adolescent mature enough to grant consent to treatment, or appoint a guardian whose consent will be legally valid if the minor is not mature.

References

Beauchamp, T.L. & Childress, J.F. (2001). *Principles of Biomedical Ethics*, 5th edn. Oxford: Oxford University Press.

Cardwell v. *Bechtol*, 724 S.W.2d 739 (1987).

Committee on Bioethics, American Academy of Pediatrics (1995). Informed consent, parental permission, and assent in pediatric practice. *Pediatrics*, **95**(2), 314–317.

Committee on Bioethics, American Academy of Pediatrics (1997). Religious objections to medical care. *Pediatrics*, **99**(2), 279–281.

Cummings, C.L. & Mercurio, M.R. (2010). Ethics for the pediatrician: autonomy, beneficence, and rights. *Pediatrics in Review*, **31**(6), 252–255.

Hartman, R.G. (2000). Adolescent autonomy: clarifying an ageless conundrum. *Hastings Law Journal*, **51**, 1265–1362.

In the Matter of Hauser, State of Minnesota, Brown County, Fifth Judicial District, Juvenile Division, 5/14/2009, case # JV-09-68.

In re E.G., 549 N.E.2d 322 (Ill. 1989).

Institute of Medicine (2004). *Ethical Conduct of Clinical Research Involving Children*, ed. M.J. Field & R.E. Berman. Washington, DC: National Academies Press.

Jones, R.K. & Boonstra, H. (2004). Confidential reproductive health services for minors: the potential impact of mandated parental involvement for contraception. *Perspectives on Sexual and Reproductive Health*, **36**(5), 182–191.

Meyer v. *Nebraska*, 262 US 390 (1923).

Pierce v. *Society of Sisters*, 268 US 510 (1925).

Planned Parenthood of Central Missouri v. *Danforth*, 428 US 52 (1976).

Prince v. *Massachusetts*, 321 US 158 (1944).

Rosato, J. (1996). The ultimate test of autonomy: should minors have a right to make decisions regarding life-sustaining treatment? *Rutgers Law Review*, **49**(1), 3–103.

Ross, L.F. (1997). Children as research subjects: a proposal to revise the current federal regulations using a moral framework. *Stanford Law & Policy Review*, **8**(1), 159–176.

Weithorn, L.A. & Scherer, D.G. (1994). Children's involvement in research participation decisions: psychological considerations. In *Children as Research Subjects: Science, Ethics, and Law*, ed. M.A. Grodin & L.H. Glanz. Oxford: Oxford University Press, 133–180.

Wisconsin v. *Yoder*, 406 US 205 (1972).

Chapter 3

Parental refusals of recommended medical interventions

Douglas S. Diekema

Case narrative

A 3-year-old child is brought to the emergency department by his parents who have concerns about a head injury. The day before, the child had been playing on the monkey bars when he fell about 4 feet and hit his head on the ground. He did not lose consciousness, and after about 15 minutes of crying, appeared to be fine. Today, however, he has been complaining that his head hurts and has been vomiting. He has vomited three times since arriving in the emergency department and continues to complain of a headache. The emergency department physician tells the parents that he is concerned about the possibility of intracranial bleeding and feels a CT scan of the head is essential to make a timely diagnosis and intervene if necessary. The parents are convinced that previous X-rays gave their son some learning problems, and refuse to consent to the CT scan.

Introduction

Responding to a parent who has refused a recommended diagnostic study or treatment modality presents a difficult challenge for clinicians. Clinicians must balance their assessment of the child's well-being with respect for the parent's wishes and legal rights. What are the limitations on a parent's right to refuse diagnostic testing or treatment for a child? How does a clinician resolve conflicts between the parent's values and his or her own as a medical professional? At what point should a clinician consider interfering with a parental decision to ignore the clinician's recommended course of diagnosis and/or treatment? What are the steps a clinician must take in order to justify involving state agencies to compel testing or treatment over parental objections?

Discussion of ethical issues

Clinical practice is generally guided by the principle of beneficence. The principle of beneficence states that persons have a moral obligation to contribute to the good of others. Medical professionals clearly have a duty to seek benefit for their patients. Clinicians make recommendations regarding diagnostic testing and treatment based upon what they believe will optimize the welfare of the patient. However, assessing benefit and harm is not always easy, especially when those benefits and harms may occur in only some patients. The concepts of harm, benefit, and best interests are value-laden. What seems to be a minimal harm to a medical professional may seem like a huge harm to some patients. Clinicians and patients (or a patient's legally authorized decision-maker) may disagree about whether a possible benefit from testing or treatment justifies the risk associated with the testing and treatment. In this case, for example, the clinician feels strongly that the benefit of diagnosing an intracranial bleed (or ruling it out) justifies the risks associated with radiation from the CT scan. The parents, however, have come to a different conclusion.

A clinician's assessment of the best interests of the patient is not sufficient to justify testing and treatment over a parent's objection. The clinician must also obtain consent from the patient or the patient's legally authorized decision-maker. As a general rule, minors in the United States are considered incompetent to provide legally binding consent regarding their health care. Parents (or guardians) are generally empowered to make health care decisions on behalf of their children. In most situations, parents are granted wide latitude in the decisions they make on behalf of their children, and the law has respected those decisions except where they

---

Clinical Ethics in Pediatrics: A Case-Based Textbook, ed. Douglas S. Diekema, Mark R. Mercurio and Mary B. Adam. Published by Cambridge University Press. © Cambridge University Press 2011.

place the child's health, well-being, or life in jeopardy (Hanisco, 2000).

Parental authority is not absolute, however, and when a parent or guardian fails to adequately guard the interests of a child, the state may intervene (Ross, 1998). Child abuse and neglect laws recognize that parental rights are not absolute. If a parent refuses to provide necessary care to a child, the state can assume temporary custody for the purpose of authorizing medical care under a claim of medical neglect (Hanisco, 2000).

The clinician's first duty in a case such as the one presented here is to establish whether the recommended course of action is likely to benefit the child in an important way. In this case, the child has presented with symptoms that are consistent with an intracranial bleed following a head injury. While the child's symptoms are non-specific, the possibility of a life-threatening bleed cannot be ruled out without doing a CT scan. Any other course of action would potentially delay a diagnosis and further endanger the child. While the recommendation to perform a CT scan on the child is a reasonable one with a sound basis in medical evidence and practice, the physician's assessment about what is best for the patient is not, by itself, sufficient to justify overriding the decision of a parent who disagrees with him.

A clinician's authority to interfere with parental decision-making is limited. Except in emergency situations where a child's life is threatened imminently, or a delay would result in significant suffering or risk to the child, the physician cannot do anything to a child without the permission of the child's parent or guardian. Touching (physical examination, diagnostic testing, or administering a medication or vaccine) without consent is generally considered a battery under the law.

Only the state can order a parent to comply with medical recommendations. The physician's options include either tolerating the parent's decision (while continuing to try to convince them to act otherwise) or involving a state agency to assume medical decision-making authority on behalf of the child. This can take different forms, but most frequently either includes involvement of child protective services (under a claim of medical neglect) or a court order. Both of these represent a serious challenge to parental authority and will generally be perceived as disrespectful and adversarial by parents. Such action interferes with family autonomy, can adversely affect the family's future interactions with medical professionals, and should be undertaken only after serious consideration.

How does a clinician determine when to legally challenge the decision of a parent to withhold permission? What is the threshold for when a clinician should involve state agencies in order to get permission to treat a child against the wishes of a parent?

When someone seeks to legally challenge parental decision-making they seek to invoke coercive state power, either through a court order or the action of state welfare agencies. The ethical basis for the exercise of the government's police powers lies in what has become known as the "harm principle." The harm principle holds that for the state to justifiably restrict an individual's freedom, that individual's decision or action must place another person at significant risk of serious harm, the restriction of the individual's freedom must be effective at preventing the harm in question, and no option that would be less intrusive to individual liberty would be equally effective at preventing the harm (Feinberg, 1984).

In general, parental decisions should be tolerated except in those rare cases where the decision of a parent places the child at some level of harm. The harm principle provides a basis for identifying the threshold for state action in cases where a parent refuses medical intervention on behalf of a child. State authorities may be justified in interfering with parental decisions when there is evidence that parental actions or decisions are likely to harm a child. The harm principle recognizes that society has an obligation to ensure that the basic needs of its most vulnerable members are met.

For the harm principle to be helpful, however, we must identify the level of harm to be tolerated in parental decisions. Not all harms should trigger state intervention. Parents should be granted some latitude in making decisions for their children, even when those decisions may pose some small degree of risk to the child. Parents may occasionally make decisions that "harm" one child in order to benefit the family or meet the needs of another child. Feinberg sets the harm threshold as a "significant risk of serious harm" and suggests that serious harm includes interference with interests necessary for more ultimate goals like physical health and vigor, integrity and normal functioning of one's body, absence of absorbing pain and suffering or grotesque disfigurement, minimal intellectual acuity, and emotional stability (Feinberg, 1984). Ross suggests that state intervention should be limited to cases in which children are placed at the level of harm that occurs when they are deprived of basic needs or when parental decisions to refuse a treatment place the child at high risk for serious and significant morbidity and the treatment is of proven efficacy with a high likelihood of success (Ross, 1998). Others have come to similar conclusions regarding the harm threshold for state intervention, settling on the kinds of harm that include loss of health or some other major interest, deprivation of basic needs, and deprivation of future opportunities or freedoms (Dworkin, 1982; Miller, 2003). The American Academy of Pediatrics Committee on Bioethics (1997) argues that state intervention should be a last resort, wielded only when treatment is likely to prevent substantial harm or suffering or death.

While these suggestions vary somewhat, they share the notion that state intervention should not be trivial but should be triggered when a parental decision places the child at significant risk of serious harm. For the medical professional faced with a parent refusing to consent to a suggested course of treatment, the proper question is "Does the decision made by the parents significantly increase the likelihood of serious harm as compared to other options?" Furthermore, interference is justified only if interfering with the parent's decision can prevent the harms in question. The burden rests on those challenging the parental decision to provide evidence of efficacy for the preferred intervention and demonstrate that the proposed course of action is required imminently to prevent harm (Diekema, 2004). There is a difference between a test or treatment of proven efficacy and those performed by convention (i.e., unproven standard of care). Finally, all alternatives short of state action must have been exhausted in seeking a mutually acceptable solution to the child's medical condition.

Practical summary and recommendations

Clinicians make diagnostic and treatment recommendations based upon what they consider to be in the child's best interest. Occasionally, however, a parent may disagree with those recommendations and withhold consent. In those situations, the physician's first responsibility is to try to understand the reasons for the parent's reluctance to consent, attempt to correct any misunderstandings or misperceptions related to the recommendation, and explore alternatives that might be acceptable to the parent while at the same time guarding the interests of the child. Communication and reasonable accommodation are almost always superior to the involvement of coercive state power. If

despite those efforts, the clinician cannot gain consent from the parent, the clinician must decide whether to engage state agencies or a court order to force compliance. In situations where the parent's decision to withhold consent does not place a child at substantial risk of serious harm, the physician should tolerate the parent's decision while maintaining the opportunity to further discuss the issue should things change. An example of this kind of situation might be a parent who refuses to allow routine vaccinations for a child. Likewise, interference with parental decision is not appropriate if prognosis is grave even with treatment. In situations where the child may be subjected to more serious harm by a refusal of consent, the following eight questions can be asked to help providers determine whether they should seek state action to interfere with the decision made by the parents (Diekema, 2004):

1. By refusing to consent, are the parents placing their child at significant risk of serious harm?
2. Is the harm imminent, requiring immediate action to prevent it?
3. Is the intervention that has been refused necessary to prevent the serious harm?
4. Is the intervention that has been refused of proven efficacy and, therefore, likely to prevent the harm?
5. Does the intervention that has been refused by the parents also place the child at significant risk of serious harm and do its projected benefits outweigh its projected burdens significantly more favorably than the option chosen by the parents?
6. Would any other option prevent serious harm to the child in a way that is less intrusive to parental autonomy and more acceptable to the parents?
7. Can the state intervention be generalized to all other similar situations?
8. Would most people familiar with the situation agree that the state intervention was reasonable?

In situations where state authorities must be involved to keep a child from suffering serious harm, the clinician should try to create an atmosphere of respect and concern for the child. Parents should always be informed of one's intent to notify child protective services or seek a court order.

Resolution of case and discussion

In this case, the clinician determined that the child's symptoms were consistent with an intracranial bleed, and that the possibility of an intracranial bleed placed the child at significant risk of serious harm that was imminent. A CT scan would be necessary to prevent the harm of a possible bleed, was a test of proven efficacy in making that diagnosis, and, if a bleed was present, would allow for appropriate interventions to occur that would be likely to prevent the harms often associated with an intracranial bleed. The parent's refusal of the CT scan would preclude making the diagnosis in a timely manner, and although the risk of radiation (a slight increase in the risk of brain tumor later in life) was not insignificant, it was considerably lower than the risk of death or disability from an undiagnosed intracranial bleed. The clinician also felt he would make a similar decision in other situations given the same set of facts and that most parents would agree that it was reasonable to take action despite the refusal of parental consent. The clinician was therefore prepared to involve child protective services should the parents persist in their refusal. However, before doing so, the clinician identified two alternatives to state action. The first was to explore whether an MRI, which does not involve radiation, might be acceptable to the parents and achieve the goal of making a timely diagnosis. In this situation, the MRI scanner was not an option because it was not available on an emergent basis and because it would require sedation. The final alternative was to spend the time necessary to convince the family. While there was some urgency to getting the CT scan done, the child appeared stable, and the clinician spent time talking with the family, including a frank discussion of the risks of not doing the procedure. After about an hour of discussion, the family agreed to allow the CT scan. The CT scan was normal and the child was discharged home in the care of the parents that night.

References

Committee on Bioethics, American Academy of Pediatrics (1997). Religious objections to medical care. *Pediatrics*, **99**, 279–281.

Diekema, D.S. (2004). Parental refusals of medical treatment: the harm principle as threshold for state intervention. *Theoretical Medicine and Bioethics*, **25**, 243–264.

Dworkin, G. (1982). Representation and proxy consent. In *Who Speaks for the Child: The Problems of Proxy Consent*, ed. W. Gaylin & R. Macklin. New York: Plenum Press, 190–208.

Feinberg, J. (1984). *Harm to Others: The Moral Limits of the Criminal Law.* New York: Oxford University Press.

Hanisco, C.M. (2000). Acknowledging the hypocrisy: granting minors the right to choose their medical treatment. *New York Law School Journal of Human Rights*, **16**, 899–932.

Miller, R.B. (2003). *Children, Ethics, and Modern Medicine.* Bloomington, IN: Indiana University Press.

Ross, L.F. (1998). *Children, Families, and Health Care Decision-Making.* New York: Oxford University Press.

Chapter

4

Adolescent confidentiality

Malcolm Parker

Case narrative: conflicts between confidentiality and care

Kathryn is a 16-year-old who lives with her divorced mother Stephanie. Four months ago, Kathryn was taken to the emergency department by her friend Annie, who later told Stephanie, who works full time, that Kathryn had been "like – totally bizarre," but she didn't know why. Kathryn was admitted in what appeared to be a psychotic state, and was treated with antipsychotic medication and sedation. At the time her mother was told by the attending clinician that her daughter was in a psychotic state, and that the cause of this was unclear.

Kathryn's acute psychosis resolved, but she remained withdrawn and distant. She returned home following discharge from the hospital, but after 3 weeks moved out, against her mother's strong protests, to live with two "new friends." When she asked Kathryn what the doctor thought of this idea, Kathryn replied that the doctor thought she had returned to school. She tried to reassure her mother by saying that she would continue to see the doctor every 2 weeks. Stephanie tried to contact Kathryn's doctor to discuss her concerns, but he indicated that he could not discuss Kathryn's issues in detail because of his duty to respect her confidentiality. When Stephanie asked him whether he was aware that Kathryn had stopped attending school, he simply thanked her for the information.

Kathryn did not tell her mother where she was living, and answered few of her phone calls. She denied that she was taking non-prescription drugs, but Stephanie became increasingly convinced that she was. Kathryn initially turned up at home intermittently, usually asking her mother for money or food, and appearing sad and tired.

Summary of emotional, health care, and ethical issues

Kathryn's case raises a host of related ethical questions. Like all contrived cases, her story is severely limited in terms of contextual factors that would typically inform the emotional and ethical considerations taken into account by Kathryn, her mother, and her doctor. But it is sufficient to broadly illustrate the relevant ethical issues concerning adolescent confidentiality.

At the age of 16, Kathryn is growing into emotional and sexual maturity, accompanied by the tension between continuing dependence and developing independence that this developmental period encompasses. Her case is further complicated by the fact that her mother works full time and her father is no longer a part of her life. Adolescents are often impressionable, idealistic, contrary, and emotionally labile. They struggle to establish an individual identity, while in most cases fiercely conforming to group mores. They may confound their parents, who somewhat reluctantly encourage their individuation and separation, but eventually take joy in the gradual achievement of their independence. Until this has occurred, all parties struggle with the contradictions of continuing dependence and emerging autonomy, experiment and error, bravado and maturity.

In addition to health promotion and preventive health care, the adolescent years introduce new health issues related to sexual and reproductive health (including unplanned pregnancy and abortion), mental health, and smoking, excessive drinking, and other substance abuse. The tensions that exist between adolescents and their parents may manifest themselves in the health care context, raising a number of familiar ethical issues including the nature and authority

---

Clinical Ethics in Pediatrics: A Case-Based Textbook, ed. Douglas S. Diekema, Mark R. Mercurio and Mary B. Adam. Published by Cambridge University Press. © Cambridge University Press 2011.

of adolescents' competence to consent to health care; communication and trust (between health professionals and adolescent patients, professionals and parents, and between parents and the adolescents themselves); the delicate line between parental concern and undue paternalism (parental versus minors' rights); and the assurance of continuity in the adolescent's health care. The issue of confidentiality also becomes important, and represents a convergence point for all these issues.

Ethical principles and discussion

Resolving the kind of tensions evident in Kathryn's story is no simple task, and many have struggled to find an acceptable middle ground. The Convention on the Rights of the Child (UNICEF, 1989) (not ratified in the United States), as well as the vast majority of relevant Western statutes and the common law, recognize that the right to self-determination shifts increasingly to the child as the child's capacity to form his or her own views evolves and matures (Dickens & Cook, 2005). The generally accepted ethical rule is that once a minor has attained the capacity to understand a particular medical treatment plan, together with its risks and benefits, he or she ought to be attributed the ethical and legal right to make decisions concerning that treatment. In short, competent minors may consent to medical treatment, subject to some qualifications (see Chapter 2). While the laws regarding adolescent competency and age of consent vary from jurisdiction to jurisdiction, respect for autonomy stands as a fundamental ethical principle and is recognized legally in the form of statutes, judicial decisions, and common law (English & Ford, 2004; Berlan & Bravender, 2009).

As a result of this consensus on consent, mature minors – those considered to be competent to make decisions for themselves – are also afforded the protection of patient confidentiality. In our case, once Kathryn had recovered from her acute psychotic event, her doctor considered her to be competent to make her own health care decisions. Accompanying that determination was his obligation to protect her confidentiality by not divulging information to her mother without her permission. It should be noted, however, that decisions made by adolescents (and by parents on behalf of their children) may be scrutinized more closely than those made by adults, and challenged whenever they appear to place the child or adolescent at significant risk of serious harm. There is more or less universal consensus on the principle that a parent's right to make decisions on behalf of a child, including the right to consent to

or refuse medical treatment, should be in accord with the child's best interest. The same constraint applies to competent adolescents in most jurisdictions. In other words, once we judge an adolescent to be competent, we allow them to make their own medical decisions, but we insist that these must accord with what health professionals consider to be in their best medical interests. In the case of adults, of course, we allow competent adults to decide on their treatment, irrespective of whether their decision is judged by their health professionals to be in their interests. Just as adolescence is a transitional stage between childhood and adulthood, we attribute "transitional," (i.e., not full) rights to adolescents. This transitional status is the basis for some judicial decisions concerning adolescent *refusals* of treatment, where competent adolescents' decisions to refuse treatment that will preserve life or prevent serious morbidity have been overridden (see, for example, *Re M*, 1999).

The same qualification appears when we look at confidentiality. Laws in many jurisdictions, including common law (see, for example, *Gillick* v. *West Norfolk AHA*, 1986), require medical providers to encourage a competent adolescent to involve his/her parent(s) or guardian(s) in the decision-making process. This requirement allows those who still retain legal responsibility for the adolescent and who presumably care about his/her interests to participate in decision-making about her health care. While Kathryn's doctor may have encouraged Kathryn to invite her mother to his visits with Kathryn, Kathryn's refusal to involve her mother in her medical management left Stephanie somewhat stranded with regard to her ability to help her daughter. Parents often find themselves in the very difficult and stressful position of wanting to contribute support and advice to the care of their adolescent child, but feeling they are "shut out" of this participatory role on the grounds of assuring confidentiality to the young person.

Of course, there are sound ethical reasons to respect an adolescent's refusal to share certain information with parents or guardians. Such a refusal reflects the adolescent's desire to control information about him-/ herself (thereby asserting his/her developing independence). Even when respecting requests for confidentiality, it is ethically appropriate for the doctor to continue to take opportunities to encourage the adolescent patient to involve his/her parents, unless there are good reasons to think that the young person's health care and welfare would actually be threatened by such involvement.

The other major reason to respect the young person's confidentiality is because ensuring honest communication between doctor and patient, maintaining the adolescent's trust in the doctor, and assuring the adolescent's continued use of the health care system may all require that confidentiality be honored (Carlisle et al., 2006). Should Kathryn decide to refrain from seeking care because she cannot trust health care providers to maintain confidentiality it could increase her chances of entering a spiral involving drugs, unsafe sex, inadequate nutrition, and the loss of family and social support. The loss of trust between an adolescent and her doctor may also result in the adolescent becoming less willing (or unable) to take advantage of preventive health care and health promotion during a period when these visits offer an important opportunity to discuss sensitive issues and obtain advice and access to things like birth control (Stephens, 2006).

A few years ago in Australia, the federal government proposed to allow parents of minors younger than 16 access to their children's medical records without the child's consent (Bird, 2007). There was considerable public resistance to this proposal, including strong opposition from the organized medical profession, based on evidence supporting the importance of confidentiality in promoting young people's access to and utilization of health care, particularly for sensitive issues such as mental and sexual health and substance use, combined with a dearth of evidence for any benefit from mandatory parental involvement (Sanci et al., 2005).

Trust, adherence, and an honest patient–physician relationship depend on confidentiality. Given its importance, why is the duty of confidentiality to adolescents a qualified duty that may be overridden in some situations? If adolescents are competent, why shouldn't they be allowed to make choices that are not deemed to be in their best interests, and why should health practitioners still encourage them to involve their parents in decision-making? If young people are only permitted to consent to treatment that doctors think is in their interest, and are not permitted to refuse such treatment (at least in cases where a refusal will lead to significant harm or death), how can we characterize their consent or refusal as truly autonomous? One way to understand this seeming contradiction is to recognize that adolescent autonomy is not fully developed. Competence can be divided into two kinds – "occurrent" and "dispositional" – and adolescents differ from adults with regard to the second.

Occurrent competence refers to whether or not the person can "intellectually" understand what is proposed, including its risks and benefits. We infer from Kathryn's story that she was able to comprehend what the doctor told her about her condition and its management. Dispositional competence and autonomy, on the other hand, are based not only on these purely cognitive capacities, but also on the experiential knowledge accrued by the person making the decision. Dispositional competence will usually be greater in adults, since they have a degree of life experience that adolescents do not possess. However, some adolescents, especially those who have lived with a chronic disease, have taken responsibility for monitoring and treating their illness, and have become accustomed to decision-making regarding their illness, may possess more dispositional competence than some adults faced with an acute medical illness.

Determining dispositional competence can be a challenge, and most adolescents will not have had sufficient life experience to possess full dispositional competence. For that reason, even though adolescent confidentiality is usually respected, it is qualified in two ways. First, physicians should encourage adolescent patients to involve their parents. There are good reasons to think that adolescents will be better able to participate in collaborative decision-making with their doctor if their parents are also involved. Second, it may be necessary to breach confidentiality when the adolescent is about to make a decision that poses a significant and serious risk to his or her health. Even then, the physicians must be convinced that breaking confidentiality will not ultimately lead to more harm than maintaining it.

Confidentiality should only be breached in extreme cases. If the scope of exceptions becomes too broad, confidentiality loses its power to encourage patients to divulge sensitive and private information. An ethical and sometimes a legal exception to this quasi-absolute rule can be invoked in cases where breaching the patient's confidentiality is the only remaining option to prevent a serious, imminent danger to a member of the public from action by the patient – the so-called public interest exception. As discussed above, when an adolescent is involved, a breach of confidentiality may be justified when it is the only means to prevent a significant or serious harm to the minor's health (for example, when the adolescent conveys to the provider that they intend to commit suicide and have a plan).

Practical summary and recommendation

The adolescent years can be a difficult time as the young person struggles with issues of identity and independence. That search for identity and desire for independence may involve exploration and risk-taking behaviors that affect an adolescent's physical, reproductive, and mental health. It is imperative that the adolescent has a health care provider who is safe and trustworthy and from whom they can seek advice and care for preventive and health needs during this time. Some expectation that confidentiality will be respected is an important part of an adolescent's willingness to seek the counsel of a health care provider.

Emerging independence should be fostered and respected (Dickey & Deatrick, 2000). Doing so requires doctors to determine whether or not the adolescent patient has the capacity to understand and make decisions about the medical options under consideration. At the same time, doctors must take into account adolescent vulnerability and inexperience. Doctors should encourage adolescents to involve their parents, but be equally prepared to protect their emerging independence, via confidentiality, when requested. Even when an adolescent has not explicitly requested confidentiality about sensitive issues, it should be assumed until it can be clarified with the patient. Physicians often feel a duty to their adolescent patient and to the patient's parents, and the balance between these two obligations will sometimes be difficult and awkward, especially if the parent feels abandoned and frustrated. Doctors may sometimes need to think and act creatively within the parameters set by the community's ethical and legal consensus in order to minimize these difficulties. Compromises can be reached that exploit the flexibility and understanding that characterizes a maturing autonomy.

Case resolution

At the commencement of Kathryn's outpatient management, her doctor had agonized over his ethical, professional, and legal responsibilities in relation to both Kathryn and her mother. He re-read a position paper on adolescent confidentiality (Ford et al., 2004), and encouraged Kathryn to ask her mother to accompany Kathryn to some visits. The doctor felt this was important to help improve communication between Kathryn and her mother, and because involving her mother would likely benefit Kathryn in the long run and allow her mother to carry out parental responsibilities that had not been extinguished by Kathryn's strong declarations of independence (Tan et al., 2007). Although Kathryn did not return home, she obtained work in a community market garden 4 months after her hospital admission and gradually began to regain some of her energy and interest in things. Kathryn finally agreed to allow her doctor to provide some information to her mother, by way of letters, which she insisted on screening.

Finally, after 9 months, Kathryn agreed to invite her mother to a consultation. This proved to be a positive experience for both mother and daughter, but also an extremely challenging one, as they began to negotiate the next phase of Kathryn's life. One issue on which they reached early agreement with the doctor was that it would be helpful to plan a series of consultations involving them both, as well as continuing therapy for Kathryn on her own (Sawyer & Aroni, 2005).

References

Berlan, E.D. & Bravender, T. (2009). Confidentiality, consent, and caring for the adolescent patient. *Current Opinion in Pediatrics*, **21**, 450–456.

Bird, S. (2007). Adolescents and confidentiality. *Australian Family Physician*, **36**, 655–656.

Carlisle, J., Shickle, D., Cork, M., & McDonagh, A. (2006). Concerns over confidentiality may deter adolescents from consulting their doctors. A qualitative exploration. *Journal of Medical Ethics*, **32**, 133–137.

Dickens, B.M. & Cook, R.J. (2005). Adolescents and consent to treatment. *International Journal of Gynaecology and Obstetrics*, **89**, 179–184.

Dickey, S.B. & Deatrick, J. (2000). Autonomy and decision making for health promotion in adolescence. *Pediatric Nursing*, **26**, 461–467.

English, A. & Ford, C.A. (2004). The HIPAA privacy rule and adolescents: legal questions and clinical challenges. *Perspectives on Sexual and Reproductive Health*, **36**, 80–86.

Ford, C., English, A., & Sigman, G. (2004). Confidential Health Care for Adolescents: position paper for the society for adolescent medicine. *Journal of Adolescent Health*, **35**, 160–167.

Gillick v. *West Norfolk AHA* (1986). AC 112 (HL).

Re M (child: refusal of treatment) (1999). 2 FCR, 577 (HC(UK) (Fam Div)).

Sanci, L.A., Sawyer, S.M., Kang, M.S., Haller, D.M., & Patton, G.C. (2005). Confidential health care for adolescents: reconciling clinical evidence with family values. *Medical Journal of Australia*, **183**, 410–414.

Sawyer, S.M. & Aroni, R.A. (2005). Self-management in adolescents with chronic illness. What does it mean and how can it be achieved? *Medical Journal of Australia*, **183**, 405–409.

Stephens, M.B. (2006). Preventive health counseling for adolescents. *American Family Physician*, **74**, 1151–1156.

Tan, J.O., Passerini, G.E., & Stewart, A. (2007). Consent and confidentiality in clinical work with young people. *Clinical Child Psychology and Psychiatry*, **12**, 191–210.

UNICEF (1989). Convention on the Rights of the Child. Available at www.unicef.org/crc/.

5

Refusals of treatment in adolescents and young adults

Maureen Kelley

Case narrative

Kristin is a 17-year-old admitted through the emergency department of a children's hospital, where she presented with severe dehydration and abdominal pain. Her mother accompanied her to the hospital, and her father soon joined them. Kristin has a history of multiple hospital admissions for episodes of severe weight loss and dehydration. She was assigned to the general adolescent medicine service, and diagnosed with acute inflammation of the pancreas and gallbladder secondary to the diagnosis of anorexia nervosa. When asked about her daughter's medical history, Kristin's mother denied her daughter had an eating disorder. Her father explained that Kristin had always been a very driven gymnast. With a height of 5′6″ (168 cm), Kristin's weight upon admission was 79 pounds (36 kg).

Over the next week, as members of the adolescent team tried to engage Kristin directly in a discussion of her health and a treatment plan, Kristin, despite being alert and intelligent, grew agitated and angry in response to any mention of an eating disorder or anorexia, even threatening to "fire" certain providers who upset her. Kristin's mother largely stood by and asked team members not to upset her daughter. While Kristin had initially allowed nasojejunal feeds and line placement for intravenous (IV) fluids, she later questioned the nurse suspiciously when she hung a new IV bag, asking, "How many calories are in that stuff?" She demanded that the line be removed. The nurse managed to persuade Kristin that the only way she would get better was through IV rehydration and nutrition. The patient acquiesced and did not attempt to remove the line.

When a consulting surgeon recommended that Kristin's gallbladder be removed, she was allowed to consent for surgery, while her mother was in the room.

Following surgery, when Kristin regained her ability to eat by mouth, she repeatedly crossed out the items on the daily menu, leaving only broth. She began asking when she could leave the hospital. As Kristin recovered from her acute condition, the medical team became increasingly worried about her long-term health, and worried that discharging her without a plan for treatment of her underlying eating disorder would be dangerous, even life-threatening. Every attempt to persuade the patient to enter into a recovery program was rebuffed. At this point the team requested an ethics consultation to help determine whether it would be appropriate to force tube feeding against the patient's wishes.

Growing pains: of teens and a profession

While dramatic, life-and-death cases of adolescent refusals receive media attention and influence legal thinking, the case of Kristin and many young patients like her illustrate the everyday challenges clinicians now face when caring for teens and young adults in a culture that increasingly reflects the value of patient autonomy, even the imperfect, developing, inconsistent autonomy of a teenager. Nowhere is this tension more vexing than in a patient's refusal of beneficial treatment, especially when that treatment might be life-saving,. Over the past three decades, particularly in the United States, we have seen a significant shift in law and practice, giving greater voice to adolescent decision-making in high-stakes health matters (AAP, 1995; Weir & Peters, 1997; Derish & Heuvel, 2000). The move away from a paradigm that viewed parents as having absolute rights over minors until they reached the age of emancipation or legal consent is in no small part due to the work of pediatricians and child development researchers who have demonstrated that

Clinical Ethics in Pediatrics: A Case-Based Textbook, ed. Douglas S. Diekema, Mark R. Mercurio and Mary B. Adam. Published by Cambridge University Press. © Cambridge University Press 2011.

many adolescents have sufficient cognitive capacity to make decisions about their health and thereby ought to be given greater consideration for the choices they make in the clinical context (AAP, 1995; Weir & Peters, 1997). These findings have reshaped clinical pediatric practice into a more active partnership with teens, with parents involved in a supportive rather than directive role (Alderson et al., 2006).

The resulting rule-of-thumb – that pediatricians involve their patients in decision-making in a way that is developmentally appropriate – is a useful and reasonable guide for routine clinical decisions. It allows pediatricians significant flexibility in determining the capacity of particular patients in particular circumstances. While in a basic sense Piaget's categories of child development and behavioral markers remain relevant to the practicing pediatrician, we now know that fixed age categories are only an estimate for how particular children and teens will behave, reflecting significant variation in cognitive development at a given age, and in response to environment. While a 12-year-old diabetic patient may demonstrate the maturity of someone much older, given her early experience with hospitals and responsibility in managing her disease, a 17-year-old patient may react to a devastating injury by regressing and withdrawing emotionally, deferring to her parents for all decisions. With any more specificity the rule-of-thumb requiring that participation track development would be too rigid and would not account for these morally significant differences in pediatric and adolescent capacity.

That is, until the adolescent patient refuses needed and especially life-saving interventions. Bill Bartholome, pediatrician and an architect behind the American Academy of Pediatrics statement on consent and assent in pediatric decision-making, argued that in order to truly respect the developing autonomy of their older pediatric patients, clinicians would have to honor refusals of even life-saving treatment, if such refusals reflected the wishes of a patient with the capacity to understand and appreciate the implications of such a grave decision. If pediatricians only invite involvement and honor decisions when the adolescent agrees with medically recommended treatment, and fail to honor an adolescent's disagreement, such selective application of the rule would make a mockery of respect for a patient's autonomy (Bartholome, 1995). In contrast, other leaders in pediatrics have pushed back against the ethical paradigm shift, especially when a patient refuses life-saving treatment (Ross, 2010). In this latter

account, it is precisely in high-stakes decisions when the judgment of a parent is needed to inform, and even override, the less developed autonomy of a teenager or young adult when it is necessary to do so to protect her interests, or perhaps more accurately, the future interests of her older, more experienced and mature self.

Assessing adolescent capacity: the autonomy paradox

Autonomy is a muscle that must be exercised to develop, and as Aristotle, J.S. Mill, and others argued long ago, it doesn't develop in a social vacuum. This is now borne out in recent work on adolescent behavior and development (Alderson, 2007). The autonomy paradox is the paradox faced by parents. Parents need to guide children toward the right choices, but ensuring that they recognize a good choice from a bad one requires allowing a child to make choices and make mistakes, occasionally allowing them to miss the mark so as to improve their aim. One role of parents and other adult mentors is to interject and correct until a teen or young adult can make such judgments on their own. The added challenge of assessing adolescent capacity is twofold: (1) it is harder to demonstrate capacity than to demonstrate lack of capacity, and (2) it is socially difficult for minors to challenge adults, including parents or pediatricians (Alderson, 2007). With adult patients we assume capacity and only question capacity when there is clear evidence that the patient lacks it. Not so with pediatric patients. An adolescent oncology patient undergoing leukemia treatment has to overtly demonstrate the presence of capacity in order to have his/her decisions respected, particularly if they depart from what the team or the parents think reasonable, rational, or in his/her own best interests.

The empirical data that helped shift pediatrics toward a practice that was more inclusive of the pediatric patient's involvement in care decisions has also generated valuable information on the teenage brain. These data confirm what every parent of a teen knows to be true: the adolescent period of development is marked by cognitive and emotional fits and starts, sometimes skewed perception of personal risk and future consequences, and variations between genders on judgment in the face of challenges (Pasupathi et al., 2001; Gardner & Steinberg, 2005).

The case of Kristin represents the heartache faced by parents and pediatricians when a teen or young adult is making damaging and life-threatening decisions before their eyes. Heartache, not because we do not know what would be best for Kristin (entering a rehabilitation, counseling, and refeeding program), but because she is a young woman whose refusal counts for something, and represents a real and formidable barrier to our willingness to force treatment without consent. What have been somewhat overlooked in the objections to the autonomy-centered shift in pediatric ethics are the moral significance and practical challenges of forcing needed treatment on an adolescent or teenager. Beyond the physical challenges, which are not negligible, the more important consideration is the breach of trust at a developmental stage when trust of adults comes grudgingly, must be earned, and can be lost at the first betrayal.

Caring for a young adult with anorexia is one of the best illustrations of the delicate balance between maintaining trust and keeping patients from harm. Long-term success for eating disorders, much like addictions, only occurs when the patient voluntarily accepts treatment (Tan, 2003;Tan et al., 2006). Having supportive family members and a trusting relationship with care providers are essential to this process. However, when parents and providers fail to reach a patient like Kristin, is the best approach to force treatment against her will, but for the sake of her health and survival? How can Kristin's pediatrician save her from herself when control and denial are such central features of anorexia (Opel & Kelley, 2010)?

Kristin's ability to meaningfully participate in decisions about her health is undermined by the psychological characteristics of anorexia: clinical depression, a distorted body image, and the need for control. These features of the disease undermine a patient's capacity to make safe choices about her health. As is typical in patients with anorexia, Kristin's fixation on being thin may crowd out all other values, including survival. While harmful preferences are typically honored in adult patients out of respect for autonomy, more paternalistic interventions are warranted with teens and adults with mental illness to prevent self-harm (Tan, 2003; Opel & Kelley, 2010).

The trump card: are we willing to use physical force?

So if we believe it to be important for her well-being and even survival, why should we not forcibly initiate refeeding against Kristin's will? Posing the question this way helps refocus the debate over whether to respect adolescent refusals on a practical but overlooked reality: how does one physically force an adolescent patient to be treated against their will? When persuasion has failed, one is left with forcible intervention: treatment with medicated or actual restraints. It is one thing to restrain a two-year old for a vaccination, and another to insert a feeding tube into a young adult against their will. Even if the profession of pediatrics had not undergone the paradigm shift toward increasing respect for developing autonomy, this brute, practical question would remain: as a clinician, no matter how good the reasons for intervening, are you willing to force treatment on a patient?

For a patient like Kristin, the issue is subtler than a Jehovah's Witness' refusal of a life-saving blood transfusion, where a single transfusion may save a life, and the principle of not asking permission but begging forgiveness might succeed in repairing trust. When treating a chronic disease that is centrally about psychological control, a strategy of "tough love" that takes decision-making rights away from the adolescent runs the risk of undermining what trust exists between the team and the patient, and risks losing the patient to follow-up. Hope for patients like Kristin will likely be found in a strategy of compassionate but honest support, persistence, and creative but firm negotiation from the medical team and family – for example, making enrollment in an outpatient eating disorder program a condition of discharge. Clinical teams may face the difficult decision of discharging a patient who is slowly starving herself, and waiting for her to get sick enough and scared enough to voluntarily enter a treatment program (Opel & Kelley, 2010). That is the parent's lament. And that is the pediatrician's lament when faced with a young adult or teen, when the only options appear to be acquiescence or force. The hope is that by working towards a social support network that values honesty, rather than reinforcing denial, each time Kristin is confronted with a choice about treatment, she will be more likely to find the strength to make healthy decisions.

Case resolution and conclusion

The attending physician requested a psychiatric evaluation for possible involuntary commitment to an inpatient refeeding program. This was conducted at a time when Kristin's mother was not visiting. Kristin cooperated fully with the interview and evaluation. The psychiatrist determined that Kristin did not meet the criteria for involuntary commitment based on her mental status, understanding, and capacity. By this time Kristin's weight had reached 104 pounds (47 kg) and her other symptoms had cleared; she demanded to be discharged home, and the team saw no choice but to honor her request.

Cases like this one can be distressing for all involved. Health care professionals desire to benefit their patients, which may lead to attempts to force treatment against the wishes of older adolescents. While the use of force may be justifiable when a life-threatening situation can be readily reversed (such as a one-time blood transfusion in an adolescent Jehovah's Witness), it is always better to elicit the assent of the adolescent through respectful conversation and establishment of trust. While that may not always be possible, it is far better than the use of force, which shows disrespect and engenders distrust. That disrespect and distrust will likely interfere with future attempts to create an optimal care plan for adolescents with prolonged illnesses and chronic diseases. While honoring Kristin's request to go home may carry some risk to her health, it does maintain a relationship with the patient, leaving the door open for future attempts at engaging Kristin in a healthy care plan.

References

Alderson, P. (2007). Competent children? Minors' consent to health care treatment and research. *Social Science and Medicine*, **65**, 2272–2283.

Alderson, P., Sutcliffe, K., & Curtis, K. (2006). Children's competence to consent to medical treatment. *Hastings Center Report*, **36**(6), 25–34.

American Academy of Pediatrics, Committee on Bioethics (1995). Informed consent, parental permission, and assent in pediatric practice. *Pediatrics*, **95**(2), 314–317.

Bartholome, W. (1995). Letter to the Editor, in response to: Informed consent, parental permission, and assent in pediatric practice. *Pediatrics*, **95**(2), 981–982.

Derish, M.T. & Heuvel, K.V. (2000). Mature minors should have the right to refuse life-sustaining medical treatment. *Journal of Law, Medicine and Ethics*, **28**, 109–124.

Gardner, M. & Steinberg L. (2005). Peer influence on risk taking, risk preference, and risky decision making in adolescence and adulthood: an experimental study. *Developmental Psychology*, **41**(4), 625–635.

Opel, D. & Kelley, M. (2010). Denial. *Hastings Center Report*, **40**, 11–12.

Pasupathi, M., Staudinger, U.M., & Baltes, P.B. (2001). Seeds of wisdom: adolescents' knowledge and judgment about difficult life problems. *Developmental Psychology*, **37**(3), 351–361.

Ross, L.F. (2009). Against the tide: arguments against respecting a minor's refusal of efficacious life-saving treatment. *Cambridge Quarterly of Healthcare Ethics*, **18**, 302–315.

Tan, J.O. (2003). Conduct and compassion: the anorexia talking? *Lancet*, **362**, 1246.

Tan, J.O., Hope, T., Stewart, A., & Fitzpatrick, R. (2006). Competence to make treatment decisions in anorexia nervosa: thinking processes and values. *Philosophy, Psychiatry, and Psychology*, **13**(4), 267–282.

Weir, R.F. & Peters, C. (1997). Affirming the decisions adolescents make about life and death. *Hastings Center Report*, **27**(6), 29–40.

Chapter

6

Family beliefs and the medical care of children

Roger Worthington and Mark R. Mercurio

Case narrative

Richard, a 15-year-old living with his parents and younger sister, has recently been diagnosed with Hodgkin disease after having been brought into the hospital by a school nurse. He enjoyed good health prior to his diagnosis, having previously experienced no major illnesses or need for surgery. After an initial evaluation, Richard and his parents meet with the hematologist/oncologist to discuss the diagnosis and treatment. They are told that with appropriate treatment, including chemotherapy, his chances of long-term survival are better than 90%. However, side effects of treatment are significant, including marked fatigue, nausea, and vomiting. While long-term sequelae may result from the disease and the treatment, Richard could live for decades with the recommended regimen and be able to fulfill his dream of becoming a pilot. His parents ask what the outcome would be if they decline the recommended treatment and are told that his chances of survival would be extremely low, possibly zero.

The parents appear genuinely concerned for their son and seem to understand what is at stake. They thank the physician for the information and then politely say that the decision they have reached is to pray for healing, and not to give permission for their son's medical treatment. They say that this decision is in keeping with long-held family beliefs and they feel confident that their son is going to be "fine." Richard, who seems bright if slightly immature, says he agrees with his parents' decision and that "it's about respecting family beliefs and tradition."

Introduction of ethical issues

This case raises several important questions. Perhaps the primary ethical issue concerns parental authority, particularly the question of when parents can refuse potentially life-saving medical treatment on behalf of a minor on grounds of religious, cultural, or personal beliefs. In this case, Richard appears to agree with his parents, which also requires an exploration of his own authority (particularly when supported by his parents) to make life-altering decisions about his health care. These questions are accompanied by several additional questions:

- *How mature is Richard and how much does he understand?* Though Richard may have partial autonomy, it might not be appropriate to respect his refusal of life-saving treatment. Given the serious consequences that will result from a decision to forgo recommended treatment, demonstration of a high level of maturity and capacity would be required before the decision of a minor would be respected.

- *Does it matter if the family's objection is based solely on religion?* Many pediatricians (including MM) would argue that the analysis is essentially the same – prioritize the child's fundamental rights and administer treatments that are likely to save a child's life – regardless of whether the parent's objection to recommended medical treatment is based on religious, philosophical, or other beliefs.

- *To what extent does it matter that a religion is well established as opposed to something that is less well understood? What does "prayer" really mean?* Prayer alone does not imply any organized religion, merely that the family is in some sense "religious." The degree to which their religious beliefs are shared by others (i.e., is theirs a mainstream religion or not) should not be determinative. What matters more is the relationship between parental rights, Richard's

Clinical Ethics in Pediatrics: A Case-Based Textbook, ed. Douglas S. Diekema, Mark R. Mercurio and Mary B. Adam. Published by Cambridge University Press. © Cambridge University Press 2011.

right to be treated, and the obligations of the clinical team.

- *Does it make a difference that Richard lives at home with his parents and therefore may be subject to "coercion" in expressing his opinion? If coerced, consent is normally invalidated.* Richard lives at home with his parents and so is not an "emancipated minor." His independent views may not be well established, and even if they were, that fact might not determine the final decision on whether or not he has medical treatment.

Ethical principles and discussion

Based on respect for autonomy (the principle of self-determination), it is generally accepted that a mentally competent adult has a right to refuse recommended medical or surgical treatment, even if that refusal results in death. For children, respect for autonomy is not always feasible or reasonable as it requires a level of understanding and reasoning ability that the child may not possess. If a child lacks sufficient maturity to be able to play a decisive role in decision-making, a surrogate decision-maker (usually the parents) will decide on the child's behalf (Mercurio, 2010). In this case, the parents and Richard are in agreement, but given the risk to benefit ratio not everyone would agree that the family's decision should be respected. Richard's right to have his life and future prospects protected may trump respect for the autonomy of the family.

Parents have responsibility for but do not *own* their children, and they can and should gradually cede autonomy to their children as they grow up. When determining the extent to which a given child or adolescent is permitted to decide, it must be recognized that children mature at different rates and that medical interventions carry varying degrees of risk. While the quality of the relationship between physician and family is pivotal, so too is that between parent and child, and although parents may want to influence choices that their children make, it is not guaranteed that from a child's perspective parental influence is always benign. While questions of consent and assent are dealt with elsewhere in this text, it should be emphasized that young people must not be excluded from the decision-making process, and a responsible teenager is entitled to hold his/her independent views, including views on matters of belief. Such views may not be determinative but they should never be ignored, and situations such as this require careful handling.

Questions of rights

Rights are an important element in making medical decisions for and with minors. Though rights have the characteristic of being concerned with overarching principles, rights can equally apply to the specifics of a given case. For instance, if parents ask a physician to act in a way that appears *not* to be in a child's best interests, the physician may have a duty not to comply, if it helps protect a child from harm. While parents generally have a right to determine what is done to or for their child, including on matters of religious and cultural belief, the rights of the child (e.g., to receive effective treatment) trump those of the parents. Children have personhood and human rights independently of their parents, and sometimes physicians and others need to assume the role of advocate.

Children's rights generally need more protection than parental rights, irrespective of questions of religion, and in the present case, the issue is whether treatment refusal is justified and whether alternative measures being advocated are reasonable and appropriate. In short, the harm of allowing Richard to die may not be outweighed by the benefit of respecting family beliefs. If the clinical team makes a determination based on the child's best interests, they need to question the preference shared by Richard and his parents and establish what *genuinely* is in his best interests, while recognizing that elements of subjectivity are necessarily entailed in making that judgment.

Whilst basic principles of freedom to practice belief free from external interference are not in dispute, where medical decisions have to be made on behalf of a child, such freedoms are not without limit. In this situation, the question is whether the team, backed up by the courts if need be, could be justified in going against the wishes of the family in order to guarantee that Richard has necessary and appropriate medical treatment. While the answer here is probably "yes," it may be helpful to consider another, less controversial case.

A secondary case

A 29-year-old woman is brought in to the emergency department after an auto accident with internal injuries and hemorrhage. She is conscious and gives consent for surgery; however, when told that she will almost certainly need a transfusion, she withdraws consent based on her religious belief. Her husband is present and confirms that this decision is consistent with her beliefs. Subsequently, another ambulance brings in their 3-year-old son with similar injuries. The parents give consent for surgery on their son but not for transfusion on the same basis of religion.

- *Should the woman be transfused over her own objection once in the operating room?*
- *Does she have sufficient capacity to make this decision, and if so, does her right to autonomy mean that her decision must be respected?*
- *Could the husband override her refusal?*
- *Should the child be transfused over the parents' objection?*
- *What if one parent consents but not the other?*

In this situation a judgment has to be made based on the likely outcomes of doing surgery without transfusion, doing surgery with transfusion, and doing no surgery at all. This will be done by the attending physician in consultation with members of the team, often with reference to a formal protocol for handling similar cases. Her refusal may have to be respected, even though she is a mother with responsibility for a young child. However, her mental capacity may be compromised due to the accident, making it difficult for her to reach a proper decision. While her prior wishes are clear, in this situation a second opinion might be needed in order to establish her level of capacity. If she is mentally competent the mother's refusal of her own transfusion has to be honored, and her husband has no legal right to oppose that decision.

If the parents disagree with each other about their son, and/or if the parents both object to him having a transfusion, physicians should seek a court order in order to protect the life and well-being of this 3-year-old. Physicians are in any case justified in proceeding despite the parents' wishes with regard to the transfusion on the basis that this is an emergency situation requiring life-saving treatment for a vulnerable child. Questions of capacity are not relevant for the boy on account of his young age, and other questions can wait until later when there may be more time for discussion. His best interests are paramount, and they clearly point towards him having life-saving treatment, including a transfusion, should that become necessary.

To return to the main case, if reliance on prayer means refusing medical treatment, the harm principle would apply when parents refuse potentially life-saving treatment on behalf of adolescents who themselves lack capacity for making life and death decisions (i.e., possibly requiring you to involve state agencies in an attempt to intervene over parental objections). The

situation is complicated in some jurisdictions. For example, the State Code of Virginia (Virginia Code, 2007) asserts that prayer is a form of treatment. The State Code does not have federal jurisdiction, and such claims are controversial though not without precedent (Mercurio, 2007). The Virginia state law was passed in response to the case of an adolescent named Abraham Cherrix, who, with his parents in agreement, refused additional chemotherapy for Hodgkin disease. The Cherrix case, which has similarities with Richard's case, had to be resolved in court, resulting in a compromise agreement whereby Abraham was directed to receive radiotherapy but without chemotherapy. The family was not prevented from continuing to use prayer and herbal remedies, but they were not permitted to rely solely on prayer for his treatment. He was a minor, and until he turned 18 he had to keep the court informed about his medical progress. This was viewed by some as overly intrusive on the family's freedom. Subsequently, with the passage in Virginia of what became known as "Abraham's Law," minors 14 years old and above may be permitted to refuse medically recommended treatment in cases such as this, if parents are in agreement, and a judge feels the patient is adequately mature to make the decision.

Refusal by a child and general points of law

Refusal of treatment by a minor raises a number of issues. With young children parental wishes normally prevail, but in adolescent cases child refusal of treatment is sometimes a gray area, requiring assessment of the merits and demerits of the individual case.

A landmark US Supreme Court decision in 1944 argued that:

> Parents may be free to become martyrs themselves. But it does not follow they are free, in identical circumstances, to make martyrs of their children before they have reached the age of full and legal discretion when they can make that choice for themselves. (*Prince v. Massachusetts*, 1944)

This shows that even on matters of religion the state has power to exert control over children in a way that does not apply to adults. While there is lack of uniformity between different states (meaning that child protection measures might be invoked in some states and not others), the policy statement from the American Academy of Pediatrics (AAP) rightly makes the general point that "All legal interventions apply equally whenever children are endangered or harmed, without exemptions based on parental religious beliefs" (AAP, 1997).

The AAP position is unambiguous but it exposes tension that sometimes exists between law and ethics. While the AAP advocates that "Children, regardless of parental religious beliefs, deserve effective medical treatment when such treatment is likely to prevent substantial harm or suffering or death" (AAP, 1997/2009), this statement has no weight in law. It is an ethical opinion, and states may differ on points of law. Decisions, therefore, not only have to be clinically case specific, but they have to be addressed on the basis of the law within the jurisdiction where they occur.

The balance of harms *for* and *against* providing treatment is normally assessed against the relative risks and burdens of pursuing (or not pursuing) a given course of action, and while general principles can provide valuable frameworks, they may not provide "answers." For example, a decision to refuse available and potentially life-sustaining treatment for a minor will almost always be challenged by the clinical team or the courts. Such refusals may act as a trigger for legal measures being taken against the parents to protect a child from abuse or neglect (including choices made in the name of religion). Decisions to instigate child protection measures, however, must not be made lightly as the consequences of involving state agencies can be very far-reaching.

Summary of key points

1. *Consult, consult, consult.* Breakdown of communication is damaging to all parties, not least to a child, and dialogue is always better than confrontation, even if recourse to external decisional support is required (such as a pediatrics ethics committee or family court). In addition, when parents and/or patients disagree with treatment that the physician feels is critically important, the physician may need to consult with colleagues and invite a second opinion.
2. *The best interests principle is only a guide.* The child's best interests are always paramount, but it represents a principle, not a standard, and cases must be assessed on their merits, intervening where necessary to protect a child from harm.
3. *Children have rights.* It is sometimes but not always desirable to uphold the rights of the child over the rights of the parent(s). Specifically, the child

has a right to receive treatment likely to prevent significant harm or death (AAP 1997).

4. *Religion and culture are not necessarily the same.* Sometimes, parental objections are about cultural norms more than religious belief. Differentiate between the two, where possible, and do not be afraid to openly discuss religion if it really is pivotal. It may be helpful to involve clergy, as sometimes parents misinterpret the requirements of their religious community. The same may be true for cultural beliefs, and a community leader may be helpful in those cases. The physician must keep in mind that religious beliefs or cultural traditions may hold a position of central importance in the lives of patients and families. Problems sometimes stem not just from families misinterpreting official versions of their religion but from health professionals making wrong assumptions, such as confusing religion with cultural and social norms. Final decisions ultimately have to be based on facts, not supposition.
5. *If in doubt, seek a second opinion and/or legal advice.* Some cases are just tough, whichever way you look at them; always seek help if you need it. This help can take the form of second opinions, case conferences, ethics consultation, and consultation with legal counsel.

Resolution of the case

A boy of this age lacks maturity to reach a decision of such significance on his own. He appears to be in agreement with the surrogate decision-makers (i.e., his parents), but it would be wrong to respect these wishes without seeking some form of independent review. In this case, the situation is not an emergency and so there is plenty of time to consult. If this involved a boy or a parent with a psychiatric condition (i.e., causing "irrational" choices to be made) the process would be different; here there is no such indication. Things must always be handled with sensitivity, and while much depends on the maturity of the son and the nature of the relationship with his parents, ultimately a decision may have to be imposed on the family through state action.

Here the likely benefit of proposed treatment is so high (probably life-saving) when compared with the alternative chosen by the family (prayer alone) that the physician should not accept their refusal, regardless of whether it is based on religious, philosophical, cultural, or other grounds. If the patient and family continue to refuse after appropriate discussion and consultations, and the physician continues to believe that the recommended treatment is necessary to save the child's life, an appeal to the courts should be made. The threshold for involving the courts is relative to the extent and nature of disagreement between the parties involved. Failure to find a mutually acceptable way forward is one trigger, especially where the life of a minor is at stake, and State legal convention ultimately may be the determining factor, but it is worth remembering that in cases such as this there is time for discussion. Richard is not going to die if he does not have treatment today or tomorrow, unlike with the secondary case, where immediate transfusion was very likely to be needed and without which the child could die within a short space of time.

These decisions are always difficult for all parties. The following eight questions may be helpful in deciding when state action is indicated (Diekema, 2004):

1. By refusing to consent are the parents placing their child at significant risk of serious harm?
2. Is the harm imminent, requiring immediate action to prevent it?
3. Is the intervention that has been refused necessary to prevent the serious harm?
4. Is the intervention that has been refused of proven efficacy and, therefore, likely to prevent the harm?
5. Does the intervention that has been refused by the parents not also place the child at significant risk of serious harm and do its projected benefits outweigh its projected burdens significantly more favorably than the option chosen by the parents?
6. Would any other option prevent serious harm to the child in a way that is less intrusive to parental autonomy and more acceptable to the parents?
7. Can the state intervention be generalized to all other similar situations?
8. Would most parents agree that the state intervention was reasonable?

References

American Academy of Pediatrics, Committee on Bioethics (1997, reaffirmed 2009). Policy Statement: Religious Objections to Medical Care. *Pediatrics*, **99**, 279–281.

Diekema D.S. (2004). Parental refusals of medical treatment: the harm principle as threshold for state intervention. *Theoretical Medicine and Bioethics*, **25**(4), 243–264.

Mercurio, M.R. (2007). An adolescent's refusal of medical treatment: implications of the Abraham Cheerix case. *Pediatrics*, **120**(6), 1357–1358.

Mercurio, M.R. (2010). Adolescent parents of critically ill newborns: rights and obligations. *Journal of Pediatrics*, **157**(6), 1030–1034.

Prince v. *Massachusetts* (1944). 321 US 158 [321 US 170].

Virginia Code § 63.2–100 (2007, amended 2010). http://leg1. state.va.us/cgi-bin/legp504.exe?000+cod+63.2–100 (last accessed August 26, 2010).

Chapter

7

Fidelity and truthfulness in the pediatric setting: withholding information from children and adolescents

Christine Harrison

Case narrative

Amanda is a bright, active 12-year-old, who has been experiencing some shortness of breath and taking naps after school, something she has never done even as a toddler. After fainting during a track and field meet, her physician ordered a number of tests and diagnosed Amanda with dilated cardiomyopathy. Amanda's father died of a drug overdose before she was born. Amanda's mother, Lynn, hoping to protect Amanda from knowledge of her father's lifestyle, has told her that he died of a sudden heart attack. She is raising Amanda on her own, without family or community to support her.

At the time of Amanda's diagnosis, her pediatric cardiologist advises Lynn that Amanda will likely need a heart transplant. He suggests that the pediatric cardiology fellow, advance practice nurse, and child life specialist meet with Amanda and her mother to explain Amanda's condition, the medication she will have to take, and the likely need for surgery, in a developmentally appropriate way.

Lynn comes to the meeting without Amanda. She agrees that Amanda will have to be told that she needs to take medication, but requests that the explicit diagnosis and need for surgery not be disclosed. She insists that she knows her daughter will become depressed and "lose her right to a childhood," worrying constantly that she is about to die of a heart attack as she believes her father did.

Introduction

The parents of a child or adolescent who has a serious illness are faced with many treatment decisions. Their parenting philosophy and values may be challenged in unfamiliar ways, forcing them to reflect on the nature of their relationship with their child and their

responsibilities as parents. Health care professionals who care for children may also have their personal and professional values challenged and may experience conflicting responsibilities to their patients and their patients' parents. The health care team must decide how much information to share with a child, both at the child's initial diagnosis, and again throughout the course of her illness and treatment as new information becomes available. Parents and clinicians may hold different views about the nature of their obligations in this context. Two ethical principles that may help guide their thinking are fidelity and truthfulness.

Ethical principles: fidelity and truthfulness

Fidelity requires that we act towards others in such a way that we fulfill the commitments made and the promises implicit in the relationship we have with them. In medicine, this includes placing the patient's interests ahead of others' interests, including those of members of the patient's family, society, and oneself (Beauchamp & Childress, 2009). In pediatrics, however, the intertwined interests of the child and family often require health practitioners and parents to collaborate when determining what care is likely to be best for the child.

It is not unreasonable for parents to desire to protect their child from potentially distressing information, and, as in Amanda's case, to ask that the child not be told their explicit diagnosis. Ideally, disclosure of medical information should be guided by the principle of fidelity, but should also be appropriate to the patients' developmental capacities and independence. Decisions for younger children will be made for them by their parents (or guardians) in collaboration with

Clinical Ethics in Pediatrics: A Case-Based Textbook, ed. Douglas S. Diekema, Mark R. Mercurio and Mary B. Adam. Published by Cambridge University Press. © Cambridge University Press 2011.

the health care team; treatment decisions for older children and adolescents will more actively involve them. As minor patients increase in maturity and decision-making capacity, they should be allowed a greater role in making medical decisions, while their parents' role transitions from one of decision-making to one of support.

On first consideration it may seem obvious that physicians should be truthful with their patients and that to do otherwise would be inconsistent with values that are core to the patient–physician relationship. However, to say that one must be truthful with patients is not as straightforward as it seems. Philosophically, the notion of "truth" is the subject of considerable debate (Simmons, 2006). In health care, at minimum, we might say that being truthful means not providing inaccurate information to a patient with the intention to deceive. We might then consider questions regarding the disclosure of information, such as, how much information is enough? What format is appropriate? When is the "right" time to disclose? The answers to each of these questions will vary from case to case, especially in pediatrics where the child's or adolescent's developmental stage, emotional state and desire for knowledge, and the parents' views about how the child is likely to cope, are all relevant considerations.

Health care professionals who practice in Western settings value effective communication and truth-telling, as reflected in professional codes of ethics and the doctrine of informed consent. Interestingly, these values have not always been seen as essential to the practice of medicine. Until the mid twentieth century, most physicians believed that dismal diagnoses and prognoses should not be disclosed to patients, at least not by the physician (Katz, 1984). Some parents today, especially those from non-Western or ethnically diverse backgrounds, hold a similar view and see the decision about what information to provide children and adolescents as rightfully belonging to parents, not health care professionals (Valle, 2001; Gupta et al., 2008; Hurwitz Swota, 2008).

Pediatric associations have established standards through the development of position and policy statements stressing the importance of communicating effectively and honestly with children, while acknowledging that this may require negotiation with parents (British Medical Association, 2001; Canadian Paediatric Society Bioethics Committee, 2004; Levetown & AAP Committee on Bioethics, 2008). These guidance documents acknowledge the fact that parents may have deeply held beliefs that may be grounded in personal, religious, or cultural values that may influence their views about the disclosure of medical information to their children. In general, these beliefs should be respected. If there is concern about the child or adolescent being harmed in some way due to a decision to withhold information, those concerns should be raised with the parents in a way that focuses attention on the child's or adolescent's needs.

Requests from parents to withhold or limit information to their children should be explored with them, and discussions should include the following considerations:

- Children like Amanda have serious, lifelong health problems. They will maintain relationships with their pediatric teams until they transition to the adult system, and will require specialized care throughout their lives. The adult system presumes that the patient is the primary decision-maker and thus entitled to available information about their health condition and treatment alternatives. An important part of preparing adolescents for this transition is recognizing and supporting their role in their own health care, including decision-making about treatment.

- Health care providers can respect children and adolescents as persons by acting consistently and honestly to fulfill their commitment to these patients. There is some research to suggest that many children and adolescents want to be told the truth and to participate in decisions about their care (Ellis & Leventhal, 1993; Lyon et al., 2004; Wolfe, 2004).

- Caregivers who communicate openly and provide forthright opportunities for children and adolescents to discuss their illness may help reduce their patients' anxiety and improve coping, consistent with duties of beneficence and nonmaleficence (Turkoski, 2003; Beale et al., 2005; Goldie et al., 2005; Kouyoumdjian et al., 2005).

- Providing children and adolescents with developmentally appropriate information about their condition and treatment supports their ability and, in some cases, their right to participate in decision-making. In legal jurisdictions where there is no explicit age of consent (e.g., Ontario, Canada) the capacity to make specific treatment decisions triggers the right to do so, which also creates an obligation to ensure that legal decision-makers (in some cases the child or adolescent) are fully informed about their health condition and details of treatment options.

- Many professional codes of ethics consider good communication and the provision of information to be an ethical duty.

On the other hand, there may be reasons to honor parents' requests to withhold information from their child or adolescent. These might include the following:

- Caregivers should respect the moral and legal authority and role of parents. For example, a Canadian Supreme Court decision, *R.B. v. Children's Aid Society of Metropolitan Toronto* (1995), supported parents' rights to make decisions about issues affecting their children:

    … the common law has always, in the absence of demonstrated neglect or unsuitability, presumed that parents should make all significant choices affecting their children, and has afforded them a general liberty to do as they choose … our society is far from having repudiated the privileged role parents exercise in the upbringing of their children. This role translates into a protected sphere of parental decision-making which is rooted in the presumption that parents should make important decisions affecting their children both because parents are more likely to appreciate the best interests of their children and because the state is ill-equipped to make such decisions itself.

- While health care professionals have an independent duty to guard the interests of the child-patient, parents are usually higher standing in decisions by virtue of their personal knowledge of the child and the values by which the family lives. The consequences of decisions made are also more likely to be borne by parents than medical caretakers.

- Sometimes there exists an unspoken agreement between parents and their children to avoid speaking about distressing things. Such "mutual pretense" may serve as a coping mechanism for some patients and families (Bluebond-Langner, 1978).

- To respect parents' wishes is consistent with the philosophy of Family Centered Care, prevalent in pediatric health care institutions (Committee on Hospital Care, 2003). This philosophy recognizes the important role parents play in caring for their children, and acknowledges the significance of families' values in this context.

Amanda's mother, Lynn, has acted in the past to protect her daughter from distressing information and now wishes to prevent Amanda from learning the seriousness of her medical condition, the true cause of her father's death, and the fact that she has lied to Amanda about her father's death. Exploring these issues with Lynn may reveal that she places a higher value on beneficence than truth-telling, and that she sees her actions as protective of her daughter and consistent with her own role as a parent.

Even if Amanda's caregivers are willing to limit the information she is given about her condition and treatment, however, the physical and social environment where health care is provided makes doing so difficult or even impossible. Most attempts to keep "secrets" from patients are unsuccessful. The body language and whispering of adults combined with physician's visits, laboratory or radiologic investigations, and hospital stays that are not adequately explained lead patients, including children, to realize that something is wrong. Their imagined fears may be worse than the truth. Adolescents may find consent forms or health literature that was provided to their parents or in the waiting room that provide clues to their illness. Clinic waiting rooms, hospital play rooms, and disease-specific camps and fundraisers create opportunities for children and families to meet others who are going through similar experiences with whom they may talk. Finally, many children and adolescents use the Internet to research their health conditions. The ability to restrict and filter information that children and adolescents receive may be limited by such practicalities, and parents' wishes to protect through secrecy may not be realistically supportable in the current environment.

While Amanda's case focuses on a parent wishing to withhold information from a child who is likely to survive and do well with treatment, clinicians who care for children with life-threatening illnesses may be asked by parents to not disclose to the child when the illness has entered its terminal phase. Practically, it may be easier to carry this off if dying children are cared for at home. Changes in the care plan, such as shifting care from aggressive treatment given in the hospital to comfort measures at home, will not go unnoticed, however, and some studies suggest that, contrary to protecting children from harm in these situations, they often are well aware that they are seriously ill or dying, and their fears and anxieties may escalate if they don't have an opportunity to discuss them (Wolfe et al., 2002).

Ethics in practice

There are a number of issues that teams such as Amanda's should assess and discuss when faced with a parent's request to limit or withhold information from her child or adolescent.

Is the child or adolescent likely to experience harm if information is withheld from him or her? Team members may be uncomfortable with parents' request to limit or withhold information, yet they may be reluctant to override a parent's request at the risk of compromising the parent–provider relationship. If harm to the patient is likely, however, there is less justification for honoring the request. For example, the child might develop anxiety and depression when her questions and concerns about her health go unanswered. Children and adolescents in these situations should be carefully monitored. Some children who are seriously ill, and from whom information is withheld, may have greater anxiety than those who are able to ask questions about their condition and treatment (Turkoski, 2003; Beale et al., 2005; Goldie et al., 2005; Kouyoumdjian et al., 2005). Additionally, if there is a good chance that attempts to withhold information will fail and inadvertent disclosure occurs, this may seriously harm the child or adolescent's ability to trust her parents or the physicians in the future. Careful and sensitively planned disclosure may not eliminate this harm, but may reduce it.

Involving the multidisciplinary team. It is important that members of the multidisciplinary team participate in discussions about whether or not the team will try to limit the information that is intentionally disclosed to the child and if so, for how long. Some members spend a great deal of time with children (e.g., nurses providing bedside care and rehabilitation specialists). Children may ask these team members questions or demonstrate signs that they are confused or anxious about their condition and treatment. It is not fair to expect health care professionals to lie to their patients and doing so requires them to constantly scan the environment for risks of inadvertent disclosure.

Negotiating a plan. Teams should enter discussions with parents prepared to listen to their concerns, discuss practical and ethical reasons why secrecy may not be a realistic option, and explain their experience with other children or adolescents and their families. One model that has been developed in the context of HIV involves "partial truth-telling," i.e., gradual, developmentally appropriate disclosure. Younger children are given basic explanations about their health condition and treatment; however, the actual diagnosis and the words "HIV" or "AIDS" are not used. As the child develops and begins to indicate a desire for information, further disclosure is planned and carried out

together with families (increasing their sense of control). This strategy could be negotiated and used effectively when parents wish to withhold information from children with other conditions as well (Salter-Goldie et al., 2007).

Seeking ethics consultation. Where there is significant ethical uncertainty or conflict among team members including seemingly intractable conflict between the team and the family, pediatricians are advised to seek ethics consultation, either through an ethics committee or an ethics consultant, bioethicist, or clinical ethicist. While the roles and functions of committees and consultants may vary, they will assist clinicians in identifying and analyzing ethical issues, supporting teams and families through the facilitation of challenging negotiations, and providing information about relevant ethical norms, law, and policy considerations.

Amanda: working towards a resolution

The pediatric cardiology fellow, advance practice nurse, and child life specialist were expecting to meet with Amanda and her mother, Lynn, to begin information disclosure and education with Amanda so that her treatment might proceed and plans be set in place for a work-up towards a heart transplant. They were unprepared for her mother's request that Amanda not be given explicit information about her condition or the need for transplant. They listened to Lynn's explanation, and explained to her that her request would have to be discussed with the multidisciplinary team and the responsible physician. A follow-up appointment with Lynn was made.

Prior to this follow-up meeting, a multidisciplinary case conference was held, which included professionals from the many services who would be providing care to Amanda; the hospital bioethicist was also invited to attend. Some individuals raised concerns about the challenges of providing coordinated and complex care while constantly guarding what they said to the patient – to many this felt ethically equivalent to lying. Some were more willing to compromise than others, and after a thorough discussion over several meetings facilitated by the bioethicist, the health care team reached an agreement that the pediatric cardiologist, fellow and advance practice nurse would meet with Lynn to discuss her concerns as well as those of the team. The team's goal for the meeting was to engage Amanda's mother in a time-limited plan to identify information that would be necessary for Amanda in order to proceed with treatment, to collaborate on the most compassionate and developmentally suitable way of disclosing this information, and to decide how disclosure would occur. The team agreed to compromise, with two exceptions – they would not intentionally lie to Amanda, and they would monitor her psychological and emotional condition. If they had good reason to believe that limiting information was causing her anxiety and distress they would offer opportunities for her to raise questions and concerns with members of the team. Amanda's mother, although initially angry and reluctant to compromise, appreciated that the team respected her concerns and agreed to work together to plan staged disclosure to Amanda so that treatment could begin.

Acknowledgment

Michelle Greenwood, LLB assisted with legal research.

References

Beale, E.A., Baile, W.F., & Aaron, J. (2005). Silence is not golden: communicating with children dying from cancer. *Journal of Clinical Oncology*, **23**, 3629–3631.

Beauchamp, T.L. & Childress, J.F. (2009). *Principles of Biomedical Ethics*. New York: Oxford University Press.

Bluebond-Langner, M. (1978). *The Private Worlds of Dying Children*. Princeton, NJ: Princeton University Press.

British Medical Association (2001). *Consent, Rights and Choices in Health Care for Children and Young People*. London: BMJ Books.

Canadian Paediatric Society Bioethics Committee (2004). Treatment decisions regarding infants, children and adolescents. Canadian Paediatric Society Reference Number B04-01. *Paediatrics and Child Health*, **9**, 99–103.

Committee on Hospital Care. American Academy of Pediatrics (2003). Family-centered care and the pediatrician's role. *Pediatrics*, **112**, 691–697.

Ellis, R. & Leventhal, B. (1993). Information needs and decision-making preferences of children with cancer. *Psycho-Oncology*, **2**, 277–284.

Goldie, J., Schwartz, L., & Morrison, J. (2005). Whose information is it anyway? Informing a 12-year-old patient of her terminal prognosis. *Journal of Medical Ethics*, **31**, 427–434.

Gupta, V.B., Willert, J., Pian, M., & Stein, M.T. (2008). When disclosing a serious diagnosis to a minor conflicts with family values. *Journal of Developmental & Behavioral Pediatrics*, **29**, 231.

Hurwitz Swota, A. (2008). Cultural diversity in the clinical setting. In *Ethics By Committee: A Textbook on Consultation, Organization, and Education for Hospital Ethics Committees*, ed. D.M. Hester. Lanham, MA: Rowman & Littlefield Publishers, Inc.

Katz, J. (1984). *The Silent World of Doctor and Patient*. New York: The Free Press.

Kouyoumdjian, F.G., Meyers, T., & Mtshizana, S. (2005). Barriers to disclosure to children with HIV. *Journal of Tropical Pediatrics*, **51**, 285–287.

Levetown, M. & American Academy of Pediatrics Committee on Bioethics (2008). Communicating with children and families: from everyday interactions to skill in conveying distressing information. *Pediatrics*, **121**, E1441–1460.

Lyon, M.E., McCabe, M.A., Patel, K.M., & D'Angelo, L.J. (2004). What do adolescents want? An exploratory study regarding end-of-life decision-making. *Journal of Adolescent Health*, **35**, 529.E1–6.

R.B. v. Children's Aid Society of Metropolitan Toronto (1995). 1 SCR 315 [1994] at Para. 85.

Salter-Goldie, R., King, S.M., Smith, M.L., et al . (2007). Disclosing HIV diagnosis to infected children: a health care team's approach. *Vulnerable Children and Youth Studies*, **2**, 12–16.

Simmons, K. (2006). Truth. In *Encyclopedia of Philosophy*, ed. D. Borchert. Detroit: Macmillan Reference USA.

Turkoski, B.B. (2003). A mother's orders about truth telling. *Home Healthcare Nurse*, **21**, 81–83.

Valle, R. (2001). Cultural assessment in bioethical advocacy – toward cultural competency in bioethical practice. *Bioethics Forum*, **17**, 15–26.

Wolfe, J., Friebert, S., & Hilden, J. (2002). Caring for children with advanced cancer integrating palliative care. *Pediatric Clinics of North America*, **49**, 1043–1062.

Wolfe, L. (2004). Should parents speak with a dying child about impending death? [Comment]. *New England Journal of Medicine*, **351**, 1251–1253.

Further reading

Bok, S. (1978). *Lying: Moral Choice in Public and Private Life*. New York: Pantheon Books.

Cassidy, R. (1996). Tell all the truth? Shepherds, liberators, or educators. In *Pediatric Ethics: From Principles to Practice*, ed. R. Cassidy & A.R. Fleischman. Amsterdam: Harwood Academic Publishers.

Harrison, C. (2010). Truthtelling in pediatrics: What they don't know might hurt them. In *Pediatric Bioethics*, ed. G. Miller. New York: Cambridge University Press.

Kuther, T.L. (2003). Medical decision-making and minors: issues of consent and assent. *Adolescence*, **38**, 343–358.

Rudd, R. & Anderson, J. (2006). *The health literacy environment of hospitals and health centers. Partners for action: Making your healthcare facility literacy-friendly*. Boston: Harvard School of Public Health.

Chapter

8

Fidelity and truthfulness: disclosure of errors

David J. Loren and Thomas H. Gallagher

Case narrative: medical misadventure and the case of Chloe

Chloe is a 3-month-old infant who was brought to the emergency department by her parents after developing a fever. Over the past 18 hours, she has become increasingly fussy and refused to nurse. While Chloe was being weighed in the triage room, her parents inquired about her weight in pounds, a number quickly provided by flicking a switch on the scale that changed the reading from metric (5.4 kilograms) to English (12 pounds) units. The nursing team was about to change shift and a nurse who was recording the weight heard Chloe's weight as 12 pounds and recorded this number on the triage chart. This weight was then entered as the kilogram dose calculation weight in Chloe's electronic medical record by a medical technician. During her evaluation, Chloe appeared ill, and displayed signs of moderate dehydration. Her laboratory findings were consistent with a urinary tract infection and she was admitted for intravenous antibiotic treatment with ampicillin and gentamicin; these drugs were ordered via the computerized provider order entry system, the doses calculated based on the infant's recorded weight. During the order entry, several message boxes appeared on the computer screen providing hospital announcements. Additionally, a warning box appeared questioning the doses of both antibiotics as excessive given the age of the patient. The provider in the emergency department, who had been on-duty for 14 hours at that point, was distracted and clicked all the dialogue boxes closed, permitting the order to be signed. The ampicillin was infused while Chloe was in the emergency department; the gentamicin dose arrived at her bedside just before she was transported to her acute care inpatient room. The emergency department nurse connected the gentamicin syringe to Chloe's IV pump, and the acute

care nurse activated the pump upon arrival at Chloe's room. Over the next 12 hours, Chloe's urine output did not normalize despite appropriate fluid resuscitation efforts. While evaluating her low urine output, she was weighed again and this new weight was recorded in her nursing notes. During change of nursing shift, Chloe's nurse reviewed her charting notes and recognized that the weight being used for the medications was over twice the correct weight and realized that the two antibiotics were overdosed. Chloe's nurse then called the on-call hospitalist to report the two medication errors. Because gentamicin can cause kidney and hearing damage, the level of Chloe's gentamicin level was checked and was found to be markedly elevated at 25 mcg/ml. Her serum creatinine had increased from 0.8 on admission to 3.5 mg/dl, suggestive of rapidly worsening kidney function.

Chloe's care team is now faced with an entirely new problem in her care. They must decide how to respond to this change in her renal function, if and how to tell Chloe's parents about what happened, how to report this event to the relevant hospital operations leadership, and what to do with their own deeply unsettling feelings that they may have just participated in a sequence of events that harmed one of their patients.

Discussion of issues

Among the most fundamental of ethical precepts in medicine is the principle of primum non nocere, "first do no harm." When Chloe's care team became aware of her medication overdose and consequent kidney injury, they began to grapple with vexing ethical challenges. What exactly is a medical error? How do they balance principles of beneficence, justice, truth-telling, and informed consent? How does each team member's perception of authority gradients influence their response to Chloe's medication errors? If Chloe were

Clinical Ethics in Pediatrics: A Case-Based Textbook, ed. Douglas S. Diekema, Mark R. Mercurio and Mary B. Adam. Published by Cambridge University Press. © Cambridge University Press 2011.

an older child, would we tell her, and if so, how? Who benefits from disclosing – or concealing – the medication error? Could disclosure also be harmful to some of the parties involved? Who takes responsibility for disclosing this error given the complexity of the events that ultimately led to her medication toxicity (Wu et al., 1997; Surbone et al., 2007; Shannon et al., 2009)?

A wide spectrum of investigations over the past two decades has demonstrated the alarming frequency and toll of medical errors in terms that are both economic (lost productivity, lost actual and potential income, increased length of hospitalizations, additional procedures and testing) and human (impact on individual and public trust of health care, reduced longevity and even mortality). Despite this public and academic attention to medical errors, there remains a lack of consensus regarding a clear definition of medical error. The Institute of Medicine, in the groundbreaking 2000 publication *To Err Is Human: Building a Safer Health System*, framed medical error as the "failure of a planned action to be completed as intended or the use of a wrong plan to achieve an aim." An adverse event, "harm that is the result of the process of healthcare rather than the patient's underlying disease," is distinctly different from a medical error and refers to a specific outcome rather than a breakdown in the process of care. Many medical errors are resolved before reaching a patient and thus cause no physical harm. Furthermore, many adverse events are not anticipated yet do not arise out of medical errors. Chloe's renal failure, and potential ototoxicity from the gentamicin overdose, appears to be an adverse event resulting from a complex medical error. When Chloe's nurse alerted the care team of the error no one yet understood the cause, or the range of care providers involved in the error (Gallagher & Lucas, 2005; Espin et al., 2006).

Multiple failures within Chloe's care ultimately led to her medication overdose. Errors that occur in complex systems are often not the result of a single failure; rather they are the result of a misfortunate alignment of latent errors. The first step in mitigating these process vulnerabilities is to admit that they exist. Chloe's team could justify disclosure based on their duty to fulfill a responsibility to institutional improvement by reporting this error to the hospital. At the time these errors were recognized her attending physician had only partial information about what happened and why, and none of Chloe's providers were certain of their own responsibility, if any, in causing these events. Nevertheless, by disclosing the initial basic facts of

her overdose to Chloe's parents, her team is effectively fostering a culture of accountability, open communication, and transparency (Shapiro, 2008; Gallagher, 2009).

Chloe's team could justify disclosure within the context of justice by adhering to standards of professionalism. The Joint Commission for Accreditation of Hospital Organizations (JCAHO) Standard R1.2.90 articulates that patients and families be informed about "unanticipated outcomes" of provided care. The National Quality Forum Safe Practice #4 describes specific mechanisms to support medical error disclosure, emphasizing transparency as a core value. The American Medical Association Code of Ethics E-8.12 on professionalism (issued in 1981 and reaffirmed in 1994 and 2005) defined medical error disclosure as a "fundamental ethical requirement," further admonishing physicians to refrain from allowing fear of legal repercussions to interfere with error disclosure.

Chloe's care team members could consider disclosing the medication error within the context of informed consent. Chloe's parents need to know and understand the current status of her health in order to make fully informed decisions regarding her additional care. Their only opportunity to fully participate in informed consent is for them to comprehend the details that led to her injury. Furthermore, withholding information germane to Chloe's health care would only be interpreted as dishonesty in the eyes of her parents. Such obfuscation undermines her care team's fiduciary relationship to Chloe and her parents, further disabling her parents' ability to accept and trust any proposed care (Gallagher et al., 2003).

Chloe's care team might be motivated to disclose the error out of a desire to repair her parents' trust in both the team and in health care in general. In this context, they may perceive disclosure as an ethical imperative of truth-telling. While societal, cultural, and religious paradigms promote the general concept of truth-telling, Chloe's care team may wrestle with just exactly how much, to whom, and for what purpose do they tell the truth. Their concerns appear to be validated based on data from surveyed physicians who report skepticism that disclosure has benefits for the patient; these surveys describe concerns that disclosure may be further injurious to a patient and that *non-disclosure* may represent patient-centered care (Gallagher, 2009).

Chloe's care team may view truth-telling as an avenue to empower her parents to better participate in medical decision-making, fostering family-centered care. However, telling Chloe herself (if she were an older child) presents additional, unexplored challenges. While the tenets of assent in pediatrics promote fostering a partnership between medical care teams, parents, and the child, truth-telling to a child may only undermine this partnership. Truth-telling depends upon both the accuracy of information and the candor with which it is communicated. How much truth can be relayed when an error is first reported can be further complicated as the initial impressions of the cause of a medical error are often inaccurate. Sufficient ambiguity may also exist in the early stages of a potential error discovery that care team members are unable disaggregate an adverse event from a naturally deteriorating clinical scenario. Chloe's team had only a few simple facts about the error available to them when the medication overdose was discovered. She received over twice the appropriate dose of two antibiotics, the weight recorded in her electronic medical record was not correct, and her renal function had worsened since being admitted to the hospital. Her care team understandably pondered the etiology of her clinical condition, wondering if nature, their care, or both were responsible. What data might guide this team as they contemplated telling Chloe's parents about the error (Lantos, 1996)?

Research over the past decade with adult patients has demonstrated that virtually all want to be told about serious medical errors and most even want to be told about minor errors. Parents maintain very similar expectations regarding errors that occur with the care of their children. When told about a medical error, patients and parents want to hear an explicit statement that an error occurred, what happened and why, as well any consequences for their child's continued health care. People harmed by an error want to know that their suffering was not in vain and thus want to know how recurrences of the error will be prevented. The majority of patients also want to hear an empathetic apology recognizing the harm that they have experienced. Chloe's team sympathized with these apparently simple directives. However, they acknowledged that fulfilling these expectations might create tension between serving Chloe's needs and protecting themselves from legal and disciplinary repercussions (Gallagher et al., 2003; Loren et al., 2008; Matlow et al., 2010).

Research into physician attitudes and experiences with medical error disclosure has demonstrated that they perceive multiple barriers to error disclosure including lack of training in leading these emotionally charged conversations and fear of disciplinary actions or harm to their reputation. Lastly, many physicians express a fear of being sued after disclosing a medical error. Nurses also report challenges with error disclosure, including lack of awareness of disclosure policies and concerns related to inconsistent inclusion in planning of error disclosure conversations. Consequently, a growing number of studies in the United States and Canada have demonstrated that physicians in all medical specialties disclose medical errors at rates below what is desired by patients and families. Additionally, a physician's assessment of how much a patient knows about the error appears to influence the likelihood of disclosure. Recurrently, research in error disclosure has demonstrated that physicians disclose less frequently when a patient is not aware that a medical error had occurred in his or her care. Chloe's attending physician is hesitant at first about disclosing this error, wondering whether her parents would ever find out about the error if never specifically told. Meanwhile, Chloe's nurse is aware of the error while she performs her morning assessments, her anxiety mounting as she greets Chloe's parents who do not yet know that Chloe has been exposed to a medication overdose with potentially serious harm (Gallagher et al., 2003; Loren et al., 2008).

Potent inter-professional issues of loyalty, fidelity, and trust can be present when an error arises out of the complex interplay between personnel, clinical processes, technology, and organizational factors within a clinical setting. How does a physician disclose an error when that physician may not have been directly involved, or not involved at all in that error? How does a team decide who will lead a disclosure conversation and how can team members remain confident that they will not be unduly implicated during a disclosure conversation? Some team members providing bedside care to a child may have knowledge of an error before a family has been told, creating extreme moral distress of the kind Chloe's nurse is experiencing. Indeed, team members may not all agree that an error occurred. The authority gradients present within a multidisciplinary care team can add additional challenges to successfully resolving these dilemmas. Chloe's attending physician wanted to be forthright as soon as possible with this family; however, she was uncertain of the proportional roles that the weight and drug overdoses played in Chloe's clinical condition. Chloe's parents might never know that these errors occurred; should they be told? Considering the answers to these questions elusive,

Chloe's attending physician approached the hospital's risk manager and patient safety director, asking specifically about whether the lack of parental knowledge of the weight and dosage errors should influence the decision to reveal any details of the potential causes of her clinical condition. Both administrators recommended that the parents be told about the weight and dosage errors, specifically counseling Chloe's attending physician to relay only the basic facts along with a commitment to share additional details about the error as they become better understood (Shannon et al., 2009).

Exploring the conflicts of interest posed by the disclosure of a medical error provides insights into the nuances of truth-telling and loyalty in this setting. Disclosing a medical error places tension between a family's desire for knowledge about what happened during their child's medical care and a physician or hospital's interest for self-preservation. Contemporary developments in the relationship between risk managers and physicians may serve as an effective illustration of the changing frame of loyalties within health care settings. Historically, risk managers have been perceived as protectors of a hospital's financial interests and have counseled physicians to refrain from disclosing errors. Recently, risk managers have assumed a more proactive role in protecting the hospital and advancing the paradigm of patient safety, by encouraging adverse event reporting and disclosure of medical errors. Indeed, present experience with medical error disclosure suggests that contrary to the classical paradigm of "do no harm to the organization" (e.g., do not tell patients about any errors), open and honest communication about unanticipated outcomes may actually lead to safer health care systems and greater patient trust in those organizations (Loren et al., 2010).

Chloe's attending physician prepared for the initial disclosure to the family, attentive to her internal tension between feeling compassion and fearing that Chloe's parents might wish to find culpability within her words. She wondered if a genuine apology might be self-sacrificial. The interaction between medical error disclosure, apology, and litigation is complex. Exactly why some patients seek legal counsel against a physician is not well understood. Indeed, some authors contend that greater error disclosure could increase the rate of litigation surrounding medical errors as more patients learn about the errors that occur in their care. Other authors argue that genuine and compassionate communication can diminish both the motivation for

legal redress and the enthusiasm for an attorney to pursue a case (Lazare, 2006; Studdert et al., 2007).

Perhaps the greatest challenge faced by everyone involved in Chloe's care was the anxiety and ambivalence they felt surrounding the unfamiliar terrain of disclosing errors and the unforeseeable outcomes that could follow the initial disclosure conversation. Who was benefiting from this disclosure? Disclosing this error allowed her parents to openly admit that they had been hurt in a human enterprise. For Chloe's care team, and the hospital, disclosure began the process of forgiveness and self-reconciliation that appears to be strongly desired by health care workers who have been involved in causing a medical error. Disclosing in pediatrics may be further complicated by the possibility that we may not know that harm occurred for a prolonged period. If Chloe's renal or auditory injuries are lifelong, who will tell her how it happened, and how should that disclosure be staged over time? Indeed, what role do parents play in the disclosure to the child, and how do we address their own potential sense of guilt arising out of their belief that they may not have adequately protected their child?

The errors that occurred in Chloe's care may have caused permanent injury as well as transient but life-threatening harm, fulfilling the Institute of Medicine's characterization of a serious medical error; her care team ultimately acknowledged little uncertainty that these events deserved disclosure. Had these events unfolded somewhat differently, had the infusion of antibiotics been stopped early enough to prevent an overdose, might the obligation to disclose the error be diminished? Indeed, might some medical errors be trivial enough – causing no harm at all – to obviate the need, or expectations, for disclosure? Considering a threshold for disclosure suggests that a boundary around transparency of institutional operations can be established, and justified in the eyes of parents.

Framing the decision to disclose based on the perception of harm alone is admittedly subjective and appears to only partially account for when parents desire to be told about errors that occur in the care of their children. In one study, nearly all (98%) parents expected to be told about a harmless medical error (child received an intravenous dose of an allergenic medication but experienced no symptoms) and a majority (80%) wanted to be told about a near miss (infusion of potentially allergenic medication stopped before the dose reached the child). Indeed, almost half (41%) of the parents endorsed disclosing the near miss to the child. Parents may view disclosure as a professional and institutional prima facie obligation for truth-telling, viewing their role as a partner in the medical care team and thus expecting to learn about process failures even if they were harmless (Matlow et al., 2010).

However, revealing every procedural misadventure also has the potential to imperil parental trust of the care team. Benevolent deception – therapeutic privilege – may be one strategy care team members employ in an effort to protect parents from a litany of clinically harmless system defects – mistimed blood tests, mislabeled samples, incorrectly infused crystalloid solutions, et cetera. Aware of the alarming frequency of near misses, parents might read the hospital's marquee through the eyes of Dante's words, "All hope abandon, ye who enter here!" While care team members may be genuinely motivated by sensitivity to parents' emotional turmoil, such deception if detected can only raise parental doubt, erode trust, and undermine the therapeutic alliance. While deception may not be morally equivalent to lying, the person being deceived is rarely likely to discriminate between the two. Reversing our role with the parent could endow us with sufficient perspective to recognize benevolent deception as only self-serving. Transparency – accessibility and opportunity for scrutiny – therefore may be the institutional realization of the concept of role-reversal (Bok, 1999).

Effective disclosure of errors

Fundamental first steps to effective error disclosure are grounded in empathic, honest, and genuine communication. Although every harmful medical error is accompanied by unique circumstances, a growing body of research offers the following framework for fulfilling patient and family expectations of disclosure:

1. Attend to caring for the patient immediately, and seek out additional clinical support when appropriate (acknowledging an error may leave care team members shaken enough to impair their clinical judgment).
2. As soon as possible, familiarize yourself with your institution's error disclosure procedures. You may be directed to establish contact with a representative from your organization's office of risk management or patient safety.
3. Begin to clarify as many of the facts as possible and avoid speculation about what led to the error. Rarely are all the details available when an error is first recognized.

4. Carefully plan the initial disclosure conversation. Consider who will be present, who will lead the conversation, and how questions will be answered. Consider who might take notes for the family during the meeting.
5. When meeting with the family, assess what they know already; fill in gaps by providing basic information about the error. Describe how, and if known, why it happened and how you will manage the medical consequences of the error. Call the error what it is, an error.
6. Extend an apology that acknowledges the suffering of the child and family.
7. Describe how the error will be investigated; demonstrate a commitment to preventing recurrences of the error.
8. Offer ongoing psychological support for the family and child. Heed any request for transferring care to another provider or facility.

These conversations are multiple and can be exhausting experiences for all involved (Wu et al., 1997; Gallagher & Lucas, 2005).

Resolution of case

Within minutes of learning about the medication error, Chloe's attending physician set in motion both the disclosure and event discovery process. The nursing unit director and nursing shift administrator were both notified, ensuring that emotional support services were made available to Chloe's nursing team. Chloe's attending physician called the director of patient safety and the hospital's office of risk management, and she subsequently received guidance on crafting an initial disclosure conversation with Chloe's parents. The risk manager's counseling regarding an apology was based on her awareness of the specific state legislative codes that surround a statement of apology as well as the potential legal ramifications that may arise from the individual words offered to Chloe's parents.

Within an hour of learning about the error, the attending physician, the unit charge nurse, and a member of the family services support team met with Chloe's parents, first inquiring about what they understood about her clinical condition and then describing the medication error. Her parents were shocked; one parent was outraged, "How could such an obvious mistake be allowed to happen?" The other parent expressed guilt: "I can't believe I let her down, I've been with her ever since we got here." Their immediate questions were answered factually, candidly, and compassionately: "Will she survive?" "What happens next?" "You tell me you are going to investigate this, how can we be confident that it won't happen again before your investigation is finished?" "What will happen to the people who gave her these overdoses?" What few details were known about how the error occurred were offered (an incorrect weight in the electronic medical record, two antibiotics were provided at just over twice the appropriate dose). The attending physician and nurse both acknowledged the raw emotions of Chloe's parents, "We take this very seriously, we are so very sorry for what happened, for Chloe's suffering and for the anguish we have created for you."

Her parents were informed about the next steps necessary to appropriately manage the effects of her medication overdose, including consultation with a nephrology subspecialist and additional laboratory, ultrasound, and oto-acoustic testing. They were reassured that these services would be provided at the hospital's expense.

Within one week, a team consisting of members from each clinical service area who were directly involved in this medication error convened to review the timeline of events and to perform a root cause analysis (RCA) of the error. Their investigation identified issues related to six discrete factors: human, equipment, process and policy, communication and access to information, patient-specific, and staffing or individual competencies. From their investigation, three specific operations changes were designed that would prevent Chloe's medication error sequence from occurring again.

With guidance from the hospital's risk manager, patient safety leader, and chief medical officer, Chloe's attending physician and the nurse manager from her medical unit reviewed the RCA findings and process revisions with her parents. Still visibly shaken, Chloe's parents expressed a mixture of disappointment, anger, and appreciation for her care team's "consistent transparency about what happened." "First do no harm" may be emerging into "First, acknowledge all harm."

References

Bok, S. (1999). *Lying: Moral Choice in Public and Private and Life*, 2nd edn. New York: Vintage Books.

Espin, S., Levinson, W., Regehr, G., Baker, G.R., & Lingard L. (2006). Error or "act of God"? A study of patients' and operating room team members' perceptions of error definition, reporting, and disclosure. *Surgery*, **139**, 6–14.

Gallagher, T.H. (2009). A 62-year-old woman with skin cancer who experienced wrong-site surgery: review of medical error. *JAMA*, **302**, 669–677.

Gallagher, T.H. & Lucas, M.H. (2005). Should we disclose harmful medical errors to patients? If so, how? *Journal of Clinical Outcomes Management*, **12**, 253–259.

Gallagher, T.H., Waterman, A.D., Ebers, A.G., Fraser, V.J., & Levinson, W. (2003). Patients' and physicians' attitudes regarding the disclosure of medical errors. *JAMA*, **289**, 1001–1007.

Institute of Medicine (2000). *To Err Is Human: Building a Safer Health System*, ed. L.T. Kohn, J.M. Corrigan, & M.S. Donaldson. Washington, DC: National Academy Press.

Lantos, J. (1996). Should we always tell children the truth? *Perspectives in Biology and Medicine*, **40**, 78–92.

Lazare, A. (2006). Apology in medical practice: an emerging clinical skill. *JAMA*, **296**, 1401–1404.

Loren, D.J., Klein, E.J., Garbutt, J., et al. (2008). Medical error disclosure among pediatricians: choosing carefully what we might say to parents. *Archives of Pediatrics and Adolescent Medicine*, **162**, 922–927.

Loren, D.J., Garbutt, J., Dunagan, W.C., et al. (2010). Risk managers, physicians and disclosure of harmful medical errors. *Joint Commission Journal on Quality and Patient Safety*, **36**, 101–108.

Matlow, A.G., Moody, L., Laxer, R., et al. (2010). Disclosure of medical error to parents and paediatric patients: assessment of parents' attitudes and influencing factors. *Archives of Disease in Childhood*, **95**, 286–290.

Shannon, S.E., Foglia, M.B., Hardy, M, & Gallagher, T.H. (2009). Disclosing errors to patients: perspectives of registered nurses. *Joint Commission Journal on Quality and Patient Safety,*, **35**, 5–12.

Shapiro, E. (2008). Disclosing medical errors: best practices from the "leading edge". In *"Disclosure: What's Morally Right Is Organizationally Right,"* at the *18th Annual IHI National Forum on Quality Improvement in Health Care.* Orlando, FL, USA.

Studdert, D.M., Mello, M.M., Gawande, A.A., Brennan, T.A., & Wang, Y.C. (2007). Disclosure of medical injury to patients: an improbable risk management strategy. *Health Affairs (Millwood)*, **26**, 215–226.

Surbone, A., Rowe, M., & Gallagher, T.H. (2007). Confronting medical errors in oncology and disclosing them to patients. *Journal of Clinical Oncology*, **20**, 1463–1467.

Wu, A.W., Cavanaugh, T.A., McPhee, S.J., Lo, B., & Micco, G.P. (1997). To tell the truth: ethical and practical issues in disclosing medical mistakes to patients. *Journal of General Internal Medicine*, **12**, 770–775.

9

Requests for "non-therapeutic" interventions in children: male circumcision

E. Charlisse Caga-anan and Anthony J. Thomas, Jr.

Introduction

"Non-therapeutic" interventions are those performed or requested for reasons other than medically indicated need. Examples in the ethics literature include leg-lengthening surgery for children with achondroplastic dwarfism, or appearance-normalizing surgery for children with craniofacial abnormalities that have no functional significance (Parens, 2006). This chapter focuses on childhood male circumcision that is not medically indicated. While there are relevant differences among these cases, they demonstrate that requests for non-therapeutic interventions in children combine several complex issues for pediatric ethics: the rights and vulnerabilities of children; the boundaries of parental prerogatives; and the difficulty of defining a procedure's benefits based on social, cultural, or religious considerations. Physicians asked to perform non-therapeutic interventions on children must assess whether acceding to these requests is medically appropriate and ethically permissible.

Case narrative

During an annual check-up, the parents of a 7-year-old boy asked the pediatrician to recommend someone to circumcise their son. Having just examined the child, the pediatrician could identify no clinical indication for circumcision, and questioned the parents about why they wanted the procedure performed. They explained that their son was born in the UK, where newborns are not routinely circumcised because the National Health Service only funds circumcisions done for medical indications. Upon moving to the United States, the parents decided that they wanted their son circumcised in adherence with their culture and with

what they presumed was local custom. They believed that circumcision was the standard medical practice in the United States and that their son would feel less conspicuous among his peers.

The pediatrician was uncomfortable with the request. In her experience, circumcisions were usually performed on newborns by the delivering obstetrician at the request of their parent(s); boys the age of this patient were typically not circumcised without a medical indication. The pediatrician was concerned that, even for newborns, the procedure did not usually have any medical benefits, and in this patient, would cause unnecessary pain and pose other risks as well. She also wanted to be sensitive to the patient's family and their values. She called a urologist colleague to discuss the case.

Summary of ethical issues

Physicians have a responsibility to promote the interests of their patients while avoiding unnecessary harms. Deciding what is in a child's interests can be difficult when a procedure poses medical risks and its benefits are not based purely on medical indications, but on social, cultural, religious and/or parental beliefs. Physicians can generally assume that parents will act in their children's best interests, and parents have considerable ethical and legal authority over children's upbringing, including medical decisions. Still, there are limits to parental authority, and children who have sufficient maturity and understanding can often voice their own opinions regarding the medical procedures they undergo. Requests for non-therapeutic interventions require physicians to balance these considerations in assessing whether it is ethically supportable to perform these procedures.

Clinical Ethics in Pediatrics: A Case-Based Textbook, ed. Douglas S. Diekema, Mark R. Mercurio and Mary B. Adam. Published by Cambridge University Press. © Cambridge University Press 2011.

Background on circumcision

History

The precise origin of male circumcision is unknown. Throughout history and across cultures it has been considered an important practice for reasons of religion, custom, and health. The oldest pictorial evidence of circumcision is found on an Egyptian tomb dating back circa 2400 BCE. Circumcision was accorded honor by ancient Egyptians as a religious and social practice, and may have signified cleanliness for a culture attentive to health and hygiene (Gollaher, 2000, pp. 1–6).

Among the major religions, circumcision continues to be practiced by people of Jewish and Muslim faiths. In Judaism, circumcision embodies the covenant between God and Abraham: the Torah states that God promised, "I will make of you a great nation," and in exchange Abraham and his male descendants would circumcise themselves. The bris (from the Hebrew word for "covenant") takes place on the eighth day of an infant boy's life; traditionally a *mohel* (a person trained to do circumcisions) performs the procedure. Circumcision marks the child's entrance into the Jewish community (Gollaher, 2000, pp. 6–29).

Though the Qur'an is silent about circumcision, its importance in Islam is drawn from the *hadith*, the sayings of the prophet Muhammad that ground much of Islamic law and practice. Muhammad reportedly prescribed cutting the foreskin as a *fitrah*, a means of cleanliness indicating a man's moral and mental health. Muslim clerics have never agreed on the best age to circumcise. However, males reaching puberty uncircumcised must undergo the procedure before participating in acts of worship. As Islam has spread to different continents and absorbed different cutting rituals, the act of circumcision has taken many forms (Gollaher, 2000, pp. 44–52). Beyond religion, social scientists have found extensive variations of circumcision in tribes throughout the world, and proposed that it indicated social or sexual maturity or admission into that tribal community. Attempts to interpret its meaning throughout history and across cultures have not been successful (Gollaher, 2000, pp. 53–59).

In the United States and the United Kingdom, circumcision arose as a medical intervention in the latter half of the nineteenth century, based on assertions that it was effective treatment for a variety of disorders such as epilepsy, other neurologic disorders, or even hernias. Medical reports later claimed that circumcision would also benefit healthy males. None of these "medical studies" were scientifically sound; nevertheless, doctors began to advocate that male circumcision be adopted as a routine prophylactic measure. Historical claims that circumcision curtailed masturbation and improved sanitation may also have helped make circumcision more acceptable during this period (Gollaher, 2000, pp. 73–92, 100–106). Misconceptions about circumcision continued to be reported into the mid-1900s, and neonatal circumcision became commonplace in the United States and United Kingdom. By the mid twentieth century, some physicians began to question the supposed benefits of infant circumcision and to scrutinize its burdens. The UK National Health Service stopped paying for circumcision in the 1950s, and currently only funds circumcision to treat a small number of conditions. The American Academy of Pediatrics (AAP) evaluated the available evidence and officially concluded in 1971 that there was no medical basis for routine circumcision. Nevertheless, circumcision remains common in the United States: in 1999, 65.3% of all male newborns born in hospitals were circumcised (Gollaher, 2000; CDC, 2010).

Medical risks and benefits

Some of the medical indications initially reported for circumcision were and remain legitimate today: to relieve severe phimosis, to correct paraphimosis, or to remove foreskin on which a tumor or other lesion has grown and which cannot be otherwise treated. The latter are rarely found in children, and phimosis and paraphimosis can be prevented by good hygiene and proper care of the foreskin (AAP, 1999, 2010).

Epidemiological studies have demonstrated some modest benefit to circumcision, such as a decreased incidence of urinary tract infection in circumcised versus uncircumcised boys, mostly in the first years of life. The conclusion that these studies support circumcision, however, has been subject to criticism, particularly because a large number of boys would have to undergo routine circumcision to avert a small number of potential infections. International studies have documented that circumcision can reduce a man's risk of acquiring human immunodeficiency virus (HIV), though the results and potential benefits may not be generalizable to populations with a lower risk of HIV infection than found in those studies' samples. Prevention of penile cancer is another proposed benefit, but most studies indicate that its incidence is very low, and it remains extremely rare in countries where circumcision is not done but where adequate hygiene is practiced (AAP, 1999; CDC, 2008).

The burdens of circumcision include the pain and the potential complications that accompany the procedure. Preventing the pain associated with the procedure may require a penile nerve block in newborns and mild analgesics afterward. General anesthesia is necessary when older children are circumcised and this adds risk for the child. The true incidence of complications after newborn circumcision is unknown, though reports suggest that the rate in developed countries ranges between 0.2% and 0.6%. The most frequent complication is bleeding, seen in ~0.1% of circumcisions. The need for transfusions is rare since most complications can be addressed with local measures. Infection is the second most common complication. Other complications are less common but more serious: reported cases include sepsis and surgical problems such as buried penis, urethral fistula, amputation of a portion of the glans penis, and penile necrosis. Though most of these risks are reported for newborns, many of the complications are similar in older boys. A potential harm that may be recognized later in life is diminished sexual sensation (historically considered a "benefit"). While some studies and anecdotal evidence support this claim, others do not show any significant, measurable changes in sensitivity or sexual satisfaction post-circumcision (AAP, 1999; CDC, 2008).

Ethical principles for non-therapeutic interventions

Two debates surround circumcision: (1) whether circumcision of newborns should be routine, and (2) whether non-therapeutic circumcision should be performed at all. Though both raise many of the same issues, whether circumcision should be routinely implemented for preventive purposes is also a question of public health practice and ethics (Hodges et al., 2002). This chapter focuses on the obligations that physicians must balance when they are asked to perform an apparent non-therapeutic intervention: to promote the child's interests, to respect parents making medical decisions for their children, and to respect children themselves as patients.

Physician obligations and promoting children's interests

Physicians are ethically bound to promote their patients' welfare under the principle of beneficence, and to minimize risks or burdens under the principle of nonmaleficence. Physicians thus recommend treatments that they judge as presenting the best balance of risks and benefits, and are not professionally obligated to provide interventions that they judge to offer little or no benefit and which may pose more than nominal risk. In pediatrics, this obligation is intensified by the inherent vulnerability of children, who cannot protect their own interests (Beauchamp & Childress, 2009). When the risks of a procedure are justified by a clear medical benefit, the physician's course of action is clear. For example, choosing circumcision to treat severe phimosis unresponsive to conservative management would not be ethically controversial.

For some procedures, such as circumcision, the balance of the medical risks and benefits remains uncertain. In 1999, an AAP Task Force concluded that there was potential medical benefit to circumcision, but not enough to recommend its routine performance. The AAP reaffirmed this statement in 2005, and others who have examined the evidence have reached similar conclusions (Benatar & Benatar, 2003; Diekema, 2009). The British Medical Association (BMA) similarly states that there is an "absence of unambiguously clear and consistent medical data on the implications of non-therapeutic circumcision" (2006). On the other hand, the procedure may have benefits that are not medical, but may be personally significant to the patient and/or his parents. Whether a child has undergone circumcision may determine whether he is considered to have fulfilled a covenant consistent with his family's religious beliefs or whether he can more freely participate in the religious or broader cultural life of his community.

When parents ask a physician to perform a procedure where the balance of medical risks and benefits is unclear and potential non-medical benefits are intangible, it may be difficult to determine whether acceding to the request is ethically permissible. The obligation to promote a child's well-being may be viewed by some as prohibiting physicians from performing procedures which are not shown to have clear physiological benefit. However, this interpretation may ignore other features of children's lives that may contribute to their welfare, benefits which are psychosocial in nature. Reasonable persons may disagree on how these benefits and harms should be weighed against each other regarding circumcision (Diekema, 2009).

Respecting children and parents in pediatric decision-making

The principle of respect for autonomy establishes that competent patients may make medical decisions based on their personal values, and these decisions are entitled to physicians' respect (Beauchamp & Childress, 2009). Pediatric patients challenge this framework because they are still developing as autonomous individuals, and may lack the decisional capacity to participate in the consent process. Additionally, the law may not consider pediatric patients competent to give valid informed consent (AAP, 1995).

Because most children generally lack capacity, parents are ethically and legally presumed to have the authority to make decisions for them. ("Parents" in this discussion also includes legal guardians.) This presumption acknowledges that because most parents care about their children, they may be in the best position to make decisions promoting their health and general well-being. This presumption is also justified by the parental interest in raising children according to their own personal values – such as those based in religion or culture – and transmitting those values to their children (Diekema, 2004). Physicians respect parents' role in decision-making by obtaining their informed permission to perform procedures (AAP, 1995). However, parental decisions are subject to limits. The boundaries of parental authority are clearest when parents refuse a safe, effective, and available treatment that may save a child's life. In these situations, physicians, as well as the state, are ethically justified in intervening regardless of whether the parents' choices are based on personal or religious conviction (Diekema, 2004).

Even when children are not yet fully autonomous, they are still entitled to respect as persons. Children should be able to participate along with parents in decision-making to the extent their capacity permits; as such, physicians should engage these children by obtaining their assent or their dissent. As children mature and are able to understand and rationally evaluate the information necessary to make medical decisions, the weight given to their input should correspondingly increase, even when they may not agree with their parents or physicians (AAP, 1995). In addition,

ethics and law have sometimes recognized that children's future ability to make autonomous decisions should be protected (Diekema, 2009, p. 254), especially when parental decisions would foreclose those choices entirely (Davis, 1997, pp. 9–10). Part of the objection to circumcising children when they are young is that it removes the opportunity for them to make the decision for themselves based on values they may later develop (Geisheker, 2010).

Balancing ethical considerations for non-therapeutic interventions

Ethical dilemmas may arise when it is unclear how physicians should balance their obligations to patients. In the adult world, bioethics has tended to prioritize respect for competent patients' choices over promoting their medical interests. Thus, adults can undergo procedures that are considered potentially medically harmful, provided they are competent and give informed consent. Balancing these interests is less clear in pediatrics because children are not autonomous individuals and may not have the capacity to voice their own interests. Physicians and parents must therefore make decisions on a child's behalf, based on what each judges to be in the child's best interest.

In the absence of clear medical benefit, some have interpreted the obligation to promote children's well-being as prohibiting physicians from performing circumcision when there is no medical indication (Fox & Thomson, 2005). Some would prioritize respect for children by arguing that a child's future autonomous choice regarding circumcision should be preserved, rather than permitting him to be circumcised while he is unable to fully consent. These positions often complement each other, and are also supported by pointing to circumcision's dubious history in medicine, and by claims of a child's right to bodily integrity (Geisheker, 2010). In addition, some compare male circumcision to female circumcision and call for more scrutiny of its acceptance based on religion and health. On the one hand, similarities between male circumcision and less physically damaging forms of female circumcision are also acknowledged by commentators who would not prohibit male circumcision, though they would argue that consistency may require challenging currently accepted views of both. On the other hand, this comparison may ignore relevant differences between the two: some forms of female circumcision are clearly more harmful than standard male circumcision, and further, male circumcision may present potential health benefits for certain at-risk populations (Benatar & Benatar, 2003; Abu-Sahlieh, 2006).

For some, the medical uncertainty and the historical significance surrounding circumcision argue for leaving the decision to the discretion of properly informed parents (AAP, 1999; BMA, 2006). This position does not always mean that physicians are deferring to parental authority, or abrogating their duty to promote the child's interest. Rather, it recognizes that there may be non-medical benefits motivating the request for circumcision, including those based in social, religious, or cultural tradition; parents do not necessarily ignore medical risks and benefits in their assessment, but they may give equal weight to personally significant factors which matter for their child's well-being (Benatar & Benatar, 2003; Diekema, 2009). In acknowledgment of the respect due to the child's future autonomous choice, some would also ask whether the decision to circumcise could be postponed, to the extent that the delay would not affect any non-medical benefits of the procedure and would give the child time to mature (Diekema, 2009).

As children mature and develop the capacity to make decisions, the dilemma of determining interests on their behalf may resolve itself. When they cannot make decisions for themselves, ethical and practical considerations must guide physician decisions.

Practical summary

Physicians who are asked to perform a non-therapeutic intervention must assess the request to determine whether it would be medically and ethically appropriate to do so. Physicians should engage the parents and, when appropriate, the child in a thorough discussion regarding the procedure.

Assessing requests

1. *Physicians have no ethical obligation to perform procedures they do not believe to be medically indicated or beneficial to the patient.*
   For some procedures, reasonable physicians may disagree on how to interpret the evidence regarding risks and benefits. A physician who does not believe that the medical risks of the procedure sufficiently balance the benefits can refuse to perform the procedure. However, physicians should be sensitive that they are not merely

imposing their personal values on the patient and the patient's family. As with all legally available medical services, parents may choose to seek the procedure elsewhere.

2. *If the balance of medical risks and benefits – including non-medical benefits – is uncertain, it is ethically permissible for a physician to perform the requested procedure.*
   Because a child's well-being may not depend on medical factors alone, physicians may take into account personally significant benefits, such as those based in religion or culture, in determining the child's best interest. Physicians may wish to consult others whose insight may assist in evaluating the requested procedures (e.g., religious figures, other physicians faced with similar requests, ethics committees).

3. *If the non-medical benefits of the procedure would not accrue until a later time, then the physician should attempt to persuade the family to delay the procedure.*
   The non-medical benefits of a requested procedure are less compelling when they will not affect the child until a later age. In that case, the procedure should be delayed in order to give the child more time to develop the capacity to more fully participate in decision-making.

Decision-making process

As part of respecting children and their parents, a physician who accepts a request to perform a non-therapeutic procedure should obtain the parents' informed permission and, when appropriate, the child's assent.

1. *Physicians should ensure that parents are fully informed about the procedure before obtaining their permission.*
   Parents should be informed of the procedure's short-term and long-term risks and lack of clinical benefit when not done for medical purposes. Properly informed parents, with the guidance of physicians, should be able to weigh the procedure's risks and benefits for themselves. The nature of the procedure may require the permission of both parents.

2. *Physicians should involve the child in the decision process to the extent that the child can participate.*
   Assent includes giving children information about medical procedures they will undergo, even

when they would not be able to refuse. Children who can express a considered opinion about circumcision should be part of determining their own best interest. If a child consistently refuses the procedure, the physician should not perform the procedure against the child's wishes.

Case resolution

The pediatrician and the urologist should inform the parents that their son's circumcision is not medically necessary, and further, that there is no consensus in the medical community that circumcision would be medically beneficial to their son. The physicians should also describe the various burdens of the procedure, including risks of general anesthesia for a 7-year-old to undergo the procedure, and the required recovery from the surgery. The physicians should discuss with the parents the benefits they hope their son will gain from the procedure. This may prompt the parents to more carefully weigh those benefits with the risks discussed. This may also reveal whether it is possible to delay the procedure until the son is older and can possibly make decisions regarding the procedure for himself. The circumcision should not be performed unless there is agreement between the parents regarding the decision to circumcise their son.

The physicians should also discuss circumcision with the son, and explore how he feels about the procedure and the reasons his parents are requesting it. If the son is ambivalent or refuses, the physicians may take the son's wishes into account, as it may be difficult or dangerous for the son to be circumcised even with the parents' permission. If the physicians are truly uncomfortable with providing the procedure, they should decline the request.

Conclusion

While this chapter has focused on circumcision, "nontherapeutic" interventions include a broad range of procedures. Circumcision brings to mind religious and cultural reasons for the requests, but in some circumstances parents may be motivated by other personal reasons – the belief that a procedure may afford their child an important psychosocial benefit and the wish to place their child in the best possible position to succeed in life, or the belief that a procedure may spare their child from some traumatic psychosocial harm and the desire to lessen the burdens their child already bears. The issues in these cases are made more difficult by the uncertainty surrounding most of these procedures. Though physicians and parents may want to act in the children's best interests, deciding on children's behalf is always a complicated task.

References

Abu-Sahlieh, S.A.A. (2006). Male and female circumcision: the myth of the difference. In *Female Circumcision*, ed. R.M. Abusharaf. Philadelphia: University of Pennsylvania Press, 47–72.

American Academy of Pediatrics (2010). Care for an uncircumcised penis. www.healthychildren.org/English/ages-stages/baby/bathing-skin-care/pages/Care-for-an-Uncircumcised-Penis.aspx (last accessed November 18, 2010).

American Academy of Pediatrics Committee on Bioethics (1995). Informed consent, parental permission, and assent in pediatric practice. *Pediatrics*, **95**, 314–317.

American Academy of Pediatrics Task Force on Circumcision (1999). Circumcision policy statement. *Pediatrics*, **103**, 686–693.

Beauchamp, T.L. & Childress, J.F. (2009). *Principles of Biomedical Ethics*, 6th edn. New York: Oxford University Press.

Benatar, M. & Benatar, D. (2003). Between prophylaxis and child abuse: the ethics of neonatal circumcision. *American Journal of Bioethics*, **3**, 35–48.

British Medical Association (2006). The law and ethics of male circumcision: guidance for doctors. www.bma.org.uk/ethics/consent_and_capacity/malecircumcision2006.jsp (last accessed October 31, 2010).

Centers for Disease Control and Prevention (2008). Male circumcision and risk for HIV transmission: implications for the United States. www.cdc.gov/hiv/resources/factsheets/PDF/circumcision.pdf (last accessed November 4, 2010).

Centers for Disease Control and Prevention (2010). NCHS health e-stat: trends in circumcision among newborns. www.cdc.gov/nchs/data/hestat/circumcisions/circumcisions.htm (last accessed October 31, 2010).

Davis, D.S. (1997). Genetic dilemmas and the child's right to an open future. *Hastings Center Report*, **27**, 7–15.

Diekema, D.S. (2004). Parental refusals of medical treatment: the harm principle as threshold for state intervention. *Theoretical Medicine and Bioethics*, **25**, 243–264.

Diekema, D.S. (2009). *Boldt v. Boldt*: a pediatric ethics perspective. *Journal of Clinical Ethics*, **20**, 251–257.

Fox, M. & Thomson, M. (2005). A covenant with the status quo? Male circumcision and the new BMA guidance to doctors. *Journal of Medical Ethics*, **31**, 463–449.

Geisheker, J.V. (2010). Where is the voice of the man the child will become? *Journal of Clinical Ethics*, **21**, 86–88.

Gollaher, D.L. (2000). *Circumcision: A History of the World's Most Controversial Surgery.* New York: Basic Books.

Hodges, F.M., Svoboda, J.S., & Van Howe, R.S. (2002). Prophylactic interventions on children: balancing human rights with public health. *Journal of Medical Ethics*, **28**, 10–16.

Parens, E. (ed.) (2006). *Surgically Shaping Children: Technology, Ethics, and the Pursuit of Normality.* Baltimore: Johns Hopkins University Press.

Chapter

10

Maternal–fetal conflicts

Christy L. Cummings and Mark R. Mercurio

Case narrative

LC, a 28-year-old previously healthy woman, presented to the office at 35 weeks' gestation for a routine prenatal visit. On examination the midwife became concerned about fetal distress, and sent the patient immediately to the Labor and Delivery Unit for further evaluation. On the unit, the obstetrician noted fetal bradycardia, and told the patient that an emergency cesarean section was necessary in order to avoid a very high risk of fetal death or permanent severe neurological disability. Several months ago, in what was then a normal pregnancy, LC had made prior arrangements with a midwife to deliver at home, via a carefully outlined birthing plan, and now strongly voiced those preferences to her medical team. Despite counseling and compelling persuasion from two different obstetricians and the midwife, LC refused a cesarean section. Further, she demanded that she be discharged home or she would leave against medical advice.

Summary of ethical issues

Multiple ethical issues and dilemmas can arise in the care of the pregnant woman, as illustrated by this case. The term *maternal–fetal conflict* has been widely used to describe situations when pregnant women "reject medical recommendations, use illegal drugs or engage in a range of other behaviors that have the potential to cause fetal harm" (ACOG, 2005). The ethical issues central to these difficult situations include, but are not limited to: a woman's right to autonomy ("self-rule"), the rights of the fetus and/or future child, justice for both mother and fetus, the mother's moral obligations, and the physician's moral and professional obligations. For the case described above, several questions arise. Which ethical obligation or duty takes precedence, the duty to respect LC's autonomous decision, or the duty

to benefit her viable fetus? Can the physician ensure fair treatment towards LC and still promote the well-being of her fetus? And finally, should pregnant women be punished for behavior, such as refusal of a recommended treatment, that ultimately harms their fetus or future child?

Some argue that the term *maternal–fetal conflict* should be replaced with *maternal–fetal relationship*, in order to avoid perceiving the pregnancy as an adversarial or mutually exclusive relationship between the pregnant woman and her fetus (Gilligan, 1982; Harris, 2000; Tong & Williams, 2009). Indeed, the interests of the mother and fetus are nearly always concordant. It should also be noted that the conflict could be perceived as not between the mother and fetus, but rather between the mother and physician, and some thus prefer the term *maternal–physician conflict* (Harris, 2000; ACOG, 2005). Though each of these suggestions has some validity, it must be acknowledged that there may be some cases in which the mother's refusal truly is in conflict with the interests of the fetus, or the future child. The case being considered may be one such example. For the purposes of this chapter, we will use the term maternal–fetal conflict, as it is commonly used in the literature, recognizing the limitations and connotations of the term itself.

Ethical principles and discussion

Many different methodologies may be employed in approaching these ethical dilemmas, including principlism, casuistry, feminist ethics, and the ethics of caring. Given that the issues related to maternal-fetal conflict may be best understood by a combination of methodologies that aims to respect the unique relationship between mother and fetus, what follows is a case-based approach enhanced by principlism, feminist

Clinical Ethics in Pediatrics: A Case-Based Textbook, ed. Douglas S. Diekema, Mark R. Mercurio and Mary B. Adam. Published by Cambridge University Press. © Cambridge University Press 2011.

ethics, and an ethics of caring (Gilligan, 1982; Harris, 2000; Tong & Williams, 2009).

Ethical principles and moral obligations

Starting with a traditional principle-based evaluation of this case allows for the application of the four guiding prima facie principles: respect for autonomy, nonmaleficence, beneficence, and justice (Beauchamp & Childress, 2009). The term prima facie implies that a duty is binding or obligatory, unless overridden or trumped by another duty. The ethical principles involved in the case of LC and in many maternal-fetal conflicts include: the rights of the woman, including her right to autonomy, beneficence, nonmaleficence and justice; the rights of the fetus and future child to beneficence, nonmaleficence, and justice; the mother's moral obligations; and the physician's moral and professional obligations (Harris, 2000; Beauchamp & Childress, 2009).

Respect for autonomy accords a competent adult patient the right to accept or refuse any medical treatment that is offered to her. This right was solidified by Justice Benjamin Cardozo in 1914 in *Schloendorff* v. *Society of New York Hospital*, when he penned that, "Every human being of adult years and sound mind has the right to determine what shall be done with his body; and a surgeon who performs an operation without his patient's consent commits an assault, for which he is liable in damages." Should this right to refuse recommended treatment, now widely accepted, also apply to pregnant women, or should they represent an exception?

The principle of nonmaleficence refers to the physician's obligation not to harm the patient. Thus, the physician would appear to have an obligation in this case to avoid harm to LC by not forcing an unwanted therapy. However, depending on one's views on the rights of the fetus and future child, and the physician's obligations, beneficence may require the physician to consider acting for the good of the fetus, to give the fetus a chance for life, and optimally a life without severe disability. It must be determined then, whether the ethical obligation or duty to respect LC's autonomous decision takes precedence over the duty to benefit her viable fetus (Pinkerton & Finnerty, 1996; Finnerty & Chisholm, 2003).

Should the rights or interests of the fetus be accorded the same weight as those of the pregnant woman when considering a case such as this? If moral

status generally refers to how much one's interests should count, the question becomes, what is the moral status of a fetus? Is it equal to that of a pregnant woman, or any adult, or is it something less? Some consider fetal moral status from the time of conception to be equal to that of adults. Others believe that fetuses possess a very low moral status until birth. A gradualist approach is endorsed by some, wherein the fetus's moral status gradually increases with increasing gestational age. Still others may believe that a pre-viable fetus has no rights or moral standing, while one who has reached the gestational age of viability (or the legal threshold for termination) does have rights, including the right not to be aborted. One can easily see that views about maternal-fetal conflict will be influenced by how one understands fetal moral status. Nevertheless, even among medical ethicists who perceive significant rights for a viable fetus, it is widely (though perhaps not universally) held that the fetus's rights to beneficence and to avoid harm are outweighed by the right of the woman to have her autonomy respected (Pinkerton & Finnerty, 1996; ACOG, 2005; van Bogaert & Dhai, 2008).

It could be argued that a pregnant woman who is planning to be a parent has a moral obligation to protect her fetus. Further, many claim that the physician involved in the care of the pregnant woman also has a moral obligation or duty to consider and protect the interests of the fetus as a "potential patient," despite the controversial moral status (ACOG, 2005; van Bogaert & Dhai, 2008). Is it possible to have a moral obligation to someone not yet born? The philosopher Bonnie Steinbock and others have argued that it is. For future parents, this includes preparing a safe home and, in general, optimizing the environment for their future child. Steinbock makes the point that, "just as parents have obligations to avoid exposing born children to risks of serious harm, pregnant women have comparable obligations to the children they will bear" (Steinbock, 2001). This argument applies to maternal nutrition and use of alcohol and drugs, and may be extended to certain medical treatments as well. However, even if we accept that pregnant women have such moral obligations, it does not necessarily follow that physicians have a right to enforce those obligations.

Another important ethical consideration in this case is the principle of justice, which, among other things, requires treating equals equally (Beauchamp & Childress, 2009). This case raises the possibility of a woman being forced to undergo surgery against her will, in order to save another. Even if one were to perceive the fetus at term as having moral status equal to that of an older child or adult, to perform the surgery against a competent individual's will may be fundamentally unjust. Consider whether any woman or man would be forced to undergo a procedure, such as donating bone marrow, to save a relative. While many might see a moral obligation to do so, particularly for one's own child, it seems unlikely that ethicists or physicians would consider it acceptable to force the donor to undergo such a procedure. If so, it would seem unjust to force a pregnant woman to undergo a procedure for the benefit of her fetus or future child.

After weighing all of the prima facie principles, most would respect the primacy of the pregnant woman's autonomy, while attempting to minimize the potential harm to the fetus and future child. Respect for the patient's autonomy would lead us to accept her decision, assuming that she is a capable decision-maker and has been adequately informed of and understands all reasonable treatment options. While the right of the fetus to beneficence is a strong one, especially close to term, this does not trump LC's right to have her autonomy respected. Many would not agree with her decision to refuse treatment and may even consider it unwise, immoral, or unconscionable due to the potential harm to her fetus, but would nevertheless acknowledge her right to make that decision.

While the approach described above is supportive of the pregnant woman's right to autonomy, it is interesting to consider whether that right should be absolute, or if there might be some threshold beyond which the interests of the fetus or future child might justify interfering with the woman's autonomy. It would never be appropriate to force a procedure, such as a cesarean section, on an unwilling pregnant woman for the sake of the fetus and future child. However, consider the example of a less invasive therapy that could be used once during labor, and which would ensure the health of the fetus without any side effects to the mother. Would it be acceptable to give one intravenous injection (assuming the IV is already in place) that would save the fetus? What about a one-time application of a tiny amount of skin cream to the arm, which by absorption through the skin (with no risk to the woman) would be protective of the fetus and prevent death or a lifetime of disability? Would it still be morally preferable to respect the mother's autonomy if she refused the cream?

Of course, such risk- and burden-free treatments do not exist, but some physicians and others who consider themselves advocates of maternal autonomy might also acknowledge that they would apply such a skin cream over the mother's objection. If one considers the forced cesarean section unacceptable but the skin cream acceptable, this implies that there is some threshold, perhaps difficult to locate precisely but nevertheless present, beyond which the large benefit to the fetus and/or future child outweighs the woman's right to refuse. Although this is an interesting point for ethical consideration and discussion, it must be emphasized that even if there might be such a threshold, forced invasive procedures or forced hospitalization are widely held to lie beyond it. That is, forced invasive treatments remain ethically unacceptable.

Beyond principles and rights: feminist ethics and the ethics of care

There may be limitations to the traditional principle-based approach when discussing the maternal-fetal relationship in the context of a difficult clinical case. Advocates of feminist care ethics, including Carol Gilligan and Nel Noddings, emphasize that "traditional moral theories, principles, practices, and policies are deficient to the degree they lack, ignore, trivialize, or demean values and virtues culturally associated with women" (Tong & Williams, 2009). An emphasis on relationships, and medical decisions that consider and support the importance of relationships in a patient's life, may be more appropriate than ethical analysis informed primarily by the application of fixed rules or principles.

Feminist ethics also underscores the inherent bias introduced into the principle-based approach by those that may be of a privileged, advantaged, or dominant group, such as men, for instance. It has been argued that a principlist approach neglects the "broad social and political arrangements in which clinical care occurs and in which ethical dilemmas are negotiated," specifically that sex, race, and class inequalities influence decision-making in ethics (Harris, 2000). Indeed, it is noteworthy that court-ordered obstetrical interventions have been shown in at least one review to be more likely among poor and/or minority patients (Pinkerton & Finnerty, 1996; Finnerty & Chisholm, 2003).

An alternative approach to evaluating ethical questions in pregnancy could employ relational, contextual, and equality-based moral theories, such as feminist ethics and the ethics of care. This model focuses on the mutual needs of a pregnant woman and her fetus within the context of her relationships and community, rather than on those needs (or perceived needs) that may be in conflict (Harris, 2000). Physicians are urged to consider the pregnant woman and fetus as a single entity, instead of identifying distinct obligations owed to each. Proponents also advocate prevention versus criminalization of prenatal harm. For example, rather than punishing a pregnant woman for illicit drug use and treating the addiction as a moral failing, physicians should treat her addiction as a medical and psychiatric illness, while encouraging, versus discouraging, prenatal care and successful treatment (ACOG, 2005).

Legal precedents and perspectives

A legal analysis of maternal-fetal conflict is beyond the scope of this chapter, and the expertise of the authors. In addition, court decisions, policy, and legislation do not replace ethical analyses, which is the focus of this chapter and this book. Nevertheless, it is instructive to review several relevant legal cases, as these rulings have significant implications for medical practice. We have already described above Justice Cardozo's affirmation of self-determination and the right to refuse surgical treatment in the case *Schloendorff* v. *Society of New York Hospital* (1914).

The case of AC in 1987 stands as landmark United States case law establishing the rights of pregnant women to determine their own health care (*In re A.C.*, 1987). Angela Carder was 25 weeks pregnant and suffering from a terminal recurrence of metastatic cancer. Hospital administrators requested a court hearing upon learning that Angela had decided not to have a cesarean section at 25 weeks, fearing a lawsuit by pro-life activists. Despite Angela's earlier statements that she did not want a cesarean section, and despite family and physician protests against the surgery (she was by then too sick to testify), a court order was issued for an immediate cesarean section. The baby survived for only a few hours, and Angela died 2 days later. In 1990, the decision to operate over her objections was appealed and overturned, on grounds that the order had "violated Carder's right to informed consent and her constitutional rights of privacy and bodily integrity" (*In re A.C.*, 1990).

Another important case in the reproductive history of women is that of *Baby Boy Doe* v. *Mother Doe* in 1994. In this case, the Illinois Court of Appeals declined to order a cesarean section for a woman with placental insufficiency, citing *In re A.C.* as a precedent Supreme Court case. The Illinois court stated that a woman's right to refuse invasive medical treatment is not diminished during pregnancy, and that the potential impact on the fetus is not legally relevant.

More recently, however, some court rulings have challenged these established precedents confirming the right of a pregnant woman to informed refusal of treatment. In 2004, a woman refused a cesarean section that her physicians had recommended because of feared macrosomia, despite six prior vaginal deliveries of large but healthy babies weighing close to 12 pounds (*Wyoming Valley Health Care System Hospital Inc. and Baby Doe* v. *Jane Doe and John Doe*, 2004). A court order was obtained to gain custody of the fetus and perform a cesarean section over the woman's objection. However, she moved to a different hospital, where she ultimately delivered a healthy 11-pound child vaginally (ACOG, 2005).

In the *Rowland* case in 2004, a 28-year-old woman with a history of psychiatric illness and intermittent homelessness, who had refused a timely cesarean section, delivered twins: a stillborn boy and a girl who tested positive for cocaine. She was charged with murder and child endangerment. Ultimately, she pled guilty to two counts of child endangerment (Minkoff & Paltrow, 2004). Recent cases such as this and others have prompted the American Congress of Obstetricians and Gynecologists (ACOG – formerly known as the American College of Obstetricians and Gynecologists) and other women's rights advocates to reaffirm their position statements endorsing maternal autonomy and encouraging actions and policies that promote the health of women and their fetuses through advocacy, prevention, and healthy behavior, rather than criminalization (ACOG, 2005).

Professional humility

A fundamental component of appropriate professional humility is to recognize and then to admit, to ourselves and to others, what we do not know, and when we are not certain. It has been shown that failure to follow obstetrical recommendations is a risk factor for increased neonatal morbidity and mortality (Ohel et al., 2009), and doubtless there are times when recommended obstetrical intervention can be life-saving. However, it has also been shown that some interventions that were recommended by an obstetrician and ultimately ordered by the court were, in retrospect, unnecessary (Kolder et al., 1987; Harris, 2000). Whenever faced with a pregnant patient (or any patient) who is refusing a recommended intervention, the physician does well to consider the possibility that the prognosis they have presented may be incorrect. When counseling, we need to recognize the limitations of our information, and offer clear and accurate statements regarding the clinical situation and possible outcomes with those limitations in mind.

Practical summary

When considering any case concerning maternal-fetal conflict, an approach that combines a traditional principle-based model with feminist care ethics may prove to be superior to either alone. Balancing ethical principles and rights with consideration of context and relationships will aid in the decision-making process, as will focusing on prevention of maternal and fetal harm rather than on criminalization. The medical team should realize that, more often than not, maternal and fetal interests converge rather than diverge. Often the best answer to what are termed maternal-fetal conflicts is to help the mother understand and appreciate that convergence. That is, that the recommended treatment is not only in the fetus's interest, but in hers as well. Ultimately, however, a pregnant woman's autonomous decisions should be respected. Review of the ethics committee statement put forth by the American Congress of Obstetricians and Gynecologists (ACOG) may also be worthwhile and may offer some additional guidance (ACOG, 2005). ACOG maintains that the maternal right to autonomy be respected and held absolute, and is adamant that court interventions should rarely, if ever, be sought.

The medical team should promote open communication and inquire about the patient's reasons for refusing treatment, her values and relationships, and explore her thoughts regarding her fetus. If the father, other family/friends, or anyone else the patient may trust (e.g., clergy) are readily available, it would be appropriate to ask LC whether they could be brought into the discussion, reassuring her that the final decision will remain hers. As with any disagreement between patient and physician regarding a recommended treatment, a second opinion should be sought if feasible. In this case there is clearly time pressure, but two obstetricians and a midwife are present and all agree that the procedure is indicated. An ethics consultation may prove very helpful (again depending on time pressures and feasibility), both to assist in sorting out the ethical questions and to facilitate communication.

A practical decision-making guide, described by Wallace and colleagues (1997), offers the essential elements involved in approaching a maternal-fetal case, and may serve as a useful starting point for ethical deliberation. Key elements include: medical indications (diagnosis, condition, prognosis, nature of disease, and treatment options), patient preferences (wishes, values, informed consent, competence), contextual features (religion, beliefs, culture, social/psychological factors, resources, hospital policies/concerns), quality of life (from the patient and family's perspective), and ethical principles and duties relevant to the conflict.

Resolution of case and conclusions

For the case of LC, after consideration and discussion of the factors described above, and a good-faith effort to convince her, an appropriate course of action would be to accept her decision to refuse a cesarean section, assuming that she is a capable decision-maker and has been adequately informed of and understands all reasonable treatment options. Many may not agree with her decision, citing her moral obligation to the fetus and/or future child. There may also be legitimate concerns about the clinical team's obligations to the fetus and/or future child. However, while the right of her fetus to this intervention (and thus the physician's obligation to provide it) may be strong, especially close to term, it does not trump LC's right to have her autonomy respected, and thus her right to refuse the surgery. There is no way to treat the fetus but through the woman's body, and she, like anyone else, has a right to refuse bodily intrusion.

If the medical team is unable to convince LC to undergo the cesarean section, a potential compromise could include advising her to remain hospitalized without surgical intervention in order to monitor both her and her fetus, and to optimize the care of the newborn after delivery. An ethics consultation should be sought, as time allows. It would be wise to inform the hospital's legal service of the situation, but a court order should not be sought, unless there is legitimate evidence of mental incompetence on the part of the patient – and this refusal does not by itself constitute such evidence.

References

American College of Obstetricians and Gynecologists (ACOG) (2005). ACOG Committee Opinion No. 321. Maternal decision making, ethics and the law. *Obstetrics and Gynecology*, **106**(5), 1127–1137.

Baby Boy Doe v. *Mother Doe* (1994). 632 N.E.2d 326 (Ill. App I Dist).

Beauchamp, T.L. & Childress, J.F. (2009). *Principles of Biomedical Ethics*, 6th edn. Oxford: Oxford University Press.

Finnerty, J.J. & Chisholm, C.A. (2003). Patient refusal of treatment in obstetrics. *Seminars in Perinatology*, **27**(6), 435–445.

Gilligan, C. (1982). *In a Different Voice*. Cambridge, MA: Harvard University Press.

Harris, L.H. (2000). Rethinking maternal-fetal conflict: gender and equality in perinatal ethics. *Obstetrics and Gynecology*, **96**, 786–791.

In re A.C. (1987). Dist. Col. Court of Appeals. 533 A.2D 611.

In re A.C. (1990). Dist. Col. Court of Appeals. 573 A.2D 1235–1264, *en banc*.

Kolder, V.B., Gallagher, J., & Parsons, M.T. (1987). Court-ordered obstetrical interventions. *New England Journal of Medicine*, **317**, 1223–1225.

Minkoff, H. & Paltrow, L. (2004). Melissa Rowland and the rights of pregnant women. *Obstetrics and Gynecology*, **104**(6), 1234–1236.

Ohel, I., Levy, A., Mazor, M., Wiznitzer, A., & Sheiner, E. (2009). Refusal of treatment in obstetrics – a maternal-fetal conflict. *Journal of Maternal-Fetal and Neonatal Medicine*, **22**(7), 612–615.

Pinkerton, J.V. & Finnerty, J.J. (1996). Resolving the clinical and ethical dilemma involved in fetal-maternal conflicts. *American Journal of Obstetrics and Gynecology*, **175**(2), 289–295.

Schloendorff v. *Society of New York Hospital* (1914). 211 N.Y. 125, 129.

Steinbock, B. (2001). "Mother-fetus conflict." In *A Companion to Bioethics*, ed. H. Kuhse & P. Singer. Blackwell Publishing, Blackwell Reference Online. www.blackwellreference.com/subscriber/tocnode?id=g9780631230199_chunk_g978063123019916. Last accessed October, 2010.

Tong, R. & Williams, N. (2009). Feminist ethics. In *The Stanford Encyclopedia of Philosophy*, ed. E.N. Zalta. http://plato.stanford.edu/entries/feminism-ethics/. Last accessed October, 2010.

van Bogaert, L.-J. & Dhai, A. (2008). Ethical challenges of treating the critically ill pregnant patient. *Best Practice and Research. Clinical Obstetrics and Gynaecology*, **22**(5), 983–999.

Wallace, R., Weigand F., & Warren, C. (1997). Beneficence toward whom? Ethical decision-making in a maternal-fetal conflict. *AACN Clinical Issues*, **8**(4), 586–594.

Wyoming Valley Health Care System Hospital Inc. and Baby Doe v. *Jane Doe and John Doe* (2004). Ct. Com Pl, Luzerne County, Pennsylvania, Civil Action No. 3-E 2004, Special Injunction Order and Appointment of Guardian, Judge, MT Council.

Fetal intervention and fetal care centers

Steven Leuthner

Introduction

Historically, promoting fetal well-being was not a separate endeavor from promoting maternal well-being. New imaging and sampling techniques now enhance our ability to help a woman help her fetus, and, when necessary, directly intervene with the fetus in the womb (Harrison, 2001). Some interventions are offered and recommended as preventive measures in obstetrical offices (i.e., prenatal folic acid), others are routinely provided in labor and delivery suites (i.e., antenatal antibiotics), still others are routine in perinatal specialty care (i.e., antiviral therapy). But with the development of fetal care centers, more invasive medical or surgical procedures, such as antiarrhythmics, an EXIT (ex-utero intrapartum therapy) procedure, or a skilled minimally invasive or open fetal surgery, have become possible. The difference between these newer more invasive procedures and the others seems to lie in the benefit/burden ratios to the fetus and pregnant woman. Three cases will be used to explore the ethical issues that arise from the fetal interventions performed in fetal care centers.

Case narrative 1: standard of care, potentially life-saving, chronic pediatric condition

Pam Smith is a 29-year-old, married, gravida 3 para 2 woman who otherwise has normal prenatal lab values, and has early, routine prenatal care. She has had two normal healthy pregnancies that resulted in two healthy girls, now aged 5 and 3 years. Pam and her husband are really hoping for a son with this pregnancy. At her first 18–20 week ultrasound, however, oligohydramnios was discovered, and she and her husband Bill were given the bad news that their male

fetus might have a problem. They were referred to a perinatologist, who agreed with the initial ultrasound, and also found an enlarged bladder and hydronephrosis, both classic findings in a male fetus of a bladder outlet obstruction caused by posterior urethral valves. The couple are counseled about the possibility of referral to a local fetal care center for a vesico-amniotic shunt, which entails placing a catheter with one end in the bladder and the other in the amniotic cavity. This decompresses the bladder, bypassing the valves, and allows amniotic fluid to re-accumulate. The fetal care center staff counsel the Smiths that the vesico-amniotic shunting has been shown to prevent lung hypoplasia, but has not been proven to prevent renal disease. These children may require long-term peritoneal dialysis followed by renal transplant. Not performing the procedure will likely lead to newborn death from pulmonary hypoplasia.

Case narrative 2: randomized clinical trial, searching to improve long-term quality of life (QOL), chronic pediatric condition

Pam Smith, with the obstetrical and family history as noted above, instead has a fetus diagnosed with myelomeningocele by the perinatologist. The family is informed of a fetal center that is currently involved in a clinical trial of a fetal procedure to surgically close the back. The goal of this trial is to determine whether the fetal intervention could improve long-term outcomes and quality of life. It is being offered at only three centers in the country, none local. This would require the family to travel to the center and consent to a randomized clinical trial. Participation involves transferring care to that center for both obstetrical and

Clinical Ethics in Pediatrics: A Case-Based Textbook, ed. Douglas S. Diekema, Mark R. Mercurio and Mary B. Adam. Published by Cambridge University Press. © Cambridge University Press 2011.

neonatal management, including the fetal intervention, the delivery, and the neonatal surgical care.

Case narrative 3: innovative treatment in a lethal condition, considered a life-saving attempt

Now imagine the same Pam Smith, but instead her fetus is diagnosed with a large mass at the sacrum. The perinatologist diagnoses a sacrococcygeal teratoma (SCT) and refers the couple to the local fetal care center where they confirm the SCT to be a large solid mass with significant vascular flow. Follow-up ultrasounds reveal signs of developing fetal hydrops, including fetal ascites and scalp edema. The couple are counseled that the progression is likely to end in fetal death. They are then made aware of two possible fetal interventions. One is to travel across country to a fetal center that has some experience with open fetal resection of masses. The other would entail a local innovative procedure to embolize the vascular supply to the mass in hopes of reversing the hydrops. The local procedure would be done by physicians who have performed a similar intervention in several adults with small tumors, but never performed one in a fetus.

Ethical issues in fetal intervention

The questions and thoughts that jump to the foreground in these cases might help illustrate the real ethical issues. For the *fetus* we might ask: What are the chances the procedure will work, and if it does, will a successful procedure mean improved survival or quality of life? What are the chances that the procedure itself will cause harm (e.g., preterm delivery or death) to the fetus? What are the likely outcomes if one does not proceed? How well can we prognosticate fetal death, or neonatal disease? For the *pregnant woman* we might ask: What are the risks to the mother (e.g., infection, death, etc.)? What will she have to endure (e.g., pain, time, anesthesia) for the procedure? How does an intervention now impact future pregnancies (e.g., conception, delivery method, future uterine rupture)? For the *family* we might ask: What is the family sacrifice in attempting the procedure? Will the other two children be impacted by the approach chosen? What if the woman and the father differ in their opinion? For the *professionals and institution* we might ask: Will this innovation bring notoriety and attract more patients? Will it bring financial benefit?

Can someone gain professional recognition or achieve promotion?

The cases and questions above require us to explore ethical relationships in fetal care, the fetus as a patient, a woman's autonomy as decision-maker, the father's role, and the professional and institutional interests.

Ethical relationships in fetal care

Relationships in obstetrical care are unique. Participants include the obstetrician, the pregnant woman, the fetus, and when fetal interventions are involved, we add pediatric specialists. Physicians owe both autonomy-based and beneficence-based obligations toward the pregnant woman. Medical interventions performed on the pregnant woman require her informed consent, and the autonomy of the pregnant woman should be respected. Ideally, interventions should offer a reasonable balance of potential benefit and potential risk, a calculation that should ultimately be made by the pregnant woman after she has been provided with accurate information about benefits and risks. At the same time, many of the interventions recommended in obstetric care, including fetal interventions, are based on the assumption that the pregnant woman desires a healthy newborn, leading to beneficence-based obligations toward the fetus. Finally, there may be societal expectations that a pregnant woman has beneficence-based obligations toward her fetus, obligations that extend minimally to preventing unnecessary harm to a fetus who she has chosen to bring to term. Discussions about fetal intervention seem to require balancing of obligations toward the fetus and obligations toward the pregnant woman's health and integrity.

The concept of fetus as patient

Central to every fetal intervention is the concept that the fetus is a patient. As more fetal treatment centers are being developed, collaborative multidisciplinary fetal treatment programs offer the benefit of fostering a better understanding of fetal abnormalities, the postnatal course, and long-term quality of life. However, this raises a concern about a shift of focus of care, privileging the interests and claims of the fetus over the pregnant woman. Some have claimed that obstetricians and pediatricians possess divergent professional cultural attitudes in their appraisal of fetal and maternal interests (Brown et al., 2006). Conceivably viewing both the fetus and the pregnant woman as patients can lead to ethical conflict, perhaps even gridlock about whether the moral status of the fetus is equal to that of the pregnant woman (Chervenak & McCullough, 2001).

One framework offered to help avoid this gridlock is to first acknowledge that being a patient means one can benefit from the application of the clinical skills of a physician (Chervenak & McCullough, 2001). This definition does not make a claim as to whether moral status is present or not. Of course any clinical benefit of a fetal intervention is measured by the clinical benefit that accrues to the future child that fetus becomes. There is no benefit to the fetus per se. In the framework of fetal interventions, then, the link to the future child is really dependent on a woman's autonomous decision to continue the pregnancy. In other words, the fetus has dependent moral status, and becomes a patient only when the woman chooses to proceed.

The pregnant woman as decision-maker

The primary ethical justification for respecting the pregnant woman's decision about fetal intervention is that it inevitably involves risks to her own well-being. An additional ethical justification for respecting the pregnant woman's autonomy in decision-making for fetal interventions stems from the acceptance of the fetus as a patient. Of course the fetus cannot make medical decisions. Instead, decision-making considerations in fetal treatment seem to parallel parental decision-making in determining treatment of childhood ailments. Women weigh the risks and benefits of the intervention to both themselves and to the fetus against the possible benefits and burdens without intervention. For example, in the myelomeningocele case, the woman cannot make a decision about fetal intervention without first understanding what standard obstetrical and neonatal care provides, followed by her assessment of the quality of life and best interests for her future child. If she envisions a significant burden without fetal intervention, she might consider an intervention that risks fetal death, self-harm, and family sacrifice to try to improve the future quality of life of the child she hopes to bring to term. If she foresees an acceptable quality of life without fetal intervention, she might not be willing to assume the risks of fetal intervention. Similarly, in the posterior urethral valve case, a decision to pursue a fetal intervention should be consistent with a parental decision to provide peritoneal dialysis and kidney transplantation for the future child.

If the parents have decided that they would pursue dialysis and transplant in the future, then the fetal intervention may be indicated. If they do not consider future dialysis and transplant to be acceptable, it is not clear that fetal intervention would be appropriate. While a parental decision-making model provides some justification for making these decisions, the biological framework of pregnancy means that it is not sufficient.

Any decision-making regarding fetal interventions falls within the biological framework in which the treatment of the fetus requires going through the pregnant woman, either physically or pharmacologically. Because the pregnant woman must undertake some risk, respect for her autonomy requires a thorough evaluation and discussion of her risks and harms, followed by her valid consent (Lyerly et al., 2009). The cases above illustrate different levels of maternal risk. In the case of the vesico-amniotic shunt, a needle must pierce her abdominal wall to guide a catheter. This requires some local anesthetic to reduce pain, carries a risk of causing rupture of the membranes and possible infection (a risk to both the pregnant woman and fetus) or prematurity (fetal risk). The myelomeningocele case requires a commitment to more invasive, open surgery and committing to a cesarean delivery. Risks of bleeding, hysterectomy, and future pregnancy risks, such as repeat cesarean delivery or uterine rupture with fetal and maternal death, are low, but not insignificant. Finally, one cannot ignore the sacrifice of the family in moving away from their local community for these procedures and follow-up care. The American College of Obstetrics and Gynecology states that any fetal intervention necessarily involves the pregnant woman sacrificing her bodily integrity and therefore *cannot be performed without her explicit informed consent* (American College of Obstetricians and Gynecologists, 2009). A pregnant woman's right to informed refusal must be fully respected (American College of Obstetricians and Gynecologists, 2007). So, while parental decision-making may in certain circumstances be overridden for the good of a child after birth, even the strongest evidence for fetal benefit would not ever be sufficient ethically to override a pregnant woman's decision to forgo fetal treatment (Warren, 1992; Sullivan & Douglas, 2006).

While all pregnant women undertake some risks for their fetus, women exploring a fetal intervention take on more than those normally expected. For this reason it is important to explore all factors that could influence a decision in either direction (Lyerly et al.,

2001). These could involve internal pressures, perhaps maternal feelings of guilt or a desire to make things "right." These could include external factors, such as a spouse's, extended family's, or society's expectations regarding her responsibility as a prospective mother. Finally, external pressure may come from the professionals involved in her care. Could the physicians in the SCT case be pressuring her into letting them try this innovative treatment strategy? Or could those in the clinical trial be pressuring the pregnant woman because they need participants? Finally, there is the psychosocial "therapeutic misconception," the presumption that an experimental intervention with no proof of efficacy will work merely because it is *offered*, or because it has been covered by the news media (Appelbaum et al., 1987; Sugarman et al., 1998). The informed consent process should therefore contain reasonable safeguards to prevent coercion. While a woman must be the final arbitrator of a decision, she does not typically make a difficult decision like this in a vacuum.

The role of the father

When thinking about the role of the father in these three cases, the typical presumption is that the couple will be raising this future child together, making joint decisions about health issues, and their relationship is one of shared family decision-making. It is important in these endeavors to be able to assess whether these assumptions are true, and to explore issues about decision-making with the woman alone if there are concerns. The father's perspective typically will be a struggle of balancing the health and safety of his wife, and the fetus, which in his view is his future child. In this case, the father is hoping for a boy. Will this lead him to pressure his wife to bear additional risks for the sake of his future son? Or would he dissuade her from taking additional risks because he is more concerned about her health and his living daughters? Many women look for the support of the father in making decisions, and it is important in counseling to respect and perhaps encourage the father's involvement. Pediatric care commonly involves shared decision-making between a child's mother and father, but in decisions about fetal interventions, the woman herself assumes risks and burdens associated with the decision. While it may be appropriate and helpful for the father to be involved in these decisions, to provide him with any authority to override a decision would unjustifiably erode the autonomous decision-making of the pregnant woman.

The interests of the medical team or fetal care center

To achieve the most informed decision-making, multidisciplinary teams should be assembled to oversee the care being offered. Such teams should include maternal-fetal medicine specialists and neonatologists, often the primary physicians managing the mother and baby. A complete program should include pediatric and surgical subspecialists, nurses, genetic counselors, ethicists, and family services providers.

As fetal centers are opening around the country, it is important to acknowledge the ethical issues and potential conflicts of interest that occur at an institutional level. These services can be financially lucrative and may benefit the careers of the centers' practitioners. A team of individuals may help keep these individual ambitions in check. The success of the centers themselves, however, is dependent on performing procedures. With more procedures comes greater experience and expertise. Financial gain also comes with a greater number of procedures being performed. All of these realities provide an incentive for providers at these centers to recommend and encourage the services they provide.

Some have also raised the issue of justice. Only a few women and fetuses will benefit from fetal care centers, yet the cost and resources expended on these services can be quite large. Whether this represents the best use of limited health care dollars and providers is an important question.

In addition to providing clinical care, many fetal centers also participate in research and innovation. Rapidly developing technologies may blur the boundaries between research and innovative practice. This raises concerns about the protection of pregnant women and their fetuses from the risks of unproven therapies. Although the first few uses of a new intervention (the SCT case) may be motivated by a desire to help a particular fetus, once feasibility and potential benefit have been identified, innovations should be subjected to systematic formal research as soon as possible (American College of Obstetricians and Gynecologists, 2006). Pregnant women and their fetuses are deserving of the same protections afforded to other research participants, and studies should be designed to assess the full impact of risks and benefits of these interventions on both the woman and the future child. The Management of Myelomeningocele Study (MOMS), involving fetuses diagnosed with myelomeningocele, is a research model of how interventions should proceed (Adzick et al., 2011).

Alternatives or adjunct options

Some providers in fetal care centers may erroneously believe that because a pregnant woman has been referred to them, she has already decided to pursue fetal intervention. Prospective parents may believe that there are only two possible results: success (fetal cure) or failure (fetal death). Valid informed consent, however, requires that all alternatives must be offered. Alternatives include the possibility of intervention, as well as the possibility of forgoing intervention, which means standard obstetric and neonatal care. Because of the high risk of fetal or neonatal death with many interventions, informed consent discussions should also include palliative care options (Leuthner, 2004; Munson & Leuthner, 2007). The clinical reality of serving women during pregnancy is that some women will elect pregnancy termination. Certainly each pediatrician, surgeon, and obstetrician involved in these decisions may have their own distinct views about the best course of action for any given disease entity, but these views do not suspend their duty to provide a fully informed consent that includes all reasonable and legal options. Centers offering fetal intervention should evaluate pregnant women in a timely fashion, counsel them adequately about all options, and for women who might opt for pregnancy termination, have in place appropriate mechanisms, including the ability and resources for referral, to support these women through a difficult decision. It is imperative for centers offering fetal interventions to provide care, support, and appropriate referral services for women and their families who choose an alternative to fetal intervention.

Case resolutions

Case 1: In this case, a vesico-amniotic shunt for the fetus with posterior urethral valves is considered a standard option, and with only slightly more risk to the woman than a simple amniocentesis. For this reason, the weight of the family's decision will likely focus on long-term outcomes, and the family's view on a future that involves dialysis and renal transplantation. The fetal care team should include perinatology, neonatology, nephrology and urology, and perhaps palliative care. If the family is open to fetal intervention followed by future care that includes dialysis and transplantation, the baby would presumably be aggressively

resuscitated at birth to allow for lung and kidney evaluation. If dialysis and transplant are not something the family wishes to pursue, then the fetal care team might suggest no fetal procedure and development of a palliative care plan for birth. This might include comfort from the start or some support to assure prognostic certainty.

Case 2: In this case, the fetal intervention is a randomized experimental protocol that would offer standard care versus the fetal intervention (in utero closure of the myelomeningocele). The intervention carries substantial risk for the woman and it is unknown whether the potential child would benefit from improved quality of life. There is also an increased risk of prematurity and death. The family should meet with experts in perinatology, neonatology, neurosurgery, and perhaps a myelomeningocele clinic nurse. The strength of the experimental approach is that it will occur under a well-designed multicenter research protocol, so it should provide important information for future families and centers to consider as they make similar decisions. Supporting the family's decision to choose either standard care or participation in a study seems ethically reasonable.

Case 3: In this case, the parents have been offered an innovative local procedure of no proven efficacy for the prenatal treatment of SCT. Risks of the procedure to the mother and fetus are unknown, while fetal demise is likely if nothing is done. In this situation, where an unproven fetal intervention is being offered in an attempt to avoid fetal death, palliative care services could be offered alongside the intervention. Clearly the pregnant woman would not be required to undergo this intervention, but more importantly, all conflicts of interest for those interested in attempting this procedure should to be openly discussed. The burden should fall on the fetal care center to assure that no coercion or even persuasion is used in this case. And finally, if at some point the intervention begins to look promising, the center should move toward a research-based protocol to determine efficacy and safety.

Fetal interventions are more commonplace than we realize. Outcomes have not been universally successful. Many of these interventions pose additional risk to pregnant women and fetuses. While medical progress depends on innovative approaches, it also requires that these new interventions be evaluated in the setting of well-designed clinical trials. Because most of these interventions offer uncertain benefit and pose risk to the pregnant woman, great care should be exercised to present a balanced evaluation of expected outcomes. A pregnant woman's autonomy should be respected above salvaging the fetus.

References

Adzick, S.N., Thom, E.A., Spong, C.Y., et al. for the MOMS Investigators (2011). A randomized trial of prenatal versus postnatal repair of myelomeningocele. *New England Journal of Medicine*, **364**, 993–1004.

American College of Obstetricians and Gynecologists (2006). Innovative practice: ethical guidelines. ACOG Committee Opinion No. 352. *Obstetrics and Gynecology*, **108**, 1589–1595.

American College of Obstetricians and Gynecologists (2007). Research involving women. ACOG Committee Opinion No 377. *Obstetrics and Gynecology*, **110**, 731–736.

American College of Obstetricians and Gynecologists (2009). Informed consent. ACOG Committee Opinion No. 439. *Obstetrics and Gynecology*, **114**, 401–408.

Appelbaum, P.S., Roth, L.H., Lidz, C.W., Benson, P., & Winslade, W. (1987). False hopes and best data: consent to research and the therapeutic misconception. *Hastings Center Report*, **17**(2), 20–24.

Brown, S.D., Truog, R.D., Johnson, J.A., & Ecker, J.L. (2006). Do differences in the American Academy of Pediatrics and the American College of Obstetricians and Gynecologists positions on the ethics of maternal-fetal interventions reflect subtly divergent professional sensitivities to pregnant women and fetuses? *Pediatrics*, **117**(4), 1382–1387.

Chervenak, F.A. & McCullough, L.B. (2001). Ethical considerations. In *The Unborn Patient; The Art and Science of Fetal Therapy*, 3rd edn, ed. M.R. Harrison, M.I. Evans, N.S. Adzick, & W. Holzgreve. Philadelphia: W.B. Saunders Company, 19–25.

Harrison, M.R. (2001). Professional considerations in fetal treatment. In *The Unborn Patient; The Art and Science of Fetal Therapy*, 3rd edn, ed. M.R. Harrison, M.I. Evans, N.S. Adzick, & W. Holzgreve. Philadelphia: W.B. Saunders Company, 3–9.

Leuthner, S.R. (2004). Fetal palliative care. *Clinics in Perinatology; Current Controversies in Perinatal Medicine IV*, **31**, 649–665.

Lyerly, A.D., Gates, E.A., Cefalo, R.C., & Sugarman, J. (2001). Toward the ethical evaluation and use of maternal-fetal surgery. *Obstetrics and Gynecology*, **98**, 689–697.

Lyerly, A.D., Mitchell, L.M., Armstrong, E.M., et al. (2009). Risk and the pregnant body. *Hastings Center Report*, **39**(6), 34–42.

Munson, D. & Leuthner, S.R. (2007). Palliative care for the family carrying a fetus with a life-limiting diagnosis. *Pediatric Clinics of North America*, **54**(5), 787–798.

Sugarman, J., Kass, N.E., Goodman, S.N., et al. (1998). What patients say about medical research. *IRB*, **20**(4), 1–7.

Sullivan, W.J. & Douglas, M.J. (2006). Maternal autonomy: ethics and the law. *International Journal of Obstetric Anesthesia*, **15**(2), 95–97.

Warren, M.A. (1992). The moral significance of birth. In *Feminist Perspectives in Medical Ethics*, ed. H. Bequaert Holmes & L. Purdy. Bloomington, IN: Indiana University Press, 198–215.

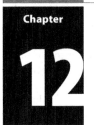
Chapter

12
Ripped from the headlines: assisted reproductive technology and multiple births

Jeffrey Ecker and Howard Minkoff

Case narrative: a case of in vitro fertilization

OM is a 34-year-old woman with two previous children born with the assistance of in vitro fertilization (IVF). In the course of IVF treatment six additional embryos were created and frozen. Now, 6 years after the birth of her second child, she plans another pregnancy using the frozen embryos. She requests that all six embryos be returned (transferred to the uterus using a trans-cervical catheter: a simple outpatient procedure) for potential implantation. She asks for this number in spite of guidelines suggesting that, for a woman of her age and health, no more than two or three be transferred. All six are transferred and she becomes pregnant with what proves to be octuplets (the pregnancy contains two sets of identical twins). After a prolonged period of maternal bed rest and hospitalization, the babies are delivered via cesarean section at 30 weeks of gestation.

Introduction

This "case" mirrors some circumstances of the 2009 California pregnancy of a woman named Nadya Suleman, quickly nicknamed "Octomom." The birth of her octuplets engendered a media storm, which included the revelation that she was a single mother who had six other children, all conceived through IVF. Many of those expressing outrage about the Suleman case questioned whether she was fit to be a parent. We have argued elsewhere that matters of fitness to parent are difficult for physicians to evaluate, and only in the most extreme and exceptional circumstances, none of which were present in the California case, should providers use such concerns to limit access to assisted reproductive technologies (Minkoff & Ecker, 2009).

This chapter will focus on a question we feel more appropriately evaluated by medical professionals: what is the right number of embryos to transfer? This discussion touches on important principles of patient autonomy and respect for autonomy, two principles we believe are related but not equivalent. We will argue that the principle of respect for patient autonomy does not require physicians to accede to any request by a patient, to consider whether the number of embryos transferred in assisted reproductive technologies should be regulated, and, if so, to reflect on the appropriate nexus for such regulation.

IVF, multiple gestations, and their risks

In the first decade of the twenty-first century, IVF accounted for 1–3% of live births in the United States and Europe, and nearly 30% of IVF cycles result in a live birth. As compared with "natural cycles," however, in vitro pregnancies are much more likely to be multiple gestations (nearly one-third) and the risk for multiples rises with the number of embryos transferred – a reality highlighted by the 2009 case of the California octuplets.

This notable (some would say notorious) case also illustrates some of the risks attendant with multiple gestations including risks to both newborns and mothers (ACOG, 2004). Babies born from multiple gestations are more likely to be premature and to suffer from associated morbidity and mortality. An average single-ton gestation lasts 40 weeks (counted from the date of the last menstrual period) while the mean duration of a twin gestation is 36 weeks and that of triplets is 33 weeks. Each additional fetus subtracts 2–3 weeks from estimated gestational length, resulting in an average duration of pregnancy that approaches the threshold

Clinical Ethics in Pediatrics: A Case-Based Textbook, ed. Douglas S. Diekema, Mark R. Mercurio and Mary B. Adam. Published by Cambridge University Press. © Cambridge University Press 2011.

of viability (23–25 weeks) with more than five fetuses. That the California octuplets were all liveborn at 30 weeks and went home from the hospital is truly exceptional (believed to be the first such case ever). However, it is important to maintain a guarded view of these children's long-term outcome as it is increasingly recognized that children born at such an early gestational age remain at risk for significant health, learning, and other developmental issues later in life.

Multiple gestations also carry important maternal risks that begin with activity restriction and medication that are often recommended as treatment for incipient preterm labor. As compared with singleton gestations, women with multiple pregnancies (and the larger associated mass of placenta) are also at risk for metabolic complications of pregnancy such as gestational diabetes and preeclampsia. Both of these conditions can compromise maternal and/or fetal well-being significantly enough to indicate premature delivery in order to forestall permanent injury or death. Finally, multiple gestations, including nearly all those of more than two fetuses, are more likely to be delivered by cesarean section and, whether vaginal or cesarean, multiple deliveries confer an increased risk for post-partum hemorrhage.

Given these risks to mother and child, why transfer more than one embryo? Although transferring two or three embryos will increase pregnancy rates (measured in a single cycle), for most women transferring more than two or three embryos does not further increase pregnancy rates, but *does* increase the rate of multiple gestations. For example, according to 1999 data for women between 30 and 34 years of age, transferring two, three, and four embryos results in live birth rates of 19%, 35%, and 36%, respectively, but multiple gestation rates of 20%, 40%, and 45% (Schieve *et al.*, 1999). Alternatives that limit the rate of multiple gestations exist: freezing embryos allows fewer to be transferred in a first cycle with stored embryos thawed and subsequently returned if the initial cycle/transfer does not result in pregnancy. In fact, in randomized studies among appropriate candidates (young, healthy, few failed previous IVF cycles), single embryo transfer followed by a second thawed cycle, if needed, produced similar cumulative pregnancy rates (39% versus 43%) but lower multiple pregnancy rates (0.8% versus 33%) as compared with a cohort who underwent transfer of multiple fresh embryos (Thurin *et al.*, 2004).

For some patients, preferences for the number of embryos transferred are driven in part by beliefs regarding the rights and respect that should be attributed to ex utero embryos. Some patients believe that frozen embryos have the same status as children, and leaving them frozen and unused is an uncomfortable or untenable option. Similarly, multifetal pregnancy reduction (using ultrasound-guided potassium injection to stop one or more fetal hearts, thereby "reducing" a triplet to a twin pregnancy) may not be an option for some patients. Even if discussed in advance of the transfer of multiple embryos, a physician can never compel a mother to undergo a fetal reduction, no matter how many gestations result from the transfer.

The ethics of IVF: making choices

Issues in reproductive ethics are often seen as balancing rights and duties owed to women and children (ACOG, 2007). For some the balance should also incorporate a consideration of the rights of the fetus, although whether such rights exist is a contentious matter that is often wrapped in the ongoing, and ultimately irreconcilable, debate about abortion. When considering IVF, however, assigning rights and weighing duties becomes even more challenging. At the time decisions are made about how many embryos to transfer, for example, there exists no pregnancy or children or fetuses, but only the potential for pregnancy. Instead of considering the rights and duties due a potential pregnancy, we argue that it is both appropriate and productive for ethicists to focus their evaluation on the woman planning a pregnancy, as her moral status is not in question. The goal of the planned pregnancy – a healthy mother and child – should inform all conversations and decisions, and these two desirable outcomes will generally lead all involved to congruent conclusions.

Even when goals are shared and uncontested, choices may still need to be made between reasonable alternative management options. Respect for autonomy requires that that patient's own evaluation of the risks and benefit of each choice should be central to decision-making. As an example, a woman with cervical cancer who is appropriately informed about the merits and perils of available options may choose between surgery, radiation therapy, or receiving no cancer treatment at all. Respect for autonomy, however, is not the same as unfettered autonomy. Patients should not and may not simply choose anything imaginable in creating a plan for care. The patient with cervical cancer may choose radiation therapy but may not choose to double or triple the usual dose of radiation because she wishes, wants, or believes that more might be better. By analogy, in considering the case presented here, it may be appropriate to think of the number of embryos transferred as a dose delivered with the goal of creating a healthy child. Respecting patient autonomy does not mean that a patient may choose whatever "dose" of embryos she desires.

These examples illustrate the difference between negative autonomy (a person's right to reject someone else's desire to do something to them) and positive autonomy (a person's right to demand that something be provided to them or done to them). Competent patients, including those who are pregnant or planning a pregnancy, are afforded almost limitless power to decline interventions, regardless of how low the risk and how great or certain the potential benefit might be to their own health. A competent woman with acute appendicitis may decline an operation. Another with pneumonia may refuse antibiotics. However, the right to decline care is not mirrored by a right to demand any or all interventions. For example, a woman without signs or symptoms of appendicitis may request an appendectomy, but a surgeon would not be obligated to provide it (and should not provide it if he or she feels it would not be in the patient's interest). Similarly, a physician is not obligated to acquiesce to a patient demanding a prescription for antibiotics when signs and symptoms offer no indication.

Providing a patient with the background and information necessary to understand the alternatives presented and their associated risks and benefits is central to respecting her autonomy. In this regard, patients planning IVF should understand how the number of embryos transferred affects (or does not affect) pregnancy rates and multiple pregnancy rates. IVF patients should be educated about the risks associated with multiple gestations, including risks of prematurity, loss before viability, and risks to a mother's health. They should understand how these risks increase even in a twin pregnancy, an outcome widely viewed as desirable and without undue risk by many hoping to become pregnant (why not get it all done at once?). These conversations should occur before undertaking treatment, as they may inform decisions regarding the techniques used and number of embryos to be created (if, for example, a parent will never want to discard/destroy any embryo). Further, anticipatory discussion avoids the awkwardness and pressure of introducing new issues at the time of transfer; a time when the goal of pregnancy (any pregnancy, higher order multiple or

not) may overwhelm other concerns. Recognizing, as argued above, that reasonable limits can be placed on the exercise of positive autonomy, it should be made clear in advance of the time of the procedure that there will be limits on the number of embryos transferred.

The principle of justice requires that persons who are similar in relevant ways – in this case all who are undergoing IVF – should be treated similarly. Professional or regulatory guidelines are helpful in assuring that all patients receive similar, evidence-based care. Guidelines may also be useful to providers who may need to defend a particular treatment plan (including placing limits on the options available to patients), such as considering how many embryos to transfer. When guidelines take the form of regulation they may have greater effect in promoting particular public health goals related to safety (e.g., offering IVF only in facilities equipped to handle anticipated complications) and other outcomes (e.g., avoiding the morbidity and health care expenses of multiple-associated prematurity). The UK, as an example, tightly regulates the number of embryos transferred during IVF and, in almost all cases, limits the transfer to no more than two to three embryos with strong preference given to single embryo transfer in appropriate candidates. Providers who fail to comply with these regulations risk sanction (HFEA, 2010).

Guidelines, but not regulation, shape IVF practices in the United States, and differences in the details are apparent when American guidelines are compared with British regulation. The American Society of Reproductive Medicine (ASRM, 2008) endorses guidelines that are slightly more liberal (i.e., endorse the transfer of more embryos) than UK policy and place less emphasis on single embryo transfer. As guidelines, compliance with ASRM regimens is voluntary and failing to follow ASRM guidelines carries no penalty. Perhaps for this reason, even though ASRM guidelines would rarely consider transfer of more than three embryos to be appropriate, the Centers for Disease Control and Prevention reported that four or more embryos were transferred in 14.3% of cycles in the United States in 2007.

The discordance between US recommendations and UK policy, and the discordance between ASRM guidelines and American IVF practice, raise questions about why practice in the United States is guided but not regulated. This question was part of the professional discussion following the case of the California octuplets. In response to the octuplet birth, contrasting editorials regarding the matter of regulation appeared in leading US obstetric and gynecology journals. Writing in *Obstetrics and Gynecology*, Dr. Ginsberg, then the President of the American Society of Reproductive Medicine, and Dr. Adamson, the organization's Past President, argued against regulation, noting that although, "(s)ome have suggested regulation … such action would ignore the success of professional standards and self-regulation … (and) would be particularly troubling in reproductive medicine …" (Adamson & Ginsburg, 2009). In an essay published just one month later in the *American Journal of Obstetrics and Gynecology* we offered another opinion, writing "… setting a limit on the number of embryos transferred is justified on ethical and medical grounds and we believe that the time has come to transform guidelines into regulation …" (Minkoff & Ecker, 2009).

While we continue to believe that regulation is warranted, there is a practical challenge associated with regulation in the United States: where would the authority for and nexus of regulation reside? In the UK, IVF practice is effectively regulated through the country's single-payer system which can regulate and license care by describing what care will be reimbursed. In contrast, in most parts of the United States, IVF costs are paid by the patient (only a very few states mandate coverage) and as a result are subject to the forces of a free market. Treated as something to be bought and sold, IVF services are for sale and customers' preferences and money may influence treatment. A patient can always threaten to take her business elsewhere if the physician refuses to transfer the requested number of embryos. Moreover, because a single cycle of IVF is so expensive (more than US$10 000), paying out of pocket may place a premium on achieving a pregnancy as quickly as possible (avoiding, for example, single embryo transfer) even if such strategies increase the risk of multiple gestation (the costs of premature newborns are covered by insurance). There is evidence to support these hypotheses: in states that mandate coverage for IVF fewer embryos are transferred per cycle and fewer multiple gestations result on average per cycle (Jain et al., 2002).

Even insurers that do not pay for IVF will pay for the care of the resulting neonates, including those who are premature. While in the abstract one can imagine insurers indicating that they will not pay for the care of neonates born prematurely in pregnancies resulting from the transfer of more than the recommended number of embryos, the ethics, mechanics, and dynamics of such a policy would be challenging at best.

Other instruments of regulation might be considered. The Food and Drug Administration could regulate IVF as a tissue therapy (sperm and ovum donation are regulated) or enforce adherence to guidelines as a requirement of licensing facilities. However, any efforts at regulation counter a deeply held aversion to the regulation of medical practice in the United States. This American ethos has long afforded great deference to provider judgment in making decisions, even those decisions that appear to diverge from usual care. Precedent supports near-complete deference to patient autonomy in decision-making when pursuing treatment plans. It is difficult for legislators and regulators to imagine every fact and circumstance that might confront providers in clinical practice. Regulation is a blunt, inflexible, and poorly adaptable tool for managing clinical practice, particularly when clinical circumstances fall outside the usual. Regulation is also subject to political, religious, and other considerations; influences that are usually held separate from the patient–provider relationship. Reproductive medicine has long been an area where legislation and regulation have limited patient choices in matters of abortion, contraceptive counseling, and other contentious issues. Physicians practicing reproductive health have often decried past regulatory efforts, arguing that legislation has placed important limitations on choices available to them and their patients (Minkoff & Marshall, 2009). This experience no doubt makes them reluctant to consider regulation of IVF practice.

Conclusions: what is to be done?

Despite these concerns about regulatory solutions, there are situations (protecting the health, safety, and welfare of citizens) in which society sets boundaries on its citizens' activities. If we mandate seatbelts, why should we not mandate safe IVF? Medicine is already heavily regulated; physician licensure and the regulation of health care facilities are just two examples. With regard to IVF, we would ask whether there are some limits that fall so far outside of acceptable practice (exceeding ASRM guidelines, for example) and some goals that are so widely shared (a healthy mother, babies born beyond the risks of extreme prematurity) that regulation should be considered. In such cases, we believe patients and providers will see the wisdom of imposed limits not as inappropriate restrictions on autonomy, but as wise thresholds designed to achieve the end that all desire: a healthy pregnancy and child.

No doubt there will not be a simple answer or quick debate here. And even though we favor regulation, as discussed, we are hard-pressed in our current health care system to identify a ready instrument or nexus for such regulation. But rather than halting any consideration of regulation, that fact should animate a broader discussion of the appropriateness and means of regulation. In the meantime we recognize that cases in which outrageous numbers of embryos are transferred during IVF are the exception. Informed, considerate, and ethical patient and provider teams, working together, will, left alone, generally make reasonable decisions. As one of us wrote, "… we hope for the continued good health of the California mother and her (octuplets). But we will also hope that such cases only rarely – maybe never – happen again" (Ecker, 2010).

References

ACOG (American College of Obstetricians and Gynecologists), Obstetric Practice Bulletins Committee (2004). ACOG Practice Bulletin 56: Multiple gestation: complicated twin, triplet and higher-order multifetal pregnancy. Washington, DC: American College of Obstetricians and Gynecologists.

ACOG (American College of Obstetricians and Gynecologists), Ethics Committee (2007). ACOG Committee Opinion 390: Ethical decision making in obstetrics and gynecology. Washington, DC: American College of Obstetricians and Gynecologists.

Adamson, D. & Ginsburg, E. (2009). The octuplets tragedy. *Obstetrics and Gynecology*, **113**, 970–971.

ASRM (American Society of Reproductive Medicine), Practice Committee (2008). Guidelines on the number of embryos transferred. *Fertility and Sterility*, **90**, S163–S164.

Centers for Disease Control and Prevention, American Society for Reproductive Medicine, Society for Assisted Reproductive Technology (2007). *Assisted Reproductive Technology Success Rates: National Summary and Fertility Clinic Reports*. Atlanta: US Department of Health and Human Services, Centers for Disease Control and Prevention.

Ecker, J.L. (2010). It's not easy/eight is enough. Room for debate. *New York Times*. Available at: http://roomfordebate.blogs.nytimes.com/2009/01/27/eight-is-enough/. Last accessed October 14, 2010.

HFEA (Human Fertilisation and Embryo Authority) (2010). Guidance note: Multiple births. Available at: www.hfea.gov.uk/docs/2010_FEB_multiple_births_FIN.pdf. Last accessed October 14, 2010.

Jain, T., Harlow, B.L., & Hornstein, M.D. (2002). Insurance coverage and outcomes of in vitro fertilization. *New England Journal of Medicine*, **347**, 661–666.

Minkoff, H. & Ecker, J. (2009). The California octuplets and the duties of reproductive endocrinologists. *American Journal of Obstetrics and Gynecology*, **201**(1), 15.e1–e3.

Minkoff, H. & Marshall, M. (2009). Scripted consents: when ethics and law collide. *Hastings Center Report*, **39**(5), 21–23.

Schieve, L.A., Peterson, H.B., Meikle, S.F., et al. (1999). Live-birth rates and multiple-birth risk using in vitro fertilization. *JAMA*, **282**, 1832–1838.

Thurin, A., Hausken, J., Hillensjo, T., et al. (2004). Elective single-embryo transfer versus double-embryo transfer in in vitro fertilization. *New England Journal of Medicine*, **346**, 731–737.

13

Preimplantation and prenatal genetic testing for inherited diseases, dispositions, and traits

Jeffrey R. Botkin

Case narrative

Jack Garrod is a 2-week-old infant who is new to your pediatric practice. Christina Garrod's pregnancy was full term and uncomplicated. Although she is only 26 years of age, she and her husband pursued prenatal diagnosis early in the pregnancy through the analysis of fetal DNA circulating in her blood. The test was expensive but effective in providing the couple with a complete DNA sequence on Jack. The testing service provided an analysis of 65 genes associated with health conditions and screened the sample for copy number variants. It was revealed that Jack has a relative risk of colon cancer in adulthood of 2.2 and for type II diabetes of 1.8. Fortunately his relative risk for nicotine addiction is 0.6. However, the screen also detected copy number variants in four regions of the genome and these particular variants have not been characterized. Therefore, it is uncertain whether these will produce significant health problems. The Garrods decided not to terminate the pregnancy based on this information but are anxious and eager for you to assess the baby and manage his health based on this genetic information.

Prenatal diagnosis

This case is, of course, science fiction, but a similar story is likely to be within technical reach in the next decade. Prenatal diagnosis – available since the 1960s – enables couples to diagnose genetic or anatomic abnormalities in a fetus prior to birth. The purposes of prenatal diagnosis are to offer an informed choice about whether to continue the pregnancy, make appropriate preparations for a child with special needs or, rarely, to intervene prenatally with therapeutic measures. Prenatal ultrasound examination is now used routinely by most obstetricians to evaluate gestational age

and fetal anatomy, although its efficacy in improving pregnancy outcomes remains controversial. Invasive measures like amniocentesis and chorionic villus sampling are conducted on a more selective basis. These are largely safe and effective tools but they leave some couples with difficult decisions about abortion if a significant abnormality is identified. To circumvent some of the ethical difficulties of prenatal diagnosis, pre-implantation genetic diagnosis (PGD) was developed in the 1990s as in vitro fertilization (IVF) became more technically efficient and available. PGD involves the genetic analysis of embryos in vitro to enable a choice of which embryos to transfer into the uterus. Other prenatal diagnostic approaches, such as isolating fetal DNA from the maternal circulation, are actively being developed. The general trend over recent decades is for less invasive technologies to be used more broadly in pregnancy for an expanding list of conditions.

Pediatricians are only tangentially involved in pre-implantation and prenatal diagnosis. Nevertheless, there are several reasons for pediatricians to be familiar with these developments. First, the existence of prenatal diagnostic capabilities creates some legal liability for pediatricians to promptly and accurately diagnose heritable conditions for couples who may wish to prevent the birth of a second affected child. Second, prenatal or preimplantation genetic diagnosis will increasingly provide a wealth of knowledge about the genotype of children prior to birth. The availability of this information for pediatricians may influence the nature of their clinical care for those children and their siblings. Third, new technologies will generate prenatal results of unknown clinical significance and it will be up to the pediatrician to manage the evaluation of such infants. This chapter will briefly describe existing and emerging prenatal diagnostic technologies

Clinical Ethics in Pediatrics: A Case-Based Textbook, ed. Douglas D. Diekema, Mark R. Mercurio and Mary B. Adam. Published by Cambridge University Press. (c) Cambridge University Press 2011.

and comment on the implications of these capabilities for pediatricians.

Maternal serum screening

Neural tube defects, including spina bifida and anencephaly, are relatively common forms of congenital malformation in children. Investigators in the 1960s recognized that neural tube defects in the fetus are associated with elevated levels of alpha-fetoprotein (AFP) in the maternal circulation. Routine screening for AFP has become common in the United States by the 1980s. The American College of Obstetrics and Gynecology (ACOG) currently recommends that all pregnant women be offered non-invasive prenatal diagnosis, including maternal serum AFP screening (MSAFP) (American College of Obstetrics and Gynecology, 2007). MSAFP screening will detect approximately 75% of fetuses with a neural tube defect (Wang et al., 2009). Of note, increased AFP is associated with an increased incidence of pregnancy loss in the absence of identifiable fetal anomalies, for reasons that remain to be fully clarified (Gagnon et al., 2008).

In due course, investigators recognized that common forms of trisomy are associated with *low* maternal AFP levels. Additionally, fetuses with trisomy 21 and 18 characteristically have increased nuchal translucency on ultrasound examination in the first trimester of pregnancy. Building on these findings, a relatively complex series of tests have been developed for prenatal diagnosis of neural tube defects and trisomy syndromes. The most comprehensive approach involves an ultrasound for nuchal translucency and measurement of pregnancy-associated plasma protein-A (PAPP-A) and human chorionic gonadotropin (hCG) at 11–14 weeks of pregnancy (Malone et al., 2005). During the second trimester, a "quad screen" is performed, comprised of AFP, estriol, hCG, and inhibin-A. The test results are interpreted in light of the woman's age. Abnormal screening test results may lead to amniocentesis for a definitive diagnosis of chromosomal abnormalities. The efficacy of an approach using both first and second trimester screening to identify fetuses with trisomy 21 is approximately 85–96% with a 5% false positive rate (Malone et al., 2005).

Despite the increasing utilization of accurate prenatal diagnosis and high rates of pregnancy termination following detection of trisomy syndromes, the prevalence of Down syndrome increased by over 30% from 1979 to 2003 in the United States (Shin et al.,

2009). This increase can be explained by the higher proportion of women who are having children at older ages. The rates of spina bifida in white and Hispanic women in the United States have declined by about one-third in recent years attributable, at least in part, to folic acid supplementation of enriched grain products since 1998 (Williams et al., 2005). However, the role of prenatal diagnosis in the declining incidence of neural tube defects is unknown.

Amniocentesis and chorionic villus sampling

Amniocentesis involves the sampling of amniotic fluid through needle insertion into the amniotic sac and is generally performed between 15 and 20 weeks of gestation. Chorionic villus sampling (CVS) involves biopsy of the chorionic villi from the placenta between 10 and 14 weeks of pregnancy. The purpose of both techniques is to obtain cellular material directly from the developing fetus, or embryo-derived tissues in the case of the placenta, for chromosomal and genetic analysis. Amniocentesis also provides amniotic fluid that can be evaluated for biochemical abnormalities associated with certain heritable disorders. The primary advantage of CVS over amniocentesis is the earlier timing in pregnancy. In the event that the test identifies an affected fetus, CVS permits termination decisions to be made in the first trimester. When amniocentesis is performed at 18–20 weeks' gestation, termination decisions occur after "quickening" and toward the end of the legal window for abortions in many US states. Second trimester abortions are also costlier and have higher morbidity and mortality than first trimester procedures. In addition, first trimester terminations appear to result in fewer psychological burdens than second trimester terminations, although this question has not been adequately evaluated. The estimated frequency of fetal loss secondary to amniocentesis and CVS is approximately 1 in 200 procedures, although it may be much lower in experienced centers (Tabor & Alfirevic, 2010).

Several laboratory techniques are commonly used to evaluate the cells obtained from amniocentesis or CVS (South et al., 2008). Amniocytes may be cultured and used with a variety of tools to identify trisomies, monosomies, or other chromosome abnormalities. When a specific genetic defect is being targeted, DNA from amniocytes or villous cells can be analyzed for the relevant mutation to determine whether the fetus will be affected. At the present time, there are 365 genes identified in the human genome with known DNA sequence and this number is expected to increase (NCBI, 2010).

A newer genetic testing tool that is just beginning to be applied in the prenatal context is array-based comparative genomic hybridization (aCGH) (South et al., 2008). This technology has the capability of detecting small duplications or deletions in genomic DNA. Array CGH is capable of detecting deletions or duplications at a far higher resolution than traditional banded karyotypes. This technology has proven particularly useful in the evaluation of children with developmental delay but without a recognizable clinical syndrome (Shaffer et al., 2007).

A challenge with array CGH is the relatively frequent identification of copy number variants (CNV) of unknown clinical significance. If a duplication or deletion is detected that is not associated with a known clinical syndrome, then it becomes difficult to determine the appropriate clinical response. When using array CGH to test children, this circumstance can be addressed by testing each of the parents for the same copy number variant. If the parent carrying the same variant appears clinically normal, the assumption is made that the variant is probably benign. Of course, this approach is confounded by the difficulty in determining what "normal" means, particularly for developmental traits, and by the fact that the same genotype at a particular locus can be associated with different phenotypes even within the same family. Cystic fibrosis (CF), for example, can be more severe in one sibling than another, even though they share the same CF mutations and have similar genetic and environmental backgrounds.

In the context of prenatal diagnosis, findings of unknown clinical significance have different implications. News that the fetus has a DNA variant of unknown significance may lead to substantial anxiety and perhaps pregnancy termination by some couples. Because we currently have a relatively incomplete understanding of normal and abnormal copy number variants, aCGH use in prenatal diagnosis poses the risk of pregnancy terminations based on CNV findings that might ultimately prove to be benign.

Preimplantation genetic diagnosis

Preimplantation genetic diagnosis (PGD) involves a genetic analysis of an in vitro embryo or one or both polar bodies prior to transfer to the mother's uterus. This approach is used in conjunction with IVF and has

been available since the early 1990s. For a couple at risk of conceiving a child with cystic fibrosis, for example, PGD involves harvesting a number of oocytes from the mother followed by IVF. The viable embryos undergo biopsy to determine which are not homozygous for the CF mutation. Unaffected embryos then would be eligible for transfer to the mother's uterus, or frozen for future attempts at pregnancy. Homozygous embryos would be discarded or donated for research purposes. The genetic analysis of a polar body will indicate whether the oocyte carries the mutation of concern to the couple. Analysis of polar bodies is applicable to recessive conditions or to dominant conditions when the mother carries the dominant mutation.

Preimplantation genetic diagnosis was developed initially for the diagnosis of single gene disorders affecting children. The most common single gene disorders prompting PGD include CF, sickle cell disease, spinal muscular atrophy, beta-thalassemia, myotonic dystrophy, Huntington disease, Charcot–Marie–Tooth disease, fragile X, Duchenne muscular dystrophy, and hemophilia (Geraedts & Wert, 2009). However, in recent years this technology has been used commonly to screen embryos for aneuploidy prior to transfer in couples without known genetic conditions. Couples with advanced maternal age, recurrent implantation failure, or recurrent pregnancy loss have been good candidates for this approach given the higher possibility of aneuploidy in these circumstances. The term preimplantation genetic screening (PGS) refers to the screening of embryos for this purpose, in contrast to PGD of embryos from at-risk couples (American Society for Reproductive Medicine, 2008). While PGS is theoretically attractive, recent controlled trials indicate that PGS does not improve pregnancy outcomes and, in fact, may reduce pregnancy rates per cycle. The American Society of Reproductive Medicine currently does not support the use of PGS for the indications noted above (American Society for Reproductive Medicine, 2008).

A primary advantage of PGD is the ability to select embryos prior to the pregnancy, thereby eliminating the need for a pregnancy termination (at least for the genetic conditions targeted by PGD). For those who believe that the embryo does not have the same moral status as a fetus, PGD substantially reduces the ethical challenges associated with prenatal diagnosis (Botkin, 1998). For those who believe embryos have full moral status, PGD actually presents greater problems than more traditional prenatal diagnosis. For each pregnancy established through PGD, numerous embryos are created and either destroyed or cryopreserved for an uncertain future. Therefore the total loss of prenatal life is typically greater through PGD than through prenatal diagnosis. Yet PGD, like IVF generally, has not been the focus of significant social controversy in the United States. Current evidence does not indicate that PGD increases the probability of congenital malformation in the child, although additional study of this issue is warranted (Simpson, 2010).

Within the scholarly and clinical communities, controversy surrounding PGD is related to the scope of its use. Should PGD be used for detecting conditions that are not severe pediatric disorders (Botkin, 1998)? That is, should PGD be used for conditions like genetic risk for adult-onset breast/ovarian cancer or colon cancer? Professional organizations in the United States have not taken a stand on this issue and in recent years PGD has been used for families with these types of adult-onset cancer syndromes (Sagi et al., 2009). Fears also were raised about the future use of PGD for extensive embryo selection for non-health attributes like intelligence, body build, personality traits, etc., once genetic correlates for such traits were identified (Botkin, 2000). But as the complexity of genetic information has become more apparent, in tandem with the current inability to identify significant genetic attributes associated with even common multifactorial traits like diabetes and atherosclerotic heart disease, concerns about extensive selection of embryos based on non-health related traits have diminished.

Another prominent controversy regarding PGD involves its use in the deliberate selection of a future child that will be a good tissue match for a previous child with a fatal condition. These so-called "savior siblings" have received prominent coverage in the media. This situation arises when a child with fatal condition amenable to treatment with a bone marrow transplant does not have a suitable living donor (Samuel et al., 2009). If the parents are of reproductive age, a sibling can be selected through PGD that is an appropriate HLA match. Once the child is born, bone marrow is harvested from the donor sibling for transplant. This approach has been successful for conditions including Fanconi anemia, Blackfan–Diamond syndrome, and beta-thalassemia. The ethics of this approach have been debated at some length (Dickens, 2005). In general, the concerns over the "designer baby" aspects of this approach have not outweighed the potential life-saving benefits for a few children and their families

through the use of this technology, at least in the eyes of the general public (Hudson, 2006).

From the pediatrician's perspective, PGD technology offers the opportunity to thoroughly evaluate the genetic status of an embryo at its earliest stage of development. Currently, blastomeres can be evaluated for single gene disorders, chromosome abnormalities, or copy number variants through aCGH. As costs for DNA sequencing fall, the prospect of extensive or even full sequencing of embryonic DNA will emerge. Presumably this information will be available for the pediatrician. The implications of these potential developments will be discussed below.

Fetal DNA in maternal circulation

Human fetal cells were first isolated in the maternal circulation in 1990 (Bianchi et al., 1990). Isolation of fetal cells in the maternal circulation raised the prospect of prenatal genetic diagnosis of the fetus through a simple blood draw from the pregnant woman. However, this approach has not proven fruitful for prenatal diagnosis for several reasons, including the low number of fetal cells in maternal circulation, challenges with enriching fetal cells, and technical difficulties with DNA analysis from these types of cells (Wright & Burton, 2009). Remarkably, it was recognized that cells continue to circulate in the maternal blood from previous pregnancies, in addition to the current pregnancy, and fetal cells have been detected in the mother's system up to 27 years after pregnancy (Bianchi et al., 1996). Nests of fetal cells may be sequestered in a woman's body during pregnancy and continue to shed cells into her system for years. While this is a fascinating phenomenon of uncertain clinical significance for the mother, it further complicates the ability to conduct prenatal diagnosis using this technology.

But in the late 1990s, investigators identified fetal cell-free DNA in the maternal blood in low concentration (Lo et al., 1997). It is estimated that about 3–6% of cell-free DNA circulating in a pregnant woman's blood is fetal DNA (Lo et al., 1998). There are a number of challenges in isolating and analyzing cell-free fetal DNA for prenatal diagnosis (Wright & Burton, 2009). First, the DNA exists in low concentration compared with maternal DNA. Second, the fetus shares half of its genome with the mother and therefore distinguishing fetal DNA from maternal DNA is a significant challenge. Detection of Y chromosome markers in the presence of a male fetus is most easily performed.

There are several clinical applications of this approach that are in development. Sex determination of the fetus using Y chromosome targets is useful in the context of X-linked diseases like Duchenne muscular dystrophy. A non-invasive determination of sex early in the pregnancy would reduce the number of invasive procedures in at-risk pregnancies by potentially eliminating the need for further evaluations when a female fetus is identified. Single gene disorders can be detected through this approach when the allele is paternally inherited. A third application under active development is in the management of pregnancy-related risks such as rhesus (Rh) incompatibility. If the fetus is determined to be RhD negative in an RhD negative woman, then Rh prophylaxis need not be conducted. Finally, there is work toward the ability to detect aneuploidy through cell-free DNA by analyzing the relative concentration of relevant fetal DNA sequences circulating in the mother's system (Wright & Burton, 2009).

Fetal DNA in the maternal circulation is highly fragmented and it has been unclear until recently whether the full fetal genome is represented. However, Lo and colleagues recently isolated a whole fetal genome from maternal blood, indicating that full sequence analysis may be possible in the future from a non-invasive test (Lo et al., 2010). This is remarkable work that is not ready for clinical application outside the research context. However, in conjunction with anatomic screening and biochemical screening of maternal serum, it may be possible in the not-too-distant future to conduct exhaustive prenatal genetic evaluation of the fetus through essentially non-invasive means.

Implications for pediatricians

Pediatricians are not often directly involved in prenatal diagnosis, although they may be actively engaged with parents and other care providers in interpreting prenatal diagnostic results and planning for the birth of an affected child. This type of prenatal consultation would most commonly be performed by subspecialists such as pediatric geneticists or perinatologists. But other pediatric specialists may be impacted by these developments in prenatal diagnosis in several ways. First, there is potential legal liability should a physician fail to make a timely genetic diagnosis, the parents of the child conceive and give birth to a similarly affected child, and then argue that prenatal diagnosis would have allowed them the opportunity to terminate the pregnancy. Second, there are emerging prospects of extensive knowledge of the genetic traits of children. Finally, prenatal technologies may produce a volume of information of unknown clinical significance that will be challenging to manage for pediatricians.

Legal liabilities: wrongful life and wrongful birth

New capabilities often result in new responsibilities. Following the constitutional protection of abortion during the first two trimesters with the *Roe* v. *Wade* decision in 1973 and the development of prenatal diagnostic technologies, a new set of legal liabilities emerged in the United States. Given the capability of detecting an affected pregnancy and the ability to terminate, couples began to make malpractice claims when clinicians did not provide accurate or timely information about their reproductive risks. So-called "wrongful birth" suits emerged when parents brought a suit against a health care provider claiming that, but for the negligence of the provider, the parents would have been accurately informed, utilized prenatal diagnosis to identify an affected fetus, and then terminated the pregnancy (Botkin, 2003). A typical example is a pregnant woman of advanced maternal age who is not offered screening or testing for aneuploidy and has an affected child. Other examples include situations in which the parents were inaccurately informed of the heritable nature of a condition in a first child, or when the clinician fails to make a timely diagnosis in an affected child and a second affected child is born before the parents are informed of their reproductive risk.

A second type of suit brought in similar circumstances is termed a "wrongful life" suit. These are suits brought on behalf of the infant claiming negligence by health care providers leading to the child's existence in an impaired state: the child claims, but for the negligence of the clinician, that their condition would have been detected prenatally and they would not exist to suffer. The wrongful life claim presents obvious philosophical challenges and has rarely succeeded in the US legal system. However, the wrongful birth suits have been widely successful and have been supported in more than 26 states where the claims have been addressed (Botkin, 2003). The success of the wrongful birth suits clearly establishes that providers have professional obligations under the standard of care to provide a timely and accurate genetic diagnosis in order to provide parents with reproductive risk information. Note that this responsibility is different than the responsibilities directly to the child for a timely diagnosis. For example, imagine a situation in which a pediatrician fails to make a diagnosis of cystic fibrosis in a child despite suggestive symptoms. If a second child is born with CF prior to the diagnosis, the pediatrician could be liable for damages from harm to the first child from a delayed diagnosis and damages for "wrongful birth" flowing from the birth of a second affected child.

The wrongful birth suits are contingent on the ability to make a genetic diagnosis and the ability to conduct prenatal diagnosis for the condition. Therefore, as genetic knowledge and prenatal diagnostic capabilities expand, pediatricians will be obligated to keep abreast of changes in order to offer a contemporary standard of care. Take, for example, a young child who demonstrates developmental delays without a clinical history or clinical stigmata to provide a presumptive explanation. The recent emergence of aCGH as a tool to identify copy number variants in this situation means that genetic diagnosis may be feasible. And, with a genetic association in hand, the parents could pursue prenatal diagnosis through PGD, amniocentesis, CVS, or eventually through cell-free fetal DNA to detect the condition in future pregnancies. The point here is not simply that pediatricians can be sued in this situation if they fail make a timely genetic diagnosis, but that pediatricians now have an obligation to provide state-of-the-art information for families. Although aCGH is not yet state of the art for developmental delay, the whole domain of genomic analysis is rapidly progressing, requiring pediatricians to be cognizant of new capabilities for early diagnosis in children and prenatal diagnosis for their parents, should they wish to use these technologies for that purpose.

A wealth of genetic information

Diagnostic testing or screening most commonly employs tests that target specific conditions or a narrow range of conditions. A test will be positive or negative for the condition it targets (or sometimes produce indeterminate results) but also might provide surprising clues about conditions not originally targeted. A complete blood count done for concern about infection might reveal leukemia, anemia, or a thrombocytopenia that was not originally part of the justification for testing. The ethical obligation to respond to these types of unanticipated findings is usually straightforward.

But as the power of technologies expands to generate large volumes of data, our ability to respond appropriately is often uncertain and potentially overwhelming.

In the context of prenatal diagnosis, as the power of the screening technology expands, more information is generated of uncertain value. The use of aCGH is a prime example of a groundbreaking technology that produces more information that we can deal with in a clinical context at the present time. Investigators are learning that copy number variants in the genome are relatively common and that some are clearly associated with clinical abnormalities. But many other variants are benign or of uncertain association with pathology. It may take decades to catalogue and classify CNVs so that patients can be appropriately counseled when genomic analysis reveals a variant. In the meantime, clinicians, patients, and their families will be challenged to deal with this type of information. This problem will be magnified several-fold when complete genome sequencing becomes available at feasible prices.

Along with information about a specific gene being targeted by the analysis, information will be generated about a large number of other disease-associated genes. Some of these other loci may be highly predictive of future disease, such as BRCA1 mutation conferring increased risk for breast and/or ovarian cancer in an adult woman. Other markers will be of lower predictive power, such as risk information for diabetes, heart disease, or mental health disorders. Here, too, genomic variants of unknown clinical significance will be detected.

An initial question for investigators or clinicians will be to decide which results, beyond those initially targeted, should be shared with the patient or the couple in the context of prenatal diagnosis. Such information may be highly beneficial if the conditions can be ameliorated or prevented through timely interventions. For example, newborn screening is currently conducted in virtually all states to detect 29 primary and 25 secondary conditions that are amenable to intervention. Some of these conditions, like congenital hypothyroidism, are not Mendelian disorders, but many of the conditions amenable to newborn screening are autosomal recessive genetic conditions. Presently, biochemical screening is more accurate than DNA-based testing but this situation may change as more knowledge is gained about the underlying mutations associated with these conditions. If so, prenatal diagnosis using extensive genomic analysis may eliminate the need for newborn screening for those conditions. In addition, results will likely be generated prenatally that will inform the pediatrician about risks for conditions like cancer, type I diabetes, or developmental delay. Pediatricians are likely to have increasing responsibilities to record this information, interpret it appropriately, and respond in a timely way.

One category of information that presents significant ethical challenges is predictive tests for adult-onset conditions. In fact, the AAP Committee on Bioethics (2001) and the American Society of Human Genetics (1995) have published statements that discourage predictive testing of children for adult-onset conditions unless there are clinical interventions in the pediatric age range. The primary concerns relate to the psychological impact on children and on the parent–child relationship in generating risk information about conditions that cannot be addressed clinically. So, in general, children do not receive predictive genetic testing for conditions like Huntington disease, hereditary nonpolyposis colon cancer, Alzheimer disease, or breast/ovarian cancer. But as significant or complete genome sequencing information is generated through prenatal diagnosis, this information will become available. Some parents may even want to use this information in decisions about pregnancy termination or embryo selection in PGD. Therefore it may not be appropriate to withhold this information from couples while these prenatal options are available. If the information is not used for pregnancy termination or embryo selection, then presumably the parents and pediatrician will know this genetic risk information about the child. Because there has been such limited predictive testing of children for adult-onset conditions, it is hard for pediatricians to understand the potential impact on children, the clinician, or the parent-child relationship. Will such information produce a hyper-vigilance or "vulnerable child" response in parents (or perhaps in the pediatrician)? If a girl is a carrier of a BRCA1 mutation, how might that impact her attitudes about her body, puberty, self-worth generally, and ideas about marriage and reproduction? Some authors disagree with the recommended restrictions on predictive genetic testing in children for adult-onset conditions (Rhodes, 2006; Wilfond & Ross, 2009). The alternative position is to respect parental decision-making after a careful consideration of the pros and cons of testing, and to consider the broader potential psychosocial benefits of risk information beyond clinical interventions. In the context of prenatal diagnosis, this type of information generated about the child would be a secondary effect of prenatal testing, and not generally conducted for the child's welfare as the primary goal.

Finally, results of unknown significance will likely be generated with new genomic technologies. The genome is enormously complicated and variable from one individual to another. A common phenomenon in contemporary genetic testing that involves DNA sequencing is the identification of variant sequences of unknown clinical significance (Haile et al., 2010). In clinical genetic testing for BRCA1 and BRCA2 mutations, approximately 5–10% of individuals will have results of unknown clinical significance (Easton et al., 2007). If the sequence variation is a large deletion or clearly results in a non-functional protein product, then it may be assumed that the variation is deleterious. But in many situations, it cannot be determined whether the variation is benign or pathologic. This may become clear over time as experience with a particular variation is shared. But in the meantime, patients and clinicians are left with uncertainty. The literature on psychological responses to genetic information clearly illustrates that individuals with ambiguous test results often have more distress than those who test positive for a mutation (Lerman & Shields, 2004). It may be that people with positive results are better able to marshal their psychological and behavioral defenses, while those with ambiguous results are unable to respond effectively.

Case resolution and summary

We can imagine how this phenomenon might play out in the Garrod family's case presented above. An infant is born and genomic information obtained through prenatal diagnosis shows no major genetic abnormalities that are clearly associated with disease, but sequence variations of unknown clinical significance are identified in, say, four key genes. We have essentially no experience to indicate the impact of this information on the child, his parents, and the clinician. If these variations prove to be benign, we can assume that this information produced a net harm through months or years of worry. If one or more of the variations prove to be clinically significant then we can hope that interventions can be implemented to prevent or ameliorate the associated conditions. At this point, it is uncertain how many variants of unknown clinical significance will be generated through complete genome sequencing, but if BRCA1/2 testing identifies these variants in 5–10% of individuals tested for these two genes alone, we can assume that the number will be quite large.

We live in an information-rich society and we know that parents are typically eager to learn as much about their child as possible. But given the volume of information produced through sequencing, we should consider alternative ways to manage the problems associated with results of unknown clinical significance generated by predictive testing. Rather than read and interpret the genomic information as it is generated, it will be feasible to query the sequence information prenatally for only those conditions that justify prenatal diagnosis. For example, the genetic risk for type II diabetes is unlikely to be relevant to pregnancy termination or embryo selection, so perhaps this information would not be sought and analyzed from within the raw sequence data. The raw sequence data could be stored, perhaps under the control of the parent until the child reaches adulthood, and queried repeatedly for relevant information during the life span of the individual. At birth, the data could be analyzed for conditions like phenylketonuria that pose an immediate threat to the welfare of the infant. As the child approaches his or her reproductive years, the genomic data could be queried for information such as carrier status that would be relevant to reproductive decisions. This approach would reduce the concerns associated with a "data dump" on new parents of information that is alarming, ambiguous, and not actionable.

The ethical issues associated with prenatal diagnosis have been widely discussed. An enormous expansion in the amount and type of information provided through emerging prenatal diagnostic technologies will prompt further debate on basic questions over what kinds of conditions warrant prenatal diagnosis and selective termination or embryo selection. Those debates are generally beyond the scope of pediatrics. Nevertheless, the pediatric impacts and implications of information generated prenatally must be carefully considered in the implementation of these new technologies. The management of genomic information provided in large volumes will be challenging enough at any age.

References

American College of Obstetricians & Gynecologists, Committee on Practice Bulletins (2007). ACOG Practice Bulletin No. 77: Screening for fetal chromosomal abnormalities. *Obstetrics and Gynecology*, **109**, 217–227.

American Society of Human Genetics (1995). Points to consider: ethical, legal, and psychosocial implications of genetic testing in children and adolescents. *American Journal of Human Genetics*, **57**, 1233–1241.

American Society for Reproductive Medicine, Practice Committee & The Society for Assisted Reproductive Technology Practice Committee (2008). Preimplantation genetic testing: a Practice Committee Opinion. *Fertility and Sterility*, **90**(3), S136–S143. Available at: www.asrm.org/uploadedFiles/ASRM_Content/News_ and_Publications/Practice_Guidelines/Committee_ Opinions/Preimplantation_genetic_testing(1).pdf. Last accessed January 4, 2011.

Bianchi, D.W., Flint, A.F., Pizzimenti, M.F., Knoll, J.H.M., & Latt, S.A. (1990). Isolation of fetal DNA from nucleated erythrocytes in maternal blood. *Proceedings of the National Academy of Sciences USA*, **87**, 3279–3283.

Bianchi, D.W., Zickwolf, G.K., Weil, G.J., Sylvester, S., & DeMaria, M.A. (1996). Male fetal progenitor cells persist in maternal blood for as long as 27 years postpartum. *Proceedings of the National Academy of Sciences USA*, **93**, 705–708.

Botkin, J.R. (1998). Ethical issues and practical problems in preimplantation genetic diagnosis. *American Journal of Law, Medicine and Ethics*, **26**, 17–28.

Botkin, J.R. (2000). Line drawing: developing professional standards for prenatal diagnosis. In *Prenatal Testing and Disability Rights*, ed. E. Parens & A. Asch. Washington, DC: Georgetown University Press, 288–307.

Botkin, J.R. (2003). Wrongful life and wrongful birth: ethical and legal issues in prenatal diagnosis. *Florida State University Law Review*, **30**(2), 265–293.

Committee on Bioethics, American Academy of Pediatrics (2001). Ethical issues in genetic testing in pediatrics. *Pediatrics*, **107**, 1451–1455.

Dickens, B.M. (2005). Preimplantation genetic diagnosis and "savior siblings." *International Journal of Gynecologic Obstetrics*, **88**, 91–96.

Easton, D.F., Deffenbaugh, A.M., Pruss, D., et al. (2007). A systematic genetic assessment of 1,433 sequence variants of unknown clinical significance in the BRCA1 and BRCA2 breast cancer-predisposing genes. *American Journal of Human Genetics*, **81**, 873–883.

Gagnon, A., Wilson, R.D., Audibert, F., et al. (2008). Obstetrical complications associated with abnormal maternal serum markers analytes. *Journal of Obstetrics and Gynaecology Canada*, **30**(10), 918–949.

Geraedts, J.P. & Wert, G.M. (2009). Preimplantation genetic diagnosis. *Clinical Genetics*, **76**, 315–325.

Haile, B.A., Malone, K.E., Capanu, M., et al. (2010). Characterization of BRCA1 and BRCA2 deleterious mutations and variants of unknown clinical significance in unilateral and bilateral breast cancer: the WECARE study. *Human Mutation*, **31**, E1200–1240.

Hudson, K. (2006). Preimplantation genetic diagnosis: public policy and public attitudes. *Fertility and Sterility*, **85**, 1638–1645.

Lerman, C. & Shields, A.E. (2004). Genetic testing for cancer susceptibility: the promise and the pitfalls. *Nature Reviews Cancer*, **4**, 235–241.

Lo, Y.M.D., Corbetta, N., Chamberlain, P.F., et al. (1997). Presence of fetal DNA in maternal plasma and serum. *Lancet*, **350**, 485–487.

Lo, Y.M.D., Tein, M.S.C., Lau, T.K., et al. (1998). Quantitative analysis of fetal DNA in maternal plasma and serum: implications for noninvasive prenatal diagnosis. *American Journal of Human Genetics*, **62**, 768–775.

Lo, Y.M.D., Chan, K.C.A., Sun, H., et al. (2010). Maternal plasma DNA sequencing reveals the genome-wide genetic and mutational profile of the fetus. *Science Translational Medicine*, **2**, 61–91.

Malone, F.D., Canick, J.A., Ball, R.H., et al. (2005). First-trimester or second-trimester screening, or both, for Down's syndrome. *New England Journal of Medicine*, **353**, 2001–2011.

NCBI (2010). *Online Mendelian Inheritance in Man*. Available at: www.ncbi.nlm.nih.gov/Omim/mimstats.html. Last accessed January 4, 2011.

Rhodes, R. (2006). Why test children for adult-onset genetic diseases? *Mount Sinai Journal of Medicine*, **73**, 609–616.

Sagi, M., Weinberg, N., Eilat, A., et al. (2009). Preimplantation genetic diagnosis for BRCA1/2 – a novel clinical experience. *Prenatal Diagnosis*, **29**, 508–513.

Samuel, G.N., Strong, K.A., Kerridge, I., Ankeny, R.A., & Shaw, P.J. (2009). Establishing the role of pre-implantation genetic diagnosis for human leucocyte antigen typing: what place do "savior siblings" have in paediatric transplantation? *Archives of Disease in Childhood*, **94**, 317–320.

Shaffer, L.G., Bejjani, B.A., Torchia, B., et al. (2007). The identification of microdeletion syndromes and other chromosome abnormalities: cytogenetic methods of the past, new technologies for the future. *American Journal of Medical Genetics. Part C, Seminars Med Genet*, **145C**, 335–342.

Shin, M., Besser, L.M., Kucik, J.E., et al. & the Congenital Anomaly Multistate Prevalence and Survival Collaborative (2009). Prevalence of Down syndrome among children and adolescents in 10 regions of the United States. *Pediatrics*, **124**, 1565–1571.

Simpson, J.L. (2010). Children born after preimplantation genetic diagnosis show no increase in congenital anomalies. *Human Reproduction*, **25**, 6–8.

South, S.T., Chen, Z., & Brothman, A.R. (2008). Genomic medicine in prenatal diagnosis. *Clinical Obstetrics and Gynecology*, **51**, 62–73.

Tabor, A. & Alfirevic, Z. (2010). Update on procedure-related risks for prenatal diagnosis techniques. *Fetal Diagnosis and Therapy*, **27**, 1–7.

Wang, Z.P., Li, H., Hao, L.Z., & Zhao, Z.T. (2009). The effectiveness of prenatal serum biomarker screening for neural tube defects in second trimester pregnant women: a meta-analysis. *Prenatal Diagnosis*, **29**, 960–965.

Wilfond, B. & Ross, L.F. (2009). From genetics to genomics: ethics, policy, and parental decision-making. *Journal of Pediatric Psychology*, **34**, 639–647.

Williams, L.J., Rasmussen, S.A., Flores, A., Kirby, R.S., & Edmonds, L.D. (2005). Decline in the prevalence of spina bifida and anencephaly by race/ethnicity: 1995–2002. *Pediatrics*, **116**, 580–586.

Wright, C.F. & Burton, H. (2009). The use of cell-free fetal nucleic acids in maternal blood for non-invasive prenatal diagnosis. *Human Reproduction Update*, **15**, 139–151.

Chapter

14

Decision-making in the delivery room

Mark R. Mercurio

Case narrative

A 26-year-old woman is admitted to the Labor and Delivery Unit in early labor. She is at 23 weeks' gestation (based on last menstrual period and second trimester ultrasound) with a singleton female fetus, and the pregnancy has been unremarkable until today. The estimated fetal weight is 580 grams, and there are no apparent anomalies on the ultrasound done today. The perinatologist believes that the patient will deliver today, and requests that the neonatology team meet with the patient and her husband to discuss the prognosis and the management plan for the baby. Since choices surrounding care of the newborn might also influence obstetrical decisions, the meeting is requested immediately.

Summary of ethical issues

Decisions regarding newborn resuscitation are often made under great time pressure, either due to imminent delivery, thus limiting the time for discussion with the parents beforehand, or because specific actions may be required immediately after delivery if the child is to have a chance at survival. For this reason, it is essential to have considered the possible scenarios that may arise when the child is born and, as much as possible, to have worked through the ethical questions beforehand. There will be very little, if any, opportunity for ethical analysis or in-depth discussion at the time of delivery.

Difficult ethical and medical decisions made in the setting of the delivery room (DR) and newborn intensive care unit (NICU) often involve extreme prematurity or "borderline viability," and for that reason this case has been chosen for discussion. However, the ethical questions relevant to this case will be equally relevant to the management of any newborn for whom

prognosis regarding survival and/or permanent disability is significantly worse than for a normal healthy infant. Such questions include: Is the prognosis poor enough to justify a decision not to attempt resuscitation? What should prospective parents be told by the pediatric team prior to delivery? How much control should the parents have with regard to medical management? What options should they be given with regard to resuscitation and newborn care? The ethical questions faced in the management of an infant in the DR can perhaps best be summarized as follows: Which among the possible resuscitation options would be ethically impermissible, permissible, or obligatory, and how should that be determined?

Ethical principles and discussion

Honesty and fairness in considering relevant data

Though the appropriate approach for the great majority of newborns is to make every effort at resuscitation, and to provide initial intensive care measures as needed to maximize the chance of survival, there will be some newborns for whom this may not be the case. Decisions about whether or not to provide aggressive resuscitative efforts (e.g., intubation, positive-pressure ventilation, chest compressions, epinephrine, admission to the NICU) should be informed by the likelihood of survival, and the anticipated short-term and long-term morbidity. For many conditions encountered by the physician in the newborn period, these data will be a moving target, and what one read or was taught just a few short years ago may no longer be accurate. It is incumbent on those counseling the parents and participating in the decisions to be aware of current data, as well as the limitations of those data.

Clinical Ethics in Pediatrics: A Case-Based Textbook, ed. Douglas S. Diekema, Mark R. Mercurio and Mary B. Adam. Published by Cambridge University Press. © Cambridge University Press 2011.

Recent data from the National Institute of Child Health and Human Development (NICHD, 2010) report survival to discharge to be 26% for infants born at 23 completed weeks (23 weeks and 0 days to 23 weeks and 6 days) (Stoll et al., 2010). Approximately one-third of survivors will have profound neurodevelopmental impairment (severe cognitive deficits, cerebral palsy, visual impairment, and/or hearing impairment) when assessed at 18–22 months (Tyson et al., 2008; NICHD, 2010). However, follow-up studies done at 18–22 months appear to overestimate permanent disability when compared with follow-up at later ages (Hack et al., 2005). Furthermore, these outcomes come from a network of major academic centers in the United States, and may not be reflective of the hospital where this case is occurring. The physician needs to consider not just national data, but also local results as well, and should be honest and open about this when counseling parents. If transfer to a different facility with significantly greater experience and/or better outcomes is feasible, parents should be made aware of that option.

Parents must be counseled, and DR plans made, with an honest assessment of the degree of certainty regarding the prenatal diagnosis. Some plans may require flexibility, or a need to provide maximum support until the diagnosis can be confirmed. With regard to extreme prematurity, while the diagnosis is rarely in question, the accuracy of the gestational age commonly is. For this case, the gestational age could easily be off by at least a week, which could move the predicted survival up or down dramatically. Survival at 22 completed weeks was reported to be 6%, and at 24 weeks to be 55% in recent NICHD data (Stoll et al., 2010). One should consider that wide range in predicted outcomes when discussing options and counseling parents.

The self-fulfilling prophecy is a possible cause of unintentional deception and self-deception. For some disorders, reported survival data include many patients for whom resuscitation or intensive care was never attempted. Thus, predicted survival may be artificially lowered because, for that diagnosis, resuscitation is often or even typically not attempted. Extreme prematurity provides an excellent example of this. The NICHD reported survival to be 6% of all live births at 22 completed weeks. However, resuscitation was only attempted in 19%. Thus it would be misleading to say that, if attempted, the chance of a successful resuscitation at 22 weeks and survival to discharge is only 6%. This is not to say that resuscitation should necessarily be attempted at 22 weeks, but that we need to be honest about published outcomes and how they have been generated. The relevant question when considering resuscitation is not, what are the overall survival statistics for this disorder or gestational age, but rather what would be the chance of survival and intact survival *if maximal efforts were made*? Often the honest answer is that we do not know. And even if parents are not knowledgeable enough to ask the relevant question, this does not remove the physician's responsibility to consider it, and to address it with them (Mercurio, 2005).

Basing prognosis and parental counseling on gestational age alone may be needlessly inaccurate, and could lead to injustice. Gender, weight, singleton versus multiple gestation, and the presence or absence of antenatal steroids each have an independent and significant influence on likelihood of survival and neurodevelopmental impairment, leading to a wide range of predicted outcomes within a given gestational age category. A more accurate picture of prognosis can be obtained through the use of an online statistical tool based on these factors (using estimated fetal weight) and the NICHD database (Tyson et al., 2008; NICHD, 2010). This tool reveals that in certain situations a larger infant born at 22 weeks may have a higher likelihood of survival and survival without disability, than a smaller one born at 23 weeks. One can see that a policy or approach to newborn resuscitation based solely on gestational age could potentially lead to injustice, if the parents of the smaller child at 23 weeks were offered the option of resuscitation at delivery, but the parents of the larger one at 22 weeks (with a better prognosis) were not. Over time the data may change, but the importance of fairness when considering policies for provision of resuscitation will remain.

Relevant rights and patient's best interest

Parents are generally and correctly felt to have a right to determine what should be done with their children, in medical and other contexts. This right should play a central role in how the resuscitation question is approached, and the discussion about relevant ethical considerations appropriately begins here. However, their right is not absolute, and should not be confused with patient autonomy. The term autonomy literally means "self-rule," and a competent adult patient's right to control what is done to their body, in particular the right to refuse medical interventions, is widely accepted. The term "parental autonomy" seems a misnomer, in that one cannot have self-rule over someone else, even one's own child. A more appropriate term is parental authority, which should be seen as a strong right, but not an absolute one. In rare situations, parental preferences for their child may be trumped or overridden by a consideration of the child's rights.

The rights of the newborn include a right to life. If there is a reasonable chance that a procedure could save the baby's life, it would seem self-evident that he/she has a right to that procedure, including resuscitation in the DR. This may be relevant in some cases where the parents refuse resuscitative efforts. The baby also has a right to mercy, meaning a right not to be made to undergo avoidable pain that offers no chance of benefit. This may be relevant in some cases where parents demand resuscitative efforts. In addition, the baby has a right to justice, which among other things implies a right to equal treatment. That is, if he/she is to be treated differently from another patient, a relevant difference between the other patient and him/her should be identified (Beauchamp & Childress, 2001; Mercurio, 2009).

An obvious example of injustice would be to offer resuscitation to the parents of one infant but not the parents of another, when the prognoses were similar and the only difference was ethnicity. Few would consider that difference relevant. An example of a relevant difference between patients would be a marked difference in prognosis. There is evidence to suggest that resuscitation of newborns, particularly preterm newborns, is viewed by physicians and others as being less obligatory when compared with older children or adults with a similar prognosis for survival and disability (Janvier et al., 2008). It is beyond the scope of this chapter, but if this observation is valid, it is worth considering whether viewing newborns' lives as somehow more "optional" than others represents an injustice in the practice of pediatrics, or whether there are ethically valid reasons for doing so.

Most would agree that consideration of a child's rights could lead one to override a parental decision, including a decision regarding newborn resuscitation. Extreme cases make this point, such as parental refusal of resuscitation for a newborn likely to survive with little or no impairment, parental demand for resuscitation where there is no chance of survival, or parental demand for invasive and potentially painful procedures that offer no benefit to the child. The hard ethical work, however, is in the less obvious cases, and in finding the

threshold for overriding parental authority. Guidance in this regard can be found in the American Academy of Pediatrics' Guidelines on Foregoing Life-Sustaining Medical Treatment, which state that, in general, the wishes of the parents should prevail and physicians should seek to override a parental decision only when that decision is "clearly opposed" to the child's best interests (Committee on Bioethics, 1994).

Best interests are determined by weighing the benefits and burdens (short and long term) of the proposed treatment, here DR resuscitation. Burdens include such factors as the pain or discomfort of the procedure itself and the NICU course, and the disabilities with which the child may be left. Benefits would include the chance of survival, and the pleasures of life that the child may experience, both short term and long term, should he/she survive. For some cases, this will be a very subjective and difficult determination – and it will be far from clear whether either decision would be opposed to the child's interests. In such cases the decision is best left to well-informed parents. This is consistent with the Neonatal Resuscitation Guidelines of the American Heart Association, which state: "In conditions associated with uncertain prognosis in which survival is borderline, the morbidity rate is relatively high, and the anticipated burden to the child is high, parental desires concerning initiation of resuscitation should be supported" (Kattwinkel et al., 2010). Similarly, the American Academy of Pediatrics Committee on Fetus and Newborn has stated that resuscitation should be initiated if a good outcome is reasonably likely, should not be attempted if there is no chance of survival, and parents should be given the option when a good outcome is "very unlikely" (Batton et al., 2009).

Much emphasis is rightly given to the patient's best interest, but some have questioned whether the parents and physicians can also consider the interests of others affected by the decision. It is here suggested that a consideration of the family's interests is appropriate, but the interests of the patient should be given considerably more weight. Those affected by the decision may also include people beyond the family, indeed the entire society that may bear a financial burden in the case of some patients with severe disability. It has been argued that the cost of NICU treatment, and possibly treatment for a lifetime, should be considered in deciding about resuscitation. It seems inappropriate, however, for a physician to make such decisions on an individual basis. This approach would be highly vulnerable to injustice due to unequal treatment, as decisions among physicians in this regard could vary widely. If the society, or the profession, reaches a consensus on such matters, it may then be appropriate to limit care in an equitable manner. Until such time, however, it would be unjust for a given family's options to be arbitrarily limited in an effort to save societal resources.

Withholding and withdrawing

Some may believe that once intensive measures are started, they must be continued, but this is not the case. This misunderstanding could lead to withholding a trial of treatment that might be successful for fear that it would force continued aggressive care over parental objections. For many parents or staff it may be more difficult psychologically or emotionally to stop once intensive care measures have begun, and clinicians counseling parents should be aware of this. However, it is important to realize that this psychological phenomenon does not imply an ethical proscription. It is widely held that withholding and withdrawing life-sustaining medical treatment are ethically equivalent. In fact, it could be argued that for some cases it would be ethically preferable to begin intensive treatment, thus deferring the decision until more information becomes available, such as early clinical course or the results of early neurological studies, and then consider withdrawal. One possible advantage to this approach, aside from allowing for the acquisition of more information, is that it spares parents from having to make such an important decision very quickly in the midst of labor, which sometimes occurs.

Legal considerations

The focus of this discussion is ethical issues with regard to decisions in the DR. It is beyond the scope of this chapter, or the expertise of the author, to discuss relevant law. Moreover, laws vary from state to state, from nation to nation, and over time. While it is here suggested that clinicians' actions should be guided by the ethical issues outlined above, they should also be aware of the laws relevant where they practice, and seek legal counsel in their own institutions.

Practical summary

The approach to decision-making in the DR can, for practical purposes, be divided into three segments: staff discussion, meeting with the expectant parents, and decision-making at the time of birth.

In any delivery facility that cares for high-risk infants, the staff should meet periodically to discuss their overall approach to cases such as this, before a specific case is at hand. The hour of crisis is not the time for extended dialogue; an intelligent and considered approach to DR decisions will necessitate prior in-depth discussion. The discussion should include logistics (what this facility can feasibly provide), relevant data (nationally and locally), professional guidelines, and the ethical principles at play. Given the frequent overlap and cross-coverage of neonatology services, it is highly desirable for the staff to reach agreement on a policy, recognizing that deviation from that policy may be appropriate in certain cases. The plan for a given patient, or what options expectant parents are given, should not change from shift to shift or day to day.

When a specific case is at hand, the staff should first briefly discuss it amongst themselves, and then meet with the expectant parents to explain the situation and the possible outcomes in a clear and concise manner. The clinical team should initially speak to the parents alone (or mother only if no father is present) in order to respect privacy, but offer to bring anyone into the conversation that they wish. If the diagnosis is known well in advance of the delivery, the meeting with the expectant parents should ideally take place then. Relevant data and all medically reasonable options should be presented in an even-handed and non-judgmental manner. Some neonatologists prefer to remain neutral regarding which option to choose, so as not to apply undue influence. It is quite acceptable, however, and many would argue that it is preferable, for a physician to provide a recommendation and an explanation of the rationale, as long as the message is clearly conveyed to the parents that their preference (among acceptable options offered) will be supported. Their questions should be answered, and if possible they should be given a chance to discuss the situation alone, with a return visit from the pediatric team to answer further questions and to make a plan with them.

Physicians are not obligated to do whatever parents request, but a decision not to comply should be based on the assessment that the parental decision is clearly opposed to the child's best interest, or that what they have requested is not possible. Parents should be told that the clinical team might choose to deviate from the agreed-upon plan if significant new findings are apparent at birth. In addition, they should be told that if resuscitation is initiated, efforts will cease when it becomes apparent to the medical team that they cannot succeed.

In the DR, it may be appropriate for the leader of the resuscitation to deviate from the plan, but only if new information significantly changes the prognosis initially discussed (D'Angio & Mercurio, 2008). Neither the physical appearance of a newborn to be one or two weeks more or less mature than expected, nor the initial level of activity are reliable or predictive findings (Meadow, 2007), and thus they do not justify a change of plan. Further, a slow or half-hearted effort at resuscitation is not appropriate. If it was agreed that every effort would initially be put forth, then this should be done in good faith.

If a situation arises wherein it is not clear, from an ethical standpoint, how to proceed, one should generally opt for the course that is more easily reversed. In the DR, this means providing aggressive resuscitation and initial intensive care, and then reassessing the situation with the parents, and with colleagues if needed. One can withdraw life-sustaining measures afterward, but frequently one cannot as easily initiate them after a period of comfort measures only.

Resolution of case and discussion

For the case at hand, the predicted survival would be 23%, and survival without profound neurodevelopmental impairment would be 15% (NICHD, 2010). These numbers would improve with an adequate course of antenatal steroids, or if one only considers patients who were placed on mechanical ventilation, which might be a proxy for patients who were actively resuscitated. It appears that survival with resuscitation is possible, though not likely, the NICU course would be long and difficult, and if she were to survive there would be a significant risk of severe neurodevelopmental impairment. It would be hard to determine that one choice or the other is *clearly* in the child's best interest, so the parents' right to make this decision should be respected. After discussing the situation and possible outcomes, these parents should be given a choice of attempted resuscitation or comfort measures only. The neonatologist could provide guidance or opinion, after and clearly apart from an objective presentation of the data, but should ultimately defer to and support the parents' preference.

In the DR, the clinical team might reasonably deviate from the plan only if something is learned that significantly changes the prognosis. It is important to keep the lines of communication open, and to help the parents understand that if she survives the initial resuscitation, the decision-making for their child would be an ongoing process. They retain the option to withdraw intensive care measures and opt for comfort measures only. This might change over time, if she does well and her prognosis significantly improves, but for at least the first few days (and possibly much longer) withdrawal will remain an acceptable option.

References

Batton, D.G. and the Committee on Fetus and Newborn, American Academy of Pediatrics (2009). Clinical report: antenatal counseling regarding resuscitation at an extremely low gestational age. *Pediatrics*, **124**, 422–427.

Beauchamp, T.L. & Childress, J.F. (2001). *Principles of Biomedical Ethics*, 5th edn. New York: Oxford University Press, 226–282.

Committee on Bioethics, American Academy of Pediatrics (1994). Guidelines on foregoing life-sustaining medical treatment. *Pediatrics*, **93**, 532–536.

D'Angio, C.T. & Mercurio, M.R. (2008). Evidence-based ethics in the "gray zone" of neonatal viability: promises and limitations. *Pediatric Health*, **2**, 777–786.

Hack, M., Taylor, H.G., Drotar, D., et al. (2005). Poor predictive validity of the Bayley scales of infant development for cognitive function of extremely low birth weight children at school age. *Pediatrics*, **116**, 333–341.

Janvier, A., Leblanc, I., & Barrington, K.J. (2008). The best-interest standard is not applied for neonatal resuscitation decisions. *Pediatrics*, **121**, 963–969.

Kattwinkel, J., Perlman, J.M., Aziz, K., et al. (2010). Neonatal resuscitation: 2010 American Heart Association guidelines for cardiopulmonary resuscitation and emergency cardiovascular care. *Pediatrics*, **126**, e1400–e1413.

Meadow, W. (2007). Babies between a rock and a hard place – neonatologists vs parents at the edge of infant viability. *Acta Paediatrica*, **96**, 153.

Mercurio, M.R. (2005). Physicians' refusal to resuscitate at borderline gestational age. *Journal of Perinatology*, **25**, 685–689.

Mercurio, M.R. (2009). The ethics of newborn resuscitation. *Seminars in Perinatology*, **33**, 354–363.

NICHD Neonatal Research Network (NRN) (2010). Extremely preterm birth outcome data. www.nichd.nih.gov/about/org/cdbpm/pp/prog_epbo/epbo_case.cfm. Last accessed November 23, 2010.

Stoll, B.J., Hansen, N.I., Bell, E.F., et al. (2010). Neonatal outcomes of extremely preterm infants from the NICHD Neonatal Research Network. *Pediatrics*, **126**, 443–455.

Tyson, J.E., Parikh, N.A., Langer, J., et al. (2008). Intensive care for extreme prematurity – moving beyond gestational age. *New England Journal of Medicine*, **358**, 1672–1681.

Recommended reading

Byrne, S., Szyld, E., & Kattwinkel, J. (2008). The ethics of delivery-room resuscitation. *Seminars in Fetal and Neonatal Medicine*, **13**, 440–447.

Withholding and withdrawing life-sustaining intervention from neonates

Andrew C. Beckstrom and David E. Woodrum

Case narrative

Ms. Jaspreet Singh, a 34-year-old woman, was admitted to the hospital with abdominal pain during her 24th week of pregnancy. She arrived in the United States from India earlier on the day of admission with a plan to live in the area for 2 months while her husband worked for a software business on a temporary visa. Upon arrival at the hospital, she was diagnosed with a placental abruption and was taken to the labor and delivery suite for emergent cesarean section. The on-call neonatologist met with the family and briefly discussed the risks of prematurity at 24 weeks' gestation. The remainder of the conversation focused on the delivery and immediate management of the infant, the plan being to give her a "trial of therapy" in the delivery room. Although the parents had reservations, they reluctantly agreed to full resuscitation.

Baby Girl Singh was born 30 minutes later, weighing 625 grams. She had minimal respiratory effort and required aggressive resuscitation. Over the subsequent days, she had an uneventful course, considering her gestational age at birth. She required modest support, including low-level mechanical ventilation and oxygen. Her heart rate and blood pressure were within normal limits. Inotropic support was never indicated. Screening cranial ultrasound showed a small right-sided intraventricular hemorrhage (grade I).

Early in her clinical course, the parents asked the NICU team to withdraw life support measures because "people with disabilities, especially girls, are severely discriminated against in India, and there are no services for such people." They expressed their belief that "putting their daughter through an aggressive medical course is not in her best interest." At that point, her estimated chance of survival to discharge was 60% or greater; and as a survivor, there would be an estimated

50% chance of minimal to no neurodevelopment problems. The attending neonatologist and team did not feel that withdrawal of intensive care was an option due to her stable clinical status and the reasonably good estimate of long-term morbidity. Because of this conflict, an ethics consult was obtained.

Withholding and withdrawing therapy in a neonate

Since its origin in the 1960s, neonatology has experienced technological advancement, innovation, and improved patient survival. The issue of concern then and now is: *survival at what cost?* As a result, an ethical conscience has emerged, questioning whether or not "the right thing" is being done. In 1973, Duff and Campbell published in the *New England Journal of Medicine* the first description of a culture of selective withholding and withdrawing care in the NICU. This article discussed the characteristics of the patients who were allowed to die and highlighted the ethical issues – including the physician and parental perspectives of best interest and burden of care. Shortly after, leaders in neonatology and the emerging field of bioethics convened in a conference regarding *Critical Issues in Newborn Intensive Care*. The summary of the conference stated, "in the context of certain irremediable life conditions, intensive care therapy appears harmful. These conditions are ... [the] inability to survive infancy, inability to live without severe pain, and inability to participate, at least minimally, in human experience" (Jonsen et al., 1975). This was the first attempt to establish a moral framework regarding withdrawing care in the neonatal intensive care nursery.

Subsequently, the President's Commission for the Study of Ethical Problems in Medicine and Biomedical and Behavioral Research (1983) was established to,

Clinical Ethics in Pediatrics: A Case-Based Textbook, ed. Douglas S. Diekema, Mark R. Mercurio and Mary B. Adam. Published by Cambridge University Press. © Cambridge University Press 2011.

Table 15.1. Treatment options for seriously ill newborns – physician's assessment in relation to parents' preference (President's Commission, 1983)

Physician's assessment of treatment options	Parents prefer to accept treatment	Parents prefer to forgo treatment
Clearly beneficial	Provide treatment	Provide treatment during review process
Ambiguous or uncertain	Provide treatment	Forgo treatment
Futile	Provide treatment unless provider declines to do so	Forgo treatment

among other things, "re-examine the way decisions are and ought to be made about whether or not to forgo life sustaining treatment." Although the report addressed a wide spectrum of issues pertaining to end of life, special attention was paid to the seriously ill newborn. The Commission generated a table to assist parents and physicians when they are faced with the end-of-life decisions (Table 15.1).

In 1982, the issues of withholding and withdrawing care attracted public attention through media coverage of the "Baby Doe" case, involving an infant with trisomy 21, and federal policy makers responding to that event. Infant Doe's parents declined surgical treatment of an esophageal atresia and tracheoesophageal fistula on the basis of their child's potential "minimally acceptable quality of life" (Pence, 2008). The hospital administration and a local pediatrician did not agree with the parents, and challenged the decision in both the county and state courts who ruled in favor of the parents. The United States Supreme Court refused to review the case. Baby Doe died at 5 days of age. Newspapers, pro-life groups, and disability activists brought the case to the attention of the Reagan Administration, which concluded that "failure to treat disabled infants was a violation of their civil rights," based on section 504 of the Rehabilitation Act of 1973 (Pence, 2008). Subsequently, the Department of Health and Human Services issued a series of rules that required all hospitals receiving federal aid to post signs in the labor and delivery ward and the NICU advising that "anyone 'having knowledge' that a handicapped baby is being denied food or customary medical care is invited to dial the toll-free [Handicapped Infant Hotline] number," which would result in an on-site investigation within 24 hours (Society's Duty at Birth, 1983). The Department's attempt to impact parent–physician decision-making in the context of seriously ill infants was successfully challenged in the federal courts. Ultimately, a compromise was reached when Congress enacted legislation in the form of an amendment to the

Child Abuse Prevention and Treatment Act (1984). The amended legislation stated that "one must provide appropriate nutrition, hydration and medication that in the treating physician's reasonable judgment will be most likely to be effective in ameliorating or correcting the patient's condition." Notably, the legislation carried with it no criminal or civil penalties for individual physicians or hospitals (Moss, 1987). Nonetheless, the impact of the three-year debate was to significantly change the way many neonatologists approached decisions regarding the withholding and withdrawing of care from seriously ill newborn infants.

Taking this historical perspective into account, the Committee on Fetus and Newborn with the American Academy of Pediatrics (AAP) released a policy statement in 2007 related to non-initiation or withdrawal of intensive care for high-risk newborns (Bell, 2007). This policy suggests that decisions can be divided into three categories on the basis of prognosis:

1. When early death is very likely and survival would be accomplished by high risk of unacceptably severe morbidity, intensive care is not indicated.
2. When survival is likely and risk of unacceptably severe morbidity is low, intensive care is indicated.
3. When prognosis is uncertain but likely to be very poor and survival may be associated with diminished quality of life for the child … parental desires should determine the treatment approach.

In the case of Baby Girl Singh, the parents were asking to withdraw intensive care measures after a "trial of therapy" was initiated. The survival potential for this seriously ill newborn was estimated to be 60% with a 50% chance of reasonably good long-term outcome should she survive. Considering both the President's Commission (Table 15.1) and the AAP recommendations, this child's prognosis places her in either the "clearly beneficial" or possibly the "ambiguous" category. If Baby Girl Singh was truly in the "ambiguous" category, then her parents' wishes to forgo life-sustaining treatment should be respected. However, since the medical team believed that she would "clearly benefit" from the therapy and a 50% chance of moderate to severe morbidity was not deemed "unacceptable," the medical team felt the appropriate response at this juncture was to continue life-sustaining support until additional information was obtained or a change in clinical status occurred.

Parental authority and best interest

Decisions in the neonatal intensive care unit surrounding the critically ill newborn typically fall into one of three categories. The most common occurs when the parents and physicians agree to use all indicated medical therapies to treat the patient. Less commonly, there is agreement that the burden of the medical therapy far outweighs the potential benefit and both sides agree to initiate comfort care. The final decision category features disagreement between the health care team and parents regarding direction of therapy – one side desires comfort care while the other desires full therapy. This third category is the source of most ethical conflicts regarding withholding and withdrawing care in the NICU.

Critical decision-making in our autonomy-focused society ultimately falls on the individual. If an adult is rendered unable to make a decision due to illness or lack of competence, decision-making authority is transferred to a surrogate decision-maker. In situations involving a previously competent individual, the surrogate is required to make a decision based on his/her understanding of the past beliefs and desires of the individual in question. This approach is called substituted judgment (Buchanan & Brock, 1989). Substituted judgment is not applicable when dealing with a seriously ill newborn, because an infant has no history as a thinking being. Thus, the concept of autonomy does not apply. From both a legal and moral perspective, it is presumed that parents are the surrogate decision-makers for their children, unless there is a specific reason for their authority to be removed. This universal granting of parental authority is supported by the notion that parents know and care for their children, they will be concerned to ensure that the welfare of their child is maintained, and they will ultimately be affected by the decision (Buchanan & Brock, 1989). Parental authority is a unique type of surrogate decision-making that relies on the parent to choose a course of action for their child based on what a "reasonable person" would

choose. Many argue that the best interest standard is the most appropriate principle to employ in this kind of decision-making. The President's Commission (1983) states that all decisions regarding the care of the seriously newborn should focus on the best interest of the newborn only. This is "a very strict standard in that it excludes consideration of the negative effects of an impaired child's life on other persons including parents, siblings and society."

According to Buchanan and Brock (1989), the best interest standard is "a principle that expresses a positive obligation, a duty to do what best promotes someone's interests or is most conducive to his or her good." It asks the decision-makers to weigh the "net benefit" for each possible option and subtract the "net burdens" of those options. That which has the most benefit with least harm is seen as the decision made in the patient's "best interest." It takes into account quality of life judgments in decision-making. Buchanan and Brock (1989) expand "best interest" to incorporate both current and future-oriented interests.

Current interests are limited to the ability to feel pleasure and avoid pain (suffering), the latter a difficult condition to assess in the neonate. Accordingly, determination of current best interest, particularly the degree of suffering, depends on judgments made by parents and the health care team. The future-oriented interests are more crucial to identify. These include the ability to develop awareness of self, to have personal relationships, and minimization of future pain and suffering. Current population-based neonatal outcomes for extreme prematurity give infants born at 24 and 26 weeks' gestation a 58 and 75% survival rate, respectively. Many of those surviving infants will have significant morbidity (Marlow et al., 2005; Fanaroff et al., 2007). The challenge for both physicians and parents charged with predicting future-oriented interests/outcomes is the lack of accurate individualized predictability and prognostication tools. It is important to note that self-reported quality of life measures for those with significant long-term morbidity are, for the most part, similar to normal control groups (Saigal et al., 1999; Dickinson et al., 2007). Thus it is perhaps inappropriate to focus excessively on all but the most severe morbidity issues.

Others suggest that the best interest standard is not the ideal principle to be applied to the imperiled newborn. Two alternate approaches have been proposed that may better address the intricacies of this dilemma: constrained parental autonomy and the harm principle. Developed by Lainie Ross, constrained parental autonomy focuses on the child's basic needs, not best interest. Parents are granted autonomy to make health care decisions with an emphasis on the *family* interests/needs. This model differs from best interest standard by "accommodate[ing] intra-familial trade-offs provided that the basic needs of each child member are secured" (Ross, 1998). In short, constrained parental autonomy allows the basic needs of the patient to be addressed without compromising the needs of the rest of the family – something the best interest standard lacks.

The harm principle is another model that has been suggested for application to difficult decisions in the NICU. Applying the harm principle clinically, the focus is no longer to identify the therapeutic decision that is in the best interest of the individual, but to ensure the decisions being made do not cause significant harm to the patient. This theory allows more flexibility in parental decision-making and helps generate a more distinguishable threshold by which intervention outside the family unit (i.e., ethics committee, state) must be sought (Diekema, 2004). This approach also permits parents to make decisions encompassing the patient and the family unit.

Baby Girl Singh's physicians insisted that it would be in the patient's "best interest" to continue therapy, while her parents believed that it would be in the patient's "best interest" to withhold therapy. In a culture where parental authority carries great weight, the initial assessment would favor the parents' right to make the decision and allow Baby Girl Singh to die. However, with the best interest standard, an argument can be made that the potential outcomes of her disease are sufficiently "good" that withdrawal of care would not be in the "best interest" of the patient. Using the harm principle, one could argue that the parents have reached the threshold for which parental authority should no longer be granted. Based solely on Baby Girl Singh's medical condition, one could argue that choosing to allow her to die places her at significant risk of serious harm as compared with continuing aggressive therapy. However, it is critical to understand the contextual features that are embedded in this case before making a final judgment.

Contextual features

The contextual features surrounding each individual patient and/or family may be expected to impact end-of-life decision-making. Arras (1984), the author of "Toward an ethic of ambiguity," believes that it is unjust

to allow social factors to influence decision-making regarding end-of-life care. He states, "We must base our treatment decisions solely on the extent of medical disabilities. To take social factors into account is to act unjustly towards the child." In contrast, a popular ethical decision-making tool includes contextual features in case analysis and suggests they may be potentially important (Jonsen et al., 2006). Examples of contextual features that might be expected to influence a case (especially the current case) include the economic structure of the involved community with regard to health care (Partridge et al., 2005; Miljeteig et al., 2009), the society's values regarding authority for decision-making, support for persons with disability, and the individual's religious beliefs. Clearly, context often does frame decisions being made by the parents and should be considered by the health care team.

Baby Girl Singh's parents approached decisions about "best interest" of their daughter from their own contextual framework. They knew after they returned to their country of origin she would live in a society that did not support disability either from a social or an economic point of view. From their perspective, a 50% chance of disability was too great a risk to take. Notably, in India, their country of origin, economic and resource limitations are reflected in the fact that infants who are born at a gestation of less than 28 weeks are rarely resuscitated (Miljeteig et al., 2009). Additionally, their Hindu faith guided their decision-making (Firth, 2005). Like many spiritual people, the parents' religious beliefs influenced their perspective on life, death, and the afterlife. From their point of view, the potential for suffering was great and it was morally sound to proceed with withdrawal of life-sustaining treatments from their daughter. Although this context may be considered reasonable within their home country, the health care team challenged their argument because of the fact that Baby Girl Singh had a relatively good prognosis and that her birth occurred in a very different context.

Conclusion to case

The ethics team was consulted. After a full evaluation, including interviewing the medical team, parents, and reviewing the chart, the ethics team supported the medical team in their decision to continue intensive care, against the parents' wishes. Although there was a chance of severe disability, the team could not support the statement that it would be in the patient's "best interest" to discontinue ventilation based on the child's current status, no evidence of suffering, and potential good prognosis. In their consult note, the ethics team stated, "the parents' legitimate concerns for long-term morbidity do not, at this time, outweigh the infant's right to receive continued care." The parents were devastated by this news – stating that moving forward with aggressive treatment was not the standard of care in their home country. Many members of the team struggled with the failure to honor the parents' wishes, leading to increased moral distress among the NICU staff. After an additional week of intensive therapy, Baby Girl Singh's condition worsened, requiring increased ventilatory and inotropic support. At this juncture, the parents requested again that intensive care be discontinued. Both the medical team and the ethics team re-evaluated the situation. After considering the change in clinical status, the increased evidence of suffering, and the worsening prognosis, the ethics and medical teams agreed with the parents' decision to withdraw life support. Later that night, Baby Girl Singh was extubated and she died shortly thereafter in her mother's arms.

Summary and recommendations

The Baby Girl Singh case demonstrates the complexities of withholding and withdrawing care to infants in the neonatal intensive care unit. The care team and parental perspectives are deeply rooted in individual beliefs and culture, as well as medical and personal knowledge of the patient and family. Incorporating best interest, medical experience and knowledge, and contextual features, it is important to ask the question: Given *this* specific patient in *this* specific situation, is death better than continuing this existence (or future existence)?

With this in mind, the following outline is recommended for decision-making when faced with disagreeing views about withholding and withdrawing life-sustaining therapy from the neonate:

1. Determine the chance of survival and the risk of morbidity for the given patient based on the best evidence available.
2. Maintain parental authority unless the parents are unable to make appropriate decisions.
3. Parental decision-making should be honored unless their decision places the child at significant risk of serious harm compared with other options.
4. If there is consensus that the parent's decision is placing the child at significant risk of serious

harm, consider state action to remove decision-making authority from parents.
5. Consider ethics consultation at some point along the way.

References

Amendments to Child Abuse Prevention and Treatment Act (1984). Public Law 98-457. *US Statute Large* **98** (Title I Sections 101a–312a).

Arras, J.D. (1984). Toward an ethic of ambiguity. *Hastings Center Report*, **14**(2), 25–33.

Bell, E.F. (2007). Noninitiation or withdrawal of intensive care for high-risk newborns. *Pediatrics*, **119**(2), 401–403.

Buchanan, A.E. & Brock, D.W. (1989). *Deciding for Others: The Ethics of Surrogate Decision Making. Studies in Philosophy and Health Policy.* New York: Cambridge University Press, 422.

Dickinson, H.O., Parkinson, K.N., Ravens-Sieberer, U., et al. (2007). Self-reported quality of life of 8–12-year-old children with cerebral palsy: a cross-sectional European study. *Lancet*, **369**(9580), 2171–2178.

Diekema, D.S. (2004). Parental refusals of medical treatment: the harm principle as threshold for state intervention. *Theoretical Medicine and Bioethics*, **25**(4), 243–264.

Duff, R.S. & Campbell, A.G. (1973). Moral and ethical dilemmas in the special-care nursery. *New England Journal of Medicine*, **289**(17), 890–894.

Fanaroff, A.A., Stoll, B.J., Wright, L.L., et al. (2007). Trends in neonatal morbidity and mortality for very low birth-weight infants. *American Journal of Obstetrics and Gynecology*, **196**(2), 147.e1–e8.

Firth, S. (2005). End-of-life: a Hindu view. *Lancet*, **366**(9486), 682–686.

Jonsen, A.R., Phibbs, R.H., Tooley, W.H., & Garland, M.J. (1975). Critical issues in newborn intensive care: a conference report and policy proposal. *Pediatrics*, **55**(6), 756–768.

Jonsen, A.R., Siegler, M., & Winslade, W.J. (2006). *Clinical Ethics: A Practical Approach to Ethical Decisions in Clinical Medicine*, 6th edn. New York: McGraw Hill, Medical Pub. Division.

Marlow, N., Wolke, D., Bracewell, M.A., Samara, M., & the EPICure Study Group (2005). Neurologic and developmental disability at six years of age after extremely preterm birth. *New England Journal of Medicine*, **352**(1), 9–19.

Miljeteig, I., Sayeed, S.A., Jesani, A., Johansson, K.A., & Norheim, O.F. (2009). Impact of ethics and economics on end-of-life decisions in an Indian neonatal unit. *Pediatrics*, **124**(2), e322–e328.

Moss, K. (1987). The "Baby Doe" legislation: its rise and fall. *Policy Studies Journal*, **15**(4), 629–651.

Partridge, J.C., Ranchod, T.M., Ballot, D.E., et al. (2005). Intensive care for very low birthweight infants in South Africa: a survey of physician attitudes, parent counseling and resuscitation practices. *Journal of Tropical Pediatrics*, **51**(1), 11–16.

Pence, G.E. (2008). *Classic Cases in Medical Ethics: Accounts of the Cases That Have Shaped and Define Medical Ethics*, 5th edn. New York: McGraw-Hill Higher Education.

President's Commission for the Study of Ethical Problems in Medicine and Biomedical and Behavioral Research (1983). *Deciding to Forego Life Sustaining Treatment*. Washington, DC: US Government Printing Office.

Ross, L.F. (1998). *Children, Families, and Health Care Decision Making. Issues in Biomedical Ethics*. Oxford, UK & New York: Clarendon Press.

Saigal, S., Stoskopf, B.L., Feeny, D., et al. (1999). Differences in preferences for neonatal outcomes among health care professionals, parents, and adolescents. *JAMA*, **281**(21), 1991–1997.

Society's Duty at Birth (1983). *The New York Times*. April 2, 16.

Chapter

16

The role of quality of life assessments in neonatal care

John Wyatt

Case narrative

A female baby is delivered unexpectedly at 25 weeks' gestation following acute placental abruption. She is in poor condition at delivery and requires active resuscitation with endotracheal intubation. Mechanical ventilation is provided over the first 4 days of life. Routine cranial ultrasonography on day 4 indicates a large unilateral intraventricular hemorrhage with evidence of parenchymal infarction.

The findings are communicated to the parents and they are warned that there is a high possibility that the child may develop some form of cerebral palsy. The parents are distressed and horrified by this information. It appears that they have had a lifelong fear of having a disabled child. They state that they are deeply concerned that their child will have a poor quality of life, leading to lifelong distress and suffering. They are also concerned about the likely effect of the child's disability on the family, and on their marriage. The parents argue that it is morally wrong for aggressive medical interventions to be continued to ensure the survival of a child who will have such a poor quality of life, creating burdens for herself, her family, and to society.

How should predictions about future quality of life be employed in treatment decisions in neonatal care?

Background

The idea that neonatologists should be concerned about the quality of life (QOL) of their patients has obvious intuitive appeal. It seems right that physicians should not be solely interested in the indefinite prolongation of life (the "quantity" of life) but should also ensure that the life that is prolonged meets certain criteria (its "quality").

It is being increasingly suggested that some form of assessment or prediction of QOL should be employed in clinical decision-making in neonatology, including decisions about resuscitation and about withholding or withdrawing intensive life support.

The concept has also been used in several legal judgments involving neonates, such as the 1991 United Kingdom case *Re: J*, concerning a preterm infant with severe brain injury. The judgment stated, "The correct approach is for the court to judge the quality of life the child would have to endure if given the treatment and decide whether in all circumstances such a life would be so afflicted as to be intolerable to the child" (Rennie & Leigh, 2008).

The concept of QOL

Although there is an intuitive appeal to the concept of QOL, it is essential that clinicians be aware that there are very substantial logical and practical complexities in its definition, measurement, and application. Within the traditional framework of medical ethics that can be traced back to Hippocrates, physicians have always been concerned to minimize harm and to maximize the welfare and well-being of their patients. But the idea that each human life can be assigned a "quality" is a surprisingly recent innovation. The concept appears to have been unknown to philosophers and ethicists until the second half of the twentieth century and was not used in medical practice and research until the 1970s.

The English word "quality" has two distinct meanings. It can be used descriptively to mean the attributes or properties, as in "the qualities of the element chlorine", or it can have an evaluative meaning as in "the quality of this watch," implying comparison against an objective standard. Historically it seems that the evaluative meaning was applied almost exclusively to objects, particularly manufactured artifacts, rather than to people. In contrast when applied to people, the

Clinical Ethics in Pediatrics: A Case-Based Textbook, ed. Douglas S. Diekema, Mark R. Mercurio and Mary B. Adam. Published by Cambridge University Press. © Cambridge University Press 2011.

word was used almost always in its descriptive sense, as in "she has obvious leadership qualities." The conceptual novelty which appears to have commenced in the 1960s was to apply the evaluative meaning of the word "quality" to an individual human life, with the implication that it is possible to assess and quantify the unique life experience of an individual against an agreed common standard.

Definitions of QOL

The concept of QOL is alarmingly difficult to define in a logically coherent manner. It is assumed that, by performing an assessment across a series of domains such as material, physical, social, emotional, and productive well-being, a single quantitative score can be obtained. But evaluating and ranking these different aspects of a human life is highly problematic. It is not possible to rank the "goods," attributes or functions of human life in some kind of hierarchy. Is physical well-being comparable to emotional well-being? Is creativity more valuable than sensory functioning? Is mobility to be ranked with short-term memory function?

It is clearly impossible to have any consensus within our own society on these issues, and many would argue that the questions themselves are logically incoherent and meaningless. To use philosophical jargon: the different domains involved in the subjective experience of life are incommensurable.

Measurement instruments for QOL

Despite the problems of logical coherence, a wide range of measurement instruments have been developed in an attempt to quantify the life experiences of patients with chronic diseases or disabilities (Saigal & Tyson, 2008). The instruments frequently combine objective assessments of functional ability with subjective reports of positive or negative emotions. It is inevitable that attempts at evaluation tend to focus attention on easily detectable and quantifiable impairments and pay less attention to personal and relational strengths, capacities, and functions which are more difficult, if not impossible, to assess and quantify. A further difficulty is that it is self-evident that our values and preferences change as we go through life.

In summary, QOL cannot be regarded as an objective biological parameter such as the Apgar score, the grade of intraventricular hemorrhage, or the degree of impaired motor function. It involves subjective and

highly contestable value judgments involving multiple domains of an individual's life.

Self-reporting of QOL in children

One response to these conceptual problems is to place less emphasis on the attempt to quantify QOL from an external objective standpoint and instead to focus on the individual's own perceptions of their life experiences. A number of measurement tools have been developed which use self-reporting to enable individuals to weigh aspects of their health according to their own personal values – often referred to as health-related quality of life (HRQL) (Saigal & Tyson, 2008). Specialized questionnaires have been developed for self-reporting in children, using focus groups to identify particular concerns and perspectives (Ronen et al., 2001).

A major limitation of these self-reporting tools is that they cannot be used in individuals with severe cognitive disabilities or in young children. A common approach is to use parents or health professionals to provide proxy responses for severely disabled children. However, there is evidence that both parents and health professionals tend to provide lower valuations for QOL compared with the self-reported ratings of the individuals themselves (White-Koning et al., 2007; Saigal & Tyson, 2008). Parents of children with chronic diseases tend to perceive more negative consequences for emotional and social domains than do the children themselves.

A large questionnaire study of HRQL in children with cerebral palsy and their parents found that the mean child-reported scores of quality of life were significantly higher than the parent proxy reports in eight domains. Parents rated their child's quality of life lower than the children themselves in 29–57% of child-parent pairs (White-Koning et al., 2007). It seems likely that parents' perceptions of the subjective experience of illness or disability may be affected by their own experiences of providing care.

Zwicker and colleagues performed a systematic review of longitudinal studies of various measures of HRQL in children born with very low birth weights (Zwicker & Harris, 2008). They found that the effects of low birth weight on health-related quality of life appeared to diminish over time. Marked reductions in outcome measures were recorded at school age. Parents of teenagers noted significantly poorer performance in their child's global health, behavior, and physical functioning compared with peers, whereas the teenagers themselves did not. In young adulthood, differences in physical functioning remained, but self-rating of quality of life was similar to normal birth weight peers. The authors concluded that the diminution with time in the effects of low birth weight on HRQL was likely to be a consequence of differences in the child's experience versus the parents' proxy report, differing definitions of health-related quality of life, and adaptation of individuals over time to their individual circumstances.

Health professionals' perceptions

Whilst parents' perceptions of their children's quality of life tend to be more negative than those of the children themselves, there is evidence that health professionals' perceptions tend to be more negative still. In a qualitative study comparing parents' and health professionals' perceptions of quality of life in quadriplegic children, Morrow and colleagues found that health professionals often talked of the "burden" the child's condition placed on the parents, whereas parents tended to view their child's disability as a part of their lives, and viewed their child as a source of joy despite acknowledging the anxiety generated (Morrow et al., 2008). Health professionals speculated about parents' dilemmas of prolonging and curtailing life when deciding about interventions, whereas parents talked about prolonging life and the fact that they would do anything to ensure their child's well-being.

Although health professionals tend to assume that neurodevelopmental impairment in surviving preterm children will automatically lead to maternal and family difficulties, a study of the families of extremely low birth weight adults found no significant differences in marital disharmony, family dysfunction, maternal mood, state anxiety, social support, depression, and maternal physical and mental health, when compared with normal birth weight controls (Saigal et al., 2010). Mothers of extremely low birth weight adults reported that the experience of caring for their child brought their family closer together and that relatives and friends were more helpful and understanding, compared with controls. Significantly more mothers of adults with neurosensory impairments felt better about themselves for having managed their child's health.

Instead of self-reporting questionnaires, another approach to the assessment of quality of life is the use of so-called utility measures which attempt to quantify the preferences of individual patients, parents, and health professionals for a range of hypothetical health outcomes including death. The goal of this approach is to provide a score for each health outcome ranging from zero for death to 1.0 for perfect health (Saigal & Tyson, 2008). Saigal and colleagues (1999) used this approach to compare preferences for hypothetical health states in a group of ex-preterm teenagers, parents, and neonatologists and NICU nurses. They found that the health professionals tended to provide lower ratings for the severely disabling states than did teenagers and parents.

There is a tendency for health professionals to make deterministic assumptions that the presence of a biological impairment will translate automatically into reduced subjective well-being. However, these assumptions are challenged by the results of several studies that have investigated self-reported HRQL in adolescents and young adults who were born very preterm. Saigal and colleagues (2006) investigated self-reported health status and HRQL in a group of 140 adults born with extremely low birth weight compared with adults born at term. Although health status was significantly worse in the ex-preterm adults there was no significant difference in HRQL, and this finding persisted when adults with neurocognitive impairment were studied separately. It is clear that there is no simple correlation between the presence of a biological impairment and a low self-assessment for HRQL.

The "disability paradox"

This is an example of the so-called "disability paradox," the repeated finding that patients' perceptions of personal health, well-being, and life satisfaction are often discordant with external measures of objective health status and the level of disability (Albrecht & Devlieger, 1999). Many disabled people report high levels of subjective well-being despite objective evidence of significant functional impairment. The disability paradox highlights the importance of an individual's personal experience of disability in defining one's view of the world, social context, and social relationships. As a result external observers have to recognize that there are major limitations in their ability to predict the subjective experience of individuals with disabling biological impairments.

Health professionals tend to assume a "medical model" of disability in which biological impairment is the dominant feature, rather than a "social model" of disability that focuses on the social barriers, prejudice, and discrimination that disabled people experience. Yet many disabled adults state that the main factors which limit their personal well-being are not their medical impairments, such as cerebral palsy, but the prejudices and stereotypes which healthy people unthinkingly support, and the practical, social, and economic barriers which limit their involvement in normal social activities (Parens & Asch, 2000). Many of the most significant factors that impair the life experiences of children and adults are non-biological in origin.

It may therefore be unhelpful to restrict assessment of the subjective experience of disabled survivors of neonatal intensive care to health-related domains. One disadvantage of the concentration on HRQL measures is that they tend to focus attention on the individual and his or her biological impairments to the exclusion of the context of social, political, and economic policies which are of central importance to the life experience of disabled individuals.

It has been argued by disability rights activists that the very concept of quality of life as used by health professionals tends to perpetuate negative prejudices and stereotypes about the experiences of disabled people. The simplistic assumption by some clinicians that neurodevelopmental impairment necessarily translates into low subjective experience of well-being can encourage a eugenic desire to eliminate people with biological impairments from our community. It is also possible that simplistic and deterministic concepts of quality of life subtly shift the obligation for improving resources and services for disabled people away from politicians and economists. Instead they place on clinicians and parents an implicit responsibility to ensure that people who are likely to be disabled are not brought into the world.

Clinical implications

The concept of QOL is both conceptually problematic and involves subjective judgments and perceptions that are highly contested. Hence, neonatologists and pediatricians should strongly resist the simplistic assumption that it is possible to predict or evaluate the future QOL for critically ill newborns in their care. This does not imply, of course, that prognostic information is of no value in complex and difficult ethical decisions concerning the withdrawal or withholding of life-support treatments in the NICU. Instead of vague references to "poor quality of life," emphasis should

be placed on objective and empirically based assessments of the risk of death, the nature and severity of neurologic injury, and predictions of future functional ability. The development of individualized predictors of outcome for extremely premature babies based on a range of objective clinical variables at birth (Tyson et al., 2008; Parikh et al., 2010) enables informed decisions about resuscitation and intensive care. When weighing the burdens and benefits of initiating or maintaining intensive support in any individual newborn it is not possible to avoid subjective judgments about harm, risk, and long-term benefit. But wherever possible these judgments should be based on objective and empirical outcome data, which should be shared and discussed with parents, rather than on simplistic assumptions and prejudices about the life experiences of disabled children and adults.

Case resolution

In this case, the parents' concerns and perspectives should be addressed sympathetically and respectfully, but their assumptions about the life experiences of children who are born very preterm, and of their families, should be gently challenged. The nature and implications of the brain injury should be explained and discussed but it may be helpful to emphasize the degree of uncertainty in the prediction of neurodevelopmental outcome based on cranial ultrasonography, and the evidence of resilience and adaptation that empirical studies of teenage and adult survivors of neonatal intensive care have demonstrated. The assumption that functional motor impairment translates into high levels of subjective distress may be challenged by reference to relevant HRQL studies. It may be helpful to explain the concept of weighing and balancing the harms, risks, and benefits of intensive support, using individualized outcome data derived from prospective studies of preterm infants, and demonstrate how this approach can be used to aid a consensual decision about whether to continue or withhold treatment in this case.

References

Albrecht, G.L. & Devlieger, P.J. (1999). The disability paradox: high quality of life against all odds. *Social Science and Medicine*, **48**(8), 977–988.

Morrow, A.M., Quine, S., Loughlin, E.V., & Craig, J.C. (2008). Different priorities: a comparison of parents' and health professionals' perceptions of quality of life in quadriplegic cerebral palsy. *Archives of Disease in Childhood*, **93**(2), 119–125.

Parens, E. & Asch, A. (2000). The disability rights critique of prenatal genetic testing. In *Prenatal Testing and Disability Rights*, ed. E. Parens & A. Asch. Washington, DC: Georgetown University Press; 3–43.

Parikh, N.A., Arnold, C., Langer, J., & Tyson, J.E. (2010). Evidence-based treatment decisions for extremely preterm newborns. *Pediatrics*, **125**(4), 813–816.

Rennie, J.M. & Leigh, B. (2008). The legal framework for end-of-life decisions in the UK. *Seminars in Fetal and Neonatal Medicine*, **13**(5), 296–300.

Ronen, G.M., Rosenbaum, P., Law, M., & Streiner, D.L. (2001). Health-related quality of life in childhood disorders: a modified focus group technique to involve children. *Quality of Life Research*, **10**(1), 71–79.

Saigal, S. & Tyson, J. (2008). Measurement of quality of life of survivors of neonatal intensive care: critique and implications. *Seminars in Perinatology*, **32**(1), 59–66.

Saigal, S., Stoskopf, B.L., Feeny, D., et al. (1999). Differences in preferences for neonatal outcomes among health care professionals, parents, and adolescents. *JAMA*, **281**(21), 1991–1997.

Saigal, S., Stoskopf, B., Pinelli, J., et al. (2006). Self-perceived health-related quality of life of former extremely low birth weight infants at young adulthood. *Pediatrics*, **118**(3), 1140–1148.

Saigal, S., Pinelli, J., Streiner, D.L., Boyle, M., & Stoskopf, B. (2010). Impact of extreme prematurity on family functioning and maternal health 20 years later. *Pediatrics*, **126**(1), e81–e88.

Tyson, J.E., Parikh, N.A., Langer, J., Green, C., & Higgins, R.D. (2008). Intensive care for extreme prematurity – moving beyond gestational age. *New England Journal of Medicine*, **358**(16), 1672–1681.

White-Koning, M., Arnaud, C., Dickinson, H.O., et al. (2007). Determinants of child-parent agreement in quality-of-life reports: a European study of children with cerebral palsy. *Pediatrics*, **120**(4), e804–e814.

Zwicker, J.G. & Harris, S.R. (2008). Quality of life of formerly preterm and very low birth weight infants from preschool age to adulthood: a systematic review. *Pediatrics*, **121**(2), e366–e376.

Variations of practice in the care of extremely preterm infants

Annie Janvier and John D. Lantos

Introduction

A normal gestation lasts 40 weeks following the mother's last menstrual period, and prematurity is defined as a gestation lasting fewer than 37 weeks. Until the 1960s, most premature babies died. Four recent developments in neonatology – respirators, parenteral (intravenous) nutrition, antenatal corticosteroids, and surfactant replacement therapy – have improved outcomes for preterm infants. The "physiological" lower limit of viability is similar in all industrialized countries: 22 weeks gestational age with some very rare survivors at 21 weeks. There is, however, tremendous variation among countries in survival of babies at 22–25 weeks of gestation. Doctors and parents in many countries choose not to provide these infants with active interventions. Many people think that the survival rate for babies born at 22–24 weeks is too low and the rate of disabilities among survivors is too high. Some health policy makers worry about the cost of neonatal intensive care for these tiny babies. We will examine all of these issues and do so with particular attention to international variations in the treatment of extremely low gestational age neonates (ELGANs).

Case narrative

Mrs. Duran is 24 weeks pregnant. It is her first pregnancy. When she and her husband first saw the ultrasound images of their baby's heart, her fingers, and her cute profile, they decided to call her Kim. Mrs. Duran was meticulous in following the recommendations in her baby book: no alcohol, raw meat, unpasteurized cheeses, exposure to smoke, or coffee, tea, or chocolate. She exercised 4 days each week.

One night, she wakes up with tremendous pain. Upon arrival at the hospital, she learns that she is in advanced preterm labor and that Kim will probably be born in the next few hours or days.

They estimate Kim to be 24 weeks of gestational age (GA) and to weigh about 700 grams. In the delivery room, the obstetrician consults the neonatologist. The neonatologist meets the parents.

Mr. and Mrs. Duran are scared. They desire to do what is best for their daughter, their family, and themselves. They want to know what Kim's chances are. What should the neonatologist say? The answer depends on many factors.

What are Kim's chances?

Prenatal estimates of birth weight (BW) and GA have margins of error. An estimate of 24 weeks GA could be off by a week or two either way: so Kim's true gestational age lies somewhere between 22 and 26 weeks. There is a wide difference in survival at the extremes of this range.

One crucial factor in determining whether or not Kim will survive is whether she receives intensive care. Without intensive care, Kim has no chance of survival. Values of physicians, parents, and the country and hospital where Mrs. Duran gives birth will influence whether Kim will receive intensive care. With intervention, predicted survival for Kim will depend not only on her GA, but also on her birth weight (BW), whether or not she is born in a specialized center that has experience in taking care of ELGANs, her gender (girls have higher survival rates), and whether her mother gets prenatal steroids (Tyson et al., 2008). At 24 weeks, the average survival in Canada and the United States is 50–70%.

Interestingly, her GA is not very tightly correlated with the likelihood that, if she survives, she will have disabilities. Babies born at 23 weeks who survive have neurodevelopmental outcomes similar to those of babies born at 26 weeks. All babies in this range of GAs have a 50% chance of being "intact", and a 15–25% risk of major

Clinical Ethics in Pediatrics: A Case-Based Textbook, ed. Douglas S. Diekema, Mark R. Mercurio and Mary B. Adam. Published by Cambridge University Press. © Cambridge University Press 2011.

disability. In most studies, young adults who are former very low birth weight infants have slightly lower rates of educational achievements, employment, and independent living than term controls. Despite the high rates of disabilities and educational and behavioral problems encountered during their years growing up, most young adults in all studies showed surprisingly good recovery in adapting to roles of adult functioning and were doing better than had been predicted (Saigal et al., 2006).

Variations of treatment for babies similar to Kim in the industrialized world

In the early days of neonatology, physicians and policy makers were appropriately cautious about treating tiny babies (Silverman, 1992). The caution was based on the fact that long-term outcomes were unavailable, and that neonatology was one big experiment. This is no longer the case. Thirty years later, we have excellent follow-up studies about the outcomes of ELGANs, and intensive care for them is no longer an experiment.

Interestingly, different industrialized countries, with access to the same data in the medical literature, come to very different conclusions about appropriate management of ELGANs. Most use a similar framework but draw the lines within that framework differently.

ELGANs are usually classified as fitting into one of three "zones." The first zone is that in which good outcomes are likely and thus, the initiation of intensive care is generally considered morally obligatory. A second zone is often called "the gray zone." In the gray zone, outcomes are considered sufficiently ambiguous or uncertain that both intensive care and comfort care are considered two ethically defensible options. Finally, there is a third zone in which newborns are not considered viable and in which intervention is considered "non-beneficial."

In which zone does Kim fit? Unlike the physiological limit of viability, which is the same around the globe, the borders between these three zones are fuzzy, elastic, and subjective. The policies of most industrialized countries vary considerably, with the borders of the gray zone ranging somewhere between 21 and 26 weeks, depending on where the baby is born (Danish Council of Ethics, 1995; Swiss Society of Neonatologists, 2002; American Academy of Pediatrics, 2007; Kono et al., 2007; Pignotti & Donzelli, 2008; Batton, 2009; Salle & Sureau, 2010).

In some countries – including Germany, Japan, and Sweden – Kim would almost certainly receive active intervention. In Canada, the UK, and some hospitals in the United States, she would not routinely receive active intervention without prior discussion with her parents. Instead, doctors would explain to her parents the likely outcome and defer to their opinion (Canadian Paediatric Society, 1994; Nuffield Council on Bioethics, 2006). In the Netherlands (Gerrits-Kuiper et al., 2008) and in some centers in the United States (Kaempf et al., 2006), intensive care for Kim would be considered "non-beneficial" and neonatologists would recommend comfort care only.

Not surprisingly, outcomes for babies like Kim are quite different in different countries. Survival for babies born at 24 weeks is 81% in Japan, 60% in Canada, 33% in the UK, and is as low as zero in some centers in the Netherlands. In a study comparing outcomes for ELGANs in Europe, survival rates for babies born before 28 weeks ranged from 11% to 37% (Zeitlin et al., 2008). One might think that neurodevelopmental outcomes would be better overall in centers that did not save the tiniest babies. Some studies, however, have suggested the opposite. In Sweden, some centers treat more aggressively than others. Those centers reported better neurodevelopmental outcomes, with fewer cases of chronic physical or mental problems among survivors than the less aggressive centers. It seems centers that take care of greater numbers of sicker ELGANs get better at what they do.

These variations raise an interesting question about informed consent. What, exactly, should Kim's parents be told about her chances for survival? Should they be presented with only outcome data for the hospital, or the region, or the country where they live? Should they be told of the well-known international variations in standards and practices? Should doctors make a recommendation or should they simply try to provide information in a neutral, non-directive way? The discussion above about practice variation suggests that there is no neutral ground here. Whatever a doctor chooses to reveal – or to conceal – will inevitably frame the decision for parents.

Clinicians themselves may be uncomfortable conveying complex probabilistic information and may try to simplify it for the parents. As a response to uncertainty, many clinicians will say: "we do not do Y in this center" (intervene at less than 24 weeks, for example). Policy statements and guidelines that choose gestational age for ethical decision-making for ELGANs represent a comfortable option by offering an easy recipe; but are simple rules adequate for complicated decisions (Janvier et al., 2008a)? Though attractive, they may not be morally defensible.

A better response to uncertainty would be to examine the variations of practice when there is uncertainty, to feel uncomfortable, accept this discomfort, and try to learn from these variations while being honest with ourselves and our patients: "There are many ways one could view this problem. We do X here, but they do Y elsewhere (down the road, in another country ...); outcomes differ from place to place. Should we be considering Y for some of our babies? What could we improve, what works well for us, who can we learn from?" Speaking to those who do Y when one does X is what, as pediatricians and ethicists, we find most gratifying. Generally X-doers and Y-doers learn a great deal from each other.

Is practice variation between countries morally problematic?

Practice variations are common in all domains of medicine. Most are not based on explicit policies or philosophies. Instead, they seem to be either random variations or to be driven by economic incentives. By contrast, practice variations for 22- to 26-week infants are driven by explicit philosophic principles. Those who are more aggressive obviously think that intervention is ethically appropriate. Those who defend less aggressive treatment think that over-treatment is more problematic than under-treatment. Both argue that they are doing what is in the best interest of the baby and the family. Both invoke local or national policies, based on local or national outcome data, to justify their approaches.

There is an iterative relationship between values, policies, and facts. If Kim's parents are told that Kim's chances of survival are low, they will be less likely to choose treatment. If they choose comfort care, Kim will die. Kim's death, in turn, will become part of the data on outcomes. A high mortality rate for babies like Kim will be used to justify a policy of non-intervention for babies like Kim.

Policies can become self-fulfilling prophecies. The relationship between outcome studies and policies in the UK is a good example of this process. In the 1990s, British neonatologists followed a cohort of ELGANs to evaluate their outcomes. (The acronym for the study was EPICure.) This study showed that survival rates and long-term outcomes were poor. Survival at 24 weeks, *when physicians would intervene*, was 33%. A bioethics think tank, the Nuffield Council, relied upon these data to make policy recommendations (Nuffield Council on Bioethics, 2006). They recommended that treatment be discouraged below 25 weeks. These policy recommendations were followed and, in at least one center, survival rates for 23- and 24-week infants went down.

This policy parable has some interesting implications. EPICure demonstrated the outcomes for ELGANs were poor *in the UK*. What could have been adequate overall conclusions of the EPICure study? One would need to ask: were there outcomes that were better during that period in other countries? Let's compare Australia and the UK. They are both "islands" with socialized health care. During the same period, survival in Australia for 24-week infants was 55%, with better long-term outcomes. Why?

There are a number of possible explanations. Australia's system of NICU care is more successfully regionalized. There are only 22 tertiary care NICUs in Australia, compared with 137 in the UK. (There are 61 million people in the UK, compared with 21 million in Australia – so the UK has about twice as many NICUs per citizen as Australia.) In Australia, more than 90% of mothers in premature labor receive steroids (which improves outcomes). In the EPICure study, 60% of the mothers were given steroids. In the EPICure study, babies were cared for in 137 different centers, many of which had little experience in caring for ELGANs. Following the EPICure study, there have been some improvements in regionalization. On the other hand, there has not been any improvement in outcomes for babies born at 23 and 24 weeks. The Nuffield report, with GA-based guidelines, has indeed been a self-fulfilling prophecy.

The value of neonates

The Neonatal Resuscitation Program textbook, which is the standard neonatal resuscitation text used in North America states: "The ethical principles regarding resuscitation of newborns should be no different from those followed in resuscitating an older child or adult" (Zeitlin *et al.*, 2008). The Nuffield report states the same "fact" (Nuffield Council on Bioethics, 2006). The existence of policies based upon GA suggests that these principles are not followed in practice. In our study (Janvier et al., 2008b), many physicians thought that intervention was in the best interests of a 24-weeker. Interestingly, even more thought that resuscitation was in the best interests of a 2-month-old infant with meningitis, even though the 2-month-old was described as having similar outcomes (Janvier et al., 2008b). Half of those who thought resuscitation was beneficial for the 24-weeker also said that they would accept a parental decision to provide comfort care. Far fewer would accept such a parental decision for the 2-month-old. We are continuing this research and have found the same results in nine different countries, with different health care systems and cultures. Such responses suggest that decisions for tiny preterm babies are made using different values than those for older children. For resuscitation decisions, some authors think age should have an impact in decision-making, especially for the very old. Setting an upper age limit for resuscitation is not a new concept, but is very controversial. There do not appear to be official policies or professional association guidelines that suggest an age limit for resuscitation, with the exception of preterm infants.

Money

Many policies regarding NICUs invoke concerns about cost-effectiveness. Often, the high cost of saving tiny premature babies is used to justify policies of non-intervention. Indeed, NICU care for ELGANs is expensive. Surprisingly, in spite of these high costs, every study of the cost-effectiveness of NICUs shows them to be far more cost-effective than many widely accepted treatments. The standard measure of cost-effectiveness is dollars per quality-adjusted life-year (QALY). NICUs are cost-effective because most of the money is spent on babies who survive, and most survivors live a long time without serious impairments. Thus, the high initial costs are amortized over a lifetime and lead to relatively low figures for dollars/QALY. The quality-adjusted costs for life of a 24-week preterm baby will be US$7000/year. Most critical interventions for adults cost more than US$70 000/year.

One reason for this is that the babies who die in NICUs tend to die quickly: 70% of deaths occur in the first week of life (Meadow et al., 2004). Given this high mortality of ELGANs in the first week of life (Jones et al., 2005), the majority of the NICU resources are spent on survivors, and the majority of survivors do not have impairments (Meadow et al., 2004). Denying intensive care to infants born at <500 g and <600 g would lead to total NICU care savings of 0.8% and 3.2%, respectively (Stolz & McCormick, 1998). It is true that babies

who survive with disabilities will need further care and resources. But this is true for patients in every other medical domain as well, including, for example, children with cystic fibrosis or sickle cell disease, or adults who have had a myocardial infarction. The costs per QALY saved in the NICU are about 1/100th of the cost of acute adult coronary care (Doyle, 1996).

Economic analyses are utilitarian; they place a value on lives and lives saved. Because most of the premature infants in the NICU survive without major disabilities, and most extremely low birth weight babies are economically productive in follow-up studies, even when living with disability, neonatal intensive care is among the most cost-efficient of acute medical endeavors (Saigal et al., 2003, 2006). It is also noteworthy that major improvements in newborn survival have not resulted in proportionate increases in severe morbidity (Hakansson et al., 2004).

International variations in preterm rates

Just as there are variations in the treatment of ELGANs, so there are variations in the overall rate of preterm birth. About 6–8% of babies are born preterm in Europe, Canada, and Australia. The rate of preterm birth is much higher in the United States: around 13%. Many factors explain the increase in prematurity in the United States: medically induced deliveries, increasing maternal age, assisted reproductive technologies (multiple births), fear of litigation, health care system, and socioeconomic factors. How to decrease preterm births is a complex topic and would merit an entire chapter in itself. In most countries with social health care, decreasing NICU length of stay and NICU beds is desirable. In most countries with socialized health care, the government decides how many NICUs and neonatologists there are. The restrictive practices some countries apply are not related to the "budget" in those countries, but to their values and choices. Do US hospitals want to decrease NICU stay? While in most areas of pediatrics, frequency and duration of hospitalization have decreased over several years, NICU admissions have gone up mainly because of the increase in prematurity. Are NICUs economic engines that keep children's hospitals running?

Neonates in poor countries

We have focused in this chapter on the ethical dilemmas associated with active intervention or comfort care of

ELGANs. Most babies in the world do not have access to a NICU. Much worse, in many countries, babies who do not breathe immediately after birth are still left to die. Five percent of term babies need a little help to start breathing on their own. While these dilemmas are difficult, they are quite different from the dilemmas faced by neonatologists and perinatologists in "developed" (which we prefer to call industrialized) countries. The majority of neonatal deaths in the world are due to a lack of access to basic medical care. Most childhood deaths in the world are due to treatable infections and hunger. Most of these deaths occur in the first month of life. Intensive care for a baby like Kim costs about US$7000/year of life. This is extremely inexpensive compared with most adult interventions. Saving one life for a neonate in Zambia costs US$7. Such stark injustices raise issues of distributive justice that will, we predict and hope, come to the fore in the twenty-first century.

Are practice variations for ELGANs amenable to change?

With medical progress, it seems values change. It used to be the case that babies with Down syndrome and duodenal atresia were left to die without surgery. Today, in most countries, all such babies receive surgery. Standards for the treatment of premature babies may evolve in a similar way. Will our society evolve to find the death of premature infants less acceptable, the way we now find that the death of a 3-year-old "is a tragedy that is not supposed to happen?" Because neonatology is a rather new field, this might well happen. Only time will tell.

References

American Academy of Pediatrics, Committee on Fetus and Newborn (2007). Noninitiation or withdrawal of intensive care for high-risk newborns. *Pediatrics*, **119**(2), 401–403.

Batton, D.G. (2009). Committee on Fetus and Newborn. Antenatal counseling regarding resuscitation at an extremely low gestational age. *Pediatrics*, **124**(1), 422–427.

Canadian Paediatric Society, Fetus and Newborn Committee & Society of Obstetricians and Gynaecologists of Canada, Maternal-Fetal Medicine Committee (1994). Management of the woman with threatened birth of an infant of extremely low gestational age. *Canadian Medical Association Journal*, **151**(5), 547–551.

Danish Council of Ethics (1995). *Extreme Prematurity, Ethical Aspects*. Copenhagen, Denmark: Danish Council of Ethics.

Doyle, L.W. (1996). Cost evaluation of intensive care for extremely tiny babies. *Seminars in Neonatology*, **1**, 257–267.

Gerrits-Kuiper, J.A., de Heus, R., Bouwers, H.A, et al. (2008). At the limits of viability: Dutch referral policy for premature birth too reserved. *Nederlands Tijdschrift voor Geneeskunde*, **152**(7), 383–388.

Hakansson, S., Farooqi, A., Holmgren, P.A., Serenius, F., & Hogberg, U. (2004). Proactive management promotes outcome in extremely preterm infants: a population-based comparison of two perinatal management strategies. *Pediatrics*, **114**(1), 58–64.

Janvier, A., Barrington, K.J., Aziz, K., & Lantos, J. (2008a). Ethics ain't easy: do we need simple rules for complicated ethical decisions? *Acta Paediatrica*, **97**, 402–406.

Janvier, A., Leblanc, I., & Barrington, K. (2008b). The best interest standard is not applied for neonatal resuscitation decisions. *Pediatrics*, **121**(5), 963–969.

Jones, H.P., Karuri, S., Cronin, C.M., et al. (2005). Actuarial survival of a large Canadian cohort of preterm infants. *BMC Pediatrics*, **5**, 40.

Kaempf, J.W., Tomlinson, M., Arduza, C., et al. (2006). Medical staff guidelines for periviability pregnancy counseling and medical treatment of extremely premature infants. *Pediatrics*, **117**(1), 22–29.

Kono, Y., Mishina, J., Takamura, T., et al. (2007). Impact of being small-for-gestational age on survival and long-term outcome of extremely premature infants born at 23–27 weeks' gestation. *Journal of Perinatal Medicine*, **35**, 447–454.

Meadow, W., Lee, G., Lin, K., & Lantos, J. (2004). Changes in mortality for extremely low birth weight infants in the 1990s: implications for treatment decisions and resource use. *Pediatrics*, **113**(5), 1223–1229.

Nuffield Council on Bioethics (2006). Critical care decisions in fetal and neonatal medicine: ethical issues. London: Nuffield Council on Bioethics. www.nuffieldbioethics.org/neonatal-medicine.

Pignotti, M.S. & Donzelli, G. (2008). Perinatal care at the threshold of viability: an international comparison of practical guidelines for the treatment of extremely preterm births. *Pediatrics*, **121**(1), e193–e198.

Saigal, S., Pinelli, J., Hoult, L., Kim, M.M., & Boyle, M. (2003). Psychopathology and social competencies of adolescents who were extremely low birth weight. *Pediatrics*, **111**(5), 969.

Saigal, S., Stoskopf, B., Streiner, D., et al. (2006). Transition of extremely low-birth-weight infants from adolescence to young adulthood: comparison with normal birth-weight controls. *JAMA*, **295**(6), 667–675.

Salle, B. & Sureau, C. (2010). Le préma de moins de 28 SA, sa réanimation et son avenir. Rapport de l'académie de médecine, 2006, saisie dans sa séance du mardi 20 juin 2006. www.academiemedecine.fr/upload/base//

rapports_289_fichier_lie.rtf (last accessed April 3, 2010).

Silverman, W.A. (1992). Overtreatment of neonates? A personal retrospective. *Pediatrics*, **90**, 971–976.

Stolz, J. & McCormick, M. (1998). Restrictive access to neonatal intensive care: effect on mortality and economic savings. *Pediatrics*, **101**(3), 344–348.

Swiss Society of Neonatologists (2002). Recommendation for the care of infants born at the limit of viability (gestational age 22–26 weeks). www.neonet.ch/assets/doc/

Infants_born_at_the_limit_of_viability_-_english_final.pdf (last accessed April 3, 2010).

Tyson, J.E., Parikh, N.E., Langer, J., et al. (2008). Intensive care for extreme prematurity – moving beyond gestational age. *New England Journal of Medicine*, **358**, 1672–1681.

Zeitlin, J., Draper, E.S., Kollée, L., et al. (2008). Differences in rates and short-term outcome of live births before 32 weeks of gestation in Europe in 2003: results from the MOSAIC cohort. *Pediatrics*, **121**, e936–e944.

Chapter

18

End-of-life care: resolving disputes over life-sustaining interventions

Kelly Michelson and Joel Frader

Case narrative

A 7-year-old boy with recurrent medulloblastoma presents to the emergency department with seizures. He receives multiple antiepileptics and subsequently loses the ability to protect his airway. As a result, he is intubated and supported with mechanical ventilation. Over the next several days he requires high doses of benzodiazepines and barbiturates to control his seizures. Eventually, his seizures stop and physicians modify the antiepileptic agents to a maintenance regimen. He is evaluated for extubation. Because of his waxing and waning mental status and frequent apneic episodes (not related to medications) he does not meet extubation criteria. Imaging of his brain demonstrates spread of his brain tumor despite previous aggressive chemotherapy. The neuro-oncologist acknowledges that no therapeutic alternatives remain to lessen tumor burden or halt progression of the disease. The clinicians hold a meeting with the family to discuss care options and goals and create a clinical plan.

Ethical principles and discussion

Medical technologies provide the opportunity to maintain life artificially and, at times, nearly indefinitely. Most of the time life support appropriately allows time for patients to recover from complex surgery or devastating illness. However, at other times technology sustains bodily functions with no realistic possibility of cure or return to what involved parties consider a reasonable quality of life. In these situations determining when to forgo life-sustaining therapies provides clinical and emotional challenges for families and the clinicians caring for the critically ill children. While some argue that the "sanctity of life" is absolute and the full complement of available technologies should always be used to maintain life, others believe in the moral permissibility of forgoing life-sustaining therapies (FLT) in certain situations. In this chapter, we address the ethical issues posed by FLT through a discussion of the steps involved in reasoned decision making: first, recognizing criteria for considering FLT; second, deliberating about the FLT decision; and third, determining whether or not to go ahead with FLT. We also discuss the specific issues pertinent to decisions about discontinuing medically provided fluids and nutrition (MPFN). Finally, we briefly consider issues related to care of patients for whom a decision to forgo life-sustaining therapies has been made.

We begin by clarifying basic terms. We use the term *forgo* to refer to both withholding and withdrawing possible interventions. Thus our discussion considers decisions about both stopping and not starting therapies. We acknowledge that some individuals find it psychologically difficult to stop a particular therapy once begun (e.g., to extubate a patient whose breathing depends on mechanical ventilation) compared with not starting an intervention (e.g., not undertaking cardiopulmonary resuscitation for a patient with untreatable cancer). However, ethicists generally do not find a persuasive moral distinction between not starting and stopping optional or non-indicated therapies. Thus we use the term *forgo* and our discussion encompasses both withdrawing and withholding interventions.

It is also important to clarify what we mean by therapies that can sustain life. As defined by the American Academy of Pediatrics (AAP), *life-sustaining therapies* (LST) include "all interventions that may prolong the life of patients" (American Academy of Pediatrics, 1994). As such, LST can include surgical procedures like transplantation, mechanical interventions like the use of ventilators or kidney dialysis, or interventions that involve the administration of medications such as chemotherapy or antibiotics. As we will discuss, LST also include medically provided fluids and nutrition.

Criteria for FLT

In defining circumstances or criteria that justify FLT, many invoke the concept of futility. In theory, one could rationalize forgoing a treatment thought to have no purpose or to be ineffective. Thus determining whether a therapy is futile seems deceptively attractive. But defining futility remains inherently problematic and inevitably value-laden (Truog et al., 1992). In our initial case example, some might consider the use of mechanical ventilation futile because the patient's untreatable medulloblastoma will cause his death in the relatively near future, despite respiratory support. Others might argue that ventilatory support will, in fact, maintain the patient's life for some time, which should be valued for its own sake. From that perspective, each additional day or even hour of extended life has precious meaning and should be pursued.

Because of the challenge of adequately defining futility, we seek other criteria for determining the appropriateness of FLT. The President's Commission for the Study of Ethical Problems in Medicine and Biomedical and Behavioral Research provided a set of guidelines for this purpose in 1983. The Commission identified the following as warranting consideration of FLT: amount of suffering and potential for relief; severity of dysfunction and potential for restoration of function; expected duration of life; potential for the patient's personal satisfaction and enjoyment of life; and possibility of developing a capacity for self-determination (President's Commission, 1983). Thus, clinicians should not only focus on prognosis about life versus death, but also address quality of life as it pertains both to the patient's current condition and expectations about the future. Defining what constitutes a "reasonable" quality of life depends on individual circumstances and the values of those involved. Clinicians must carefully evaluate every situation based on the unique variables present. Recognizing this situational variability, the AAP recommends that consideration of FLT develops from an assessment of the benefits versus the burdens of each intervention available to the patient. The AAP's guidance reflects the classic principles of beneficence, using treatments that will benefit a patient, and nonmaleficence, avoiding treatments with potential to harm the patient (American Academy of Pediatrics, 1994).

Deliberating about FLT

The approach to deliberating about FLT differs in pediatrics from that used with adult patients. With adults, decisions about FLT typically rely on the patient's expression of his or her wishes, whether contemporaneously or with the help of advance directives (previously defined preferences for care), or substituted judgment (an impression, based on knowledge of the patient's lifestyle and values, of what the patient would want if he or she were able to participate in decision-making). In pediatrics, decision-makers are encouraged to use the "Best Interest Standard," meaning the parents or guardian must take into account all relevant information about the patient's condition, the alternative treatments (including, presumably, the resources available to obtain and maintain care), and decide, given estimates about the success of treatment, what course to follow (Frader & Michelson, 2006). While the Best Interest Standard provides some guidance, ambiguity remains. No one has proposed a clear, comprehensive, and practically useful definition of "best interests" that accounts for all the medical, psychosocial, ethical, legal, and economic factors involved. One person might consider labeling a burdensome treatment with a 1% chance of success the "best" option; another might feel that the small likelihood of success does not outweigh possible harms from the treatment and therefore conclude that the offered intervention is not in the child's best interest. The use of interventions without clearly proven benefit further complicates determinations of what is best for a particular patient. Moreover some debate the acceptability of considering "third party" or parent/family concerns, such as the cost of care, in decisions about what is best for a particular child (Frader & Michelson, 2006). Without a clear notion of what constitutes a child's best interests and agreement on what factors one may legitimately include beyond those directly affecting the child, deliberation about FLT must consider the context of each situation and the values of those involved.

Deciding to forgo life-sustaining therapies

Ultimately, deliberation must result in a decision about what to do. Some debate exists about who should make a decision about FLT. From a legal perspective, parents have presumptive decision-making authority and must give permission for treatment of their children. A few clear exceptions to this rule exist, such as when the child has status as an emancipated minor or when courts have severed parental authority because of suspected or proven child abuse. In addition, most argue that older children and adolescents should have an important, if not definitive, role in such decisions to the extent that they have the capacity to do so (American Academy of Pediatrics, 1994, 1995). Nevertheless, parents generally have the required legal authority, provided that they have adequate decision-making capacity, meaning they can understand relevant information, appreciate the differences among the available options, and incorporate values into choices they express (American Academy of Pediatrics, 1994). The AAP clearly supports active involvement of patients and physicians in end-of-life care decisions for children. Health care professionals should not just provide information about the situation; they also have an obligation to make specific recommendations about which course to follow (American Academy of Pediatrics, 1994). Many clinicians and medical ethics experts support shared decision-making which involves clinician–family collaboration and culminates in a decision arrived at through consensus of the involved groups (Charles et al., 1999).

In some cases, the parties involved may not be able to reach consensus. When that occurs, one should usually respect parents' or guardians' wishes, provided their chosen course does not definitively harm the patient (though agreeing on what constitutes "harm" may be as elusive as defining futility). While clinicians have no legal duty to provide "unnecessary" or "non-indicated" treatment requested by parents or guardians, if parents can ascribe a reasonable rationale for their requested care and the care does not add to the patient's suffering, most advocate supporting the family's wishes. In the rare cases when parents seek to continue troublingly burdensome treatment or to avoid life-sustaining therapies that jeopardize the welfare of a patient, professionals should use available avenues to usurp decisional authority by invoking a state's legal mechanisms. Diekema has cogently proposed using the "harm principle" to guide such situations. Specifically, clinicians should consider whether parental decisions "significantly increase the likelihood of serious harm for the patient as compared to other options," and if so, seek input from the relevant state agency (Diekema, 2004).

Discontinuing medically provided fluids and nutrition (MPFN)

Over the past several decades many in the medical and legal communities have agreed that forgoing MPFN does not differ substantively from discontinuing, or not starting, other forms of life support, including the provision of air via mechanical ventilation, with or without tracheostomy, or the use of medications to support circulation (Committee on Bioethics, 1994; Diekema et al., 2009). Nevertheless, the practice of forgoing MPFN remains troubling to some, perhaps especially in pediatrics. Psychological and moral reservations about forgoing MPFN arise from disparate quarters, including the recognition that the well-being of normal young children depends on adults feeding them; that death following the decision not to start or to stop MPFN may take many days, even weeks accompanied by disquieting physical changes; and recent communications from the Roman Catholic Church suggesting a moral *requirement* to provide feeding in nearly all cases (Offices of the Congregation for the Doctrine of the Faith, 2007).

We emphasize the importance of only forgoing *medically provided* fluids and nutrition. Oral feeding differs from medical administration of fluids and nutrition in several ways: those desiring to drink or eat typically have some intent or will to continue life; drinking and eating often provide feelings of pleasure for individuals; and oral feedings involve complex social and cultural meaning that differs from the provision of a medically arranged and ordered nutritional regimen. Patients who desire and can tolerate oral liquids or food should receive them, perhaps even at the risk of aspiration.

Does forgoing MPFN differ from the forgoing of other means of life support? In one crucial sense, the answer is "no." A decision to forgo any means of life support suggests the acceptability of the patient's death. The decision signals a shift in goals and priorities of patient care from life prolongation, often with the hope of cure or at least significant improvement in clinical function, to a focus on comfort and the quality of the child's remaining life. However, in another important way, forgoing MPFN differs from some other decisions about life support: assuming nothing else changes, the patient will certainly die without fluids and nutrition. At times, stopping or not starting therapies (mechanical ventilation, pharmacologic support of circulation) does not result in death, even when expected to do so.

The certainty of eventual death after forgoing MPFN leaves some uneasy, raising questions about the intent of the action: it feels like "killing."

Many parents and some health care professionals also associate forgoing MPFN with patient discomfort. One often hears the emotionally charged word "starvation." However, at least some evidence suggests dehydration alone results in loss of consciousness with rising blood urea nitrogen levels. We have good reason to believe that ketosis powerfully ablates hunger. Moreover, we believe usual measures to treat bodily discomfort, including narcotics and sedatives, can provide relief in cases where the patient is ill at ease or restless (Diekema et al., 2009).

Deciding to forgo MPFN, like deciding to forgo other means of life support, requires a balancing of the potential benefits and burdens of either going ahead with or withholding MPFN. The decision should conform to carefully considered – and articulated – goals of care for the child. Implementation of a decision to forgo MPFN will require considerable preparation, whether carried out in the hospital or at home. Those caring for the child will need an opportunity to express any reservations they have about the decision, including the potential that participation in the care will violate deeply held religious or personal values. In most cases, caregivers should have the option not to participate. Frequent sessions to support staff caring for a child may have value, especially if the child lives beyond the expected 7–10 days, and weight loss and signs of dehydration become apparent.

Whether health care professionals should initiate discussions of forgoing MPFN remains somewhat controversial. Some argue that raising the possibility conforms to the tenets of informed consent and the importance of discussing the (reasonably available) alternative courses of care. Others believe that the emotionally charged nature of forgoing MPFN dictates that professionals should wait for families to ask about the option.

Consideration of care after a decision to forgo life-sustaining therapies

Clinicians should always remember that FLT never equates to forgoing *care*. Multidisciplinary, whole-person care ought always to be the goal, particularly in cases where FLT will likely culminate in death. Please refer to Chapter 24 for a complete discussion of providing symptom management for the dying child. As it pertains to decisions about FLT, clinicians should always consider the symptoms that a patient will likely experience without a particular treatment. For example, air hunger may occur following extubation. Clinicians should set out a plan for symptom management in advance and discuss it directly with the parents, with the patient when appropriate, and with all the clinical caregivers involved.

Practical summary

Multiple factors complicate decisions about FLT. First, one cannot define universally acceptable criteria for FLT. Standards for arriving at such decisions are inherently problematic. The legal decision-maker(s) (parents or guardians) rarely determines a plan of care without input from clinicians. In light of the challenges, clinicians and family should focus on the benefits and burdens of alternative plans of care, as defined by the individual situation and the values of those involved. Ideally clinicians and families can reach consensus about the benefit/burden relationships of available life-sustaining therapies. When such consensus eludes the participants, further clarification of values supporting a particular choice may help resolve the conflict. In some cases input from a third party, such as an ethics consultant, may prove useful. Occasionally, circumstances such as concern about parental capacity or conflicts of interest require involvement of the state.

Resolution of case and discussion

The medical care team discussed the option of extubating the boy, recognizing that he would likely demonstrate respiratory insufficiency and would probably die. Because all treatments for the medulloblastoma had been exhausted, the neuro-oncologists predicted the tumor would continue to spread, causing further neurologic impairment. The family felt that the child would be more comfortable without the endotracheal tube (ETT) in place and wanted to maximize the opportunity to interact with their son before he died. They therefore requested removal of their son's ETT. In this case, the potential benefit of verbal interaction with their son and allowing him to die without the discomfort of an ETT outweighed the value of continued mechanical ventilation, a therapy that would not affect the progression of his underlying disease.

Despite the clinicians' assessment, the child was able to breathe without the support of the artificial airway or respirator. At first he was able to speak with his parents, if only intermittently. As his tumor grew he lapsed into long periods of unconsciousness. At that point, his mother questioned the need to continue nasogastric feedings. The parents and clinicians discussed the option of discontinuing all MPFN and the attending physician ended the meeting with a recommendation to do so. Three days later the parents requested the discontinuation of all MPFN. The attending physician agreed.

Many of the nurses objected to stopping MPFN and requested exemption from assignment to the patient. Over the 17 days before the patient's death, he received antipyretics for fever and morphine when he seemed uncomfortable. His mother stopped visiting. As the patient lost weight and skin turgor, many members of the care team expressed reservations about the decision to forgo MPFN.

Another unsettled question involves whether unconscious or minimally conscious patients should routinely receive analgesics or sedatives after withdrawal of MPFN. The best palliative care often involves a degree of anticipatory treatment of discomfort and scheduling medication to prevent the distress and/or suffering associated with waiting for relief after professionals recognize a need to intervene. Finally, the staff felt considerable unease about the mother's absence in the last days of the boy's life. While their distress is understandable, family member grief can manifest in many ways, and it does not seem reasonable to insist that parents witness the physical decline of their child. If family members do not visit, the clinicians still have obligations to maintain frequent and supportive contact with them.

References

American Academy of Pediatrics (1994). Guidelines on foregoing life-sustaining medical treatment. *Pediatrics*, **93**(3), 532–536.

American Academy of Pediatrics (1995). Informed consent, parental permission, and assent in pediatric practice. *Pediatrics*, **95**(2), 314–317.

Charles, C., Gafni, A., & Whelan, T. (1999). Decision-making in the physician-patient encounter: revisiting the shared treatment decision-making model. *Social Science and Medicine*, **49**(5), 651–661.

Diekema, D.S. (2004). Parental refusals of medical treatment: the harm principle as threshold for state intervention. *Theoretical Medicine and Bioethics*, **25**(4), 243–264.

Diekema, D.S., Botkin, J.R., & the Committee on Bioethics, American Academy of Pediatrics (2009). Clinical report – forgoing medically provided nutrition and hydration in children. *Pediatrics*, **124**(2), 813–822.

Frader, J. E. & Michelson, K. (2011). Ethics in pediatric intensive care. In *Pediatric Critical Care*, 4th edn, ed. B. Fuhrman & J. Zimmerman. Philadelphia, PA: Mosby Elsevier, 102–109.

Offices of the Congregation for the Doctrine of the Faith (2007). Responses to certain questions of the United States Conference of Catholic Bishops concerning artificial nutrition and hydration. Available from: www.vatican.va/roman_curia/congretations/cfaith/documents/rc_con_cfaith_doc_20070810_risposte-usa_en.html. Last accessed October 10, 2010.

President's Commission for the Study of Ethical Problems in Medicine and Biomedical and Behavioral Research (1983). Patients who lack decisionmaking capacity. In *Deciding to Forego Life-Sustaining Treatment*. Washington, DC: US Government Printing Office, 133.

Truog, R.D., Brett, A.S., & Frader, J. (1992). The problem with futility. *New England Journal of Medicine*, **326**, 1560–1564.

Chapter

19

Futility

Norman Fost

Case narrative

Carlos, age 8 months, has been in the intensive care unit, ventilator dependent with status epilepticus, almost continuously for the past 5 months. He has multifocal migrating epilepsy, with seizures originating from both hemispheres. His physicians have either ruled out all known causes of seizures or treated them empirically with no improvement. Control requires general anesthesia (propofol) or complete suppression of cortical function with barbiturate coma. The migratory multifocal origins preclude even radical surgical approaches that are sometimes considered, such as removing an entire cerebral hemisphere, or interrupting the corpus callosum. Experts from other major centers have been consulted and all agree his case is among the worst ever described, and that he has little or no prospect for recovery with meaningful neurologic function.

His single mother is insistent that everything be done to keep him alive. She does not trust the doctors and accuses them of wanting to kill Carlos because of cost concerns. She does not profess a religious faith. She seldom visits, and does not want to discuss the issue of withdrawing life-sustaining treatments any more. Carlos' father is not involved and his maternal grandmother supports Carlos' mother.

The attending physician and all members of the treatment team believe continued treatment would be futile and want to discontinue life support over the mother's objection, and allow Carlos to die comfortably. They are, however, uncertain whether it is ethically or legally justified.

What are the ethical issues?

In many cases, the ability to sustain life indefinitely may not seem to be in the interest of the patient, or the costs of such treatment may seem disproportionate to the benefits. In the vast majority of cases, physicians and parents agree on the best course. When disagreement arises, however, the physician's frustration with his/her inability to persuade the parent to make the "right" decision can lead to an understandable desire to remove the decision from the parents and make a unilateral judgment over their clear objection.

This conflicts with the generally held ethical and legal principle that patients, or their legally authorized representatives, should have nearly complete authority to make health care decisions. On the other hand, the physician believes that continuing treatment violates the duty to serve the interests of his/her patient. When discussion and persuasion have failed to resolve the disagreement, there is an understandable desire to end the discussion by asserting that continued treatment would be futile and will therefore not be continued.

The ethical and legal issues in this case cannot be fully understood without considering distinctions between killing and letting die; conscientious objection to providing medical care; rationing of limited health care resources; entitlements and immunities; and other issues, some of which are covered in other chapters in this book. This chapter will focus on the use of the concept of futility to justify unilateral withdrawal of life-sustaining treatment.

Defining futility

Futility, as used in the medical setting, is commonly framed in two distinct ways. One is called quantitative, physiologic, or medical futility. The other is called qualitative or social futility. These two versions of futility will be discussed separately.

Clinical Ethics in Pediatrics: A Case-Based Textbook, ed. Douglas S. Diekema, Mark R. Mercurio and Mary B. Adam. Published by Cambridge University Press. © Cambridge University Press 2011.

Definitional issues: quantitative or physiologic futility

Quantitative or physiologic futility refers to treatments that will not achieve the intended physiologic goal. For example, using a ventilator in an infant with pulmonary agenesis will not achieve the purpose for which the ventilator is designed; namely, exchange of oxygen and carbon dioxide. Similarly, amoxicillin will not affect the clinical course of rabies, and a physician appropriately makes a unilateral decision not to prescribe it, even in the face of a parent who demands that it be used.

Quantitative futility seems to be the less controversial version of futility, as it is based on a presumably evidence-based medical or scientific claim. It provides a pathway toward unilateral decision-making, as a physician has no obligation to offer or provide ineffective or useless treatment. In practice, however, it is more complicated (Helft et al., 2000).

There are several problems with the notion of quantitative futility. First, the claim that treatment will be ineffective may not be based on adequate evidence. Consider, for example, the claim that treatment of newborn infants below a certain weight or gestational age is futile, based on the observation that no infant below that weight has ever survived. In the 1960s, survival below 1000 grams was uncommon, and survival below 500 grams was extraordinarily rare. Today a 1000 gram infant is expected to survive with good neurologic function, and survival of 500 gram infants is common. The poor outcome in the 1960s was partly due to inadequate technology, but it was also related to the assumption that treatment would be ineffective and the consequent failure on the part of physicians to attempt to intervene. Labeling the infant "non-viable," another way of saying that treatment would be futile, was a self-fulfilling prophecy, since it was accompanied by a decision not to try to prolong survival (Mercurio, 2005; Wilkinson, 2009).

Similarly, until 2005, it was commonly stated that no one had ever survived a case of proven rabies, but this was partly related to a failure to try hard enough, as shown by Willoughby and colleagues (2005), who reported a survival with good clinical outcome. Likewise, children with trisomy 18 commonly are not treated for life-threatening problems (e.g., surgery for cardiac malformations) because of the assumption that the underlying condition is incompatible with long or meaningful survival. This approach, if widespread, can result in published data confirming the belief that the disorder is incompatible with long life. As treatment expands (rightly or wrongly), it becomes apparent that survival is possible for longer periods of time more commonly than was previously believed.

Second, the definition of "ineffective" is often ambiguous and value laden. An infant born at 16 weeks is generally considered to be non-viable, and treatment would therefore be considered futile, but only if there is agreement on what "viable" means (Fost et al., 1980). Some infants that size could be kept alive for a period of hours, and treatment is effective for that period of time.

There might be consensus that sustaining a life for that short an interval is not worthwhile, defined by cost/benefit analysis, or that it is not in the interest of the patient, but these are value judgments, not scientific or medical claims. If "viable" means "not able to survive beyond a defined period," the selection of that time period is inherently subjective. There is no objective basis for deciding which interval is sufficient to justify treatment. Thus, whether or not the treatment would be futile unavoidably involves a value judgment.

Third, the definition of "effective" might be based on the arbitrary selection of a cutoff point for probability of survival or success. Jecker and Schneiderman (1993), for example, argued that treatment should be considered ineffective or futile if it had a less than 1 in 100 probability of succeeding, but there is no scientific or medical basis for selecting 1 in 100 as the relevant cutoff, as opposed to 1 in 50 or 1 in 5000 or 1 in a million. Implicit in Jecker and Schneiderman's claim is the concern that probabilities less than 1 in 100 involve costs, or cost/benefit considerations, that are unreasonable; but here again, whether or not it is worthwhile to invest effort and cost for a small chance of success is a value judgment, not a scientific or physiologic question. A "one-in-a-million" chance of survival is not zero, and whether it is worthwhile depends, *inter alia*, on costs, the preferences of the patient or family, and whether there is societal support for it.

This is illustrated by the variable interest in rescue operations for catastrophic events, such as the search for John Kennedy, Jr. and his wife when their plane disappeared off the coast of Martha's Vineyard. There was general support for that rescue operation, though the cost/benefit ratio was enormous. The disappearance at sea of less well-known or beloved citizens is labeled "futile" much more quickly.

Fourth, there may be strong evidence that treatment was medically futile in a defined population, but the present patient may be different in an important way from the population that contributed to the evidence. In the early days of the AIDS epidemic, the mortality rate was 100%, as the diagnosis depended on clinical manifestations that became evident late in the course of the disease. Even when retroviral therapy (AZT) became available, it appeared in early studies to delay progression to death, but not to prevent ultimate mortality. It was commonly said that treatment was futile in averting death from the disease. When serologic testing allowed for diagnosis earlier in the course, it slowly became apparent that some patients did not progress to death, either because of treatment earlier in the course, or because they had a milder form of the disease that would not have progressed without treatment.

This phenomenon is common in new or rare disorders, as the first recognized cases are often the worst, leading to the impression that treatment is futile, in the sense that prolonged or meaningful survival appears unlikely. As case finding improves, milder forms of the disorder may have a different prognosis than the earlier cases, and newly discovered treatments with the potential to alter disease progression may have become available.

Fifth, diagnosis or prognosis may be in error. While a child with pulmonary agenesis cannot survive very long and a traditional ventilator will not overcome the problem, the diagnosis can be incorrect, and what appears to be "agenesis" may be "hypogenesis" with sufficient functioning lung tissue to sustain life for an uncertain period.

Finally, a claim of physiologic or quantitative futility may mask what is really a claim about qualitative futility, or a lack of clarity or disagreement about the goals of treatment. Emilio Gonzales (Moreno, 2007) was a 17-month-old "deaf, blind and terminally ill child on life support" due to Leigh's encephalopathy. The hospital sought permission to discontinue life support under a Texas statute commonly referred to as a "futile treatment" law, but the treatment was obviously effective in keeping him alive up to that point. The statute (Texas statutes, 1999), in fact, does not mention futility, but refers to "medically inappropriate" treatment instead. But this phrase is also ambiguous, failing to distinguish a claim that the treatment will be medically ineffective from a claim that it is not in the patient's interest or that it is too costly. Clarity in such cases would be served by simply stating that, in the opinion of the physicians, treatment is not in the child's interest, and explaining why they think that is

so, rather than avoiding that discussion by invoking a medical justification.

In summary, examples of quantitative or physiologic futility commonly involve value judgments about whether a low probability of success is worth the cost, or judgments about the relevance of existing evidence to the present patient. Thus, the boundary between quantitative and qualitative futility is often indistinct.

Definitional issues: qualitative futility

"Qualitative futility" refers to judgments by the physician (and other providers) that, while treatment has a reasonable prospect of medical benefit, it is not worthwhile, in monetary terms or because of suffering or because the patient's quality of life will be so poor that s/he cannot benefit from continued survival. These, of course, are value judgments, about which reasonable people may disagree. They may be justified judgments in some cases, but these are not matters of medical expertise, so the physician's claim to having superior judgment warranting unilateral action is difficult to support.

Examples of the common failure to distinguish the two senses of futility, or to misuse the word entirely, include the following:

- "The baby's long-term survival with profound cognitive disability supports our view that the treatment was futile."
  Comment: Obviously the treatment was not futile in the medical sense since it succeeded in keeping the baby alive. Whether it was futile in the qualitative sense is a disagreement that needs to be resolved.
- "CPR is futile if cardiac arrest is likely to occur again in the future."
  Comment: If cardiac arrest recurred, a heartbeat was presumably restored, however briefly. Treatment was therefore not futile in the medical sense. Whether it was worthwhile depends in part on how long normal heart function was restored; whether the patient was able to communicate between the episodes; etc.
- "Futile CPR may sometimes be undertaken if it accomplishes an important goal of the patient or family; e.g., allowing a relative time to arrive at the bedside."
  Comment: CPR is obviously not futile in the physiologic sense, since it keeps the patient alive long enough for the family to arrive. There is apparent agreement by the writer that it is also not futile in

the qualitative sense either, since it helps achieve a goal that even the person using the term considers worth the effort. It is therefore unclear why or how it is futile in any sense.

In summary, both types of futility typically involve value judgments, or disagreements about whether the potential benefits of treatment are outweighed by the costs or burdens. Use of the "F" word risks pre-empting discussion of the value questions that are at the core of the case, regardless of whether the doctor is claiming medical or qualitative futility.

Implications of abandoning "futility"

The previous discussion suggests that invoking futility as a justification for unilateral action is problematic, as it short-circuits or bypasses the difficult discussions that need to occur when physicians and parents disagree about the appropriate treatment plan.

This is not to say that physicians may never unilaterally refuse to provide life-sustaining treatment, even when the reasons are primarily social or qualitative judgments about burdens and benefits. The point is that a physician claiming that it is ethically and legally justified to refuse such treatment needs some justification other than claims of futility.

What might those justifications be? I will suggest three examples, primarily to show that abandoning the invocation of futility does not preclude unilateral refusal of possibly effective treatment.

First, treatment (which should be understood to include diagnostic studies) is appropriately withheld when it is not consistent with the patient's preferences. Respecting patient preferences in pediatrics will generally be confined to adolescents, but there are clearly mature minors capable of making their preferences known in a clear, consistent, and durable way. A 16-year-old with metastatic Ewing's sarcoma, for example, may provide clear and convincing evidence that he/she would rather die than be intubated again or admitted to an intensive care unit. If such a patient became unable to communicate and developed a potentially treatable illness requiring ICU admission, a physician could justifiably refuse a parent's insistent request that the patient be treated, not on the grounds of futility, but on the widely accepted principle of respecting the clearly stated preferences of a competent patient.

Second, medically effective treatment may be refused when it does not serve any discernible interest of the patient. A child reliably diagnosed as being in a permanent vegetative state is, by definition, incapable of experiencing life. (Footnote: We will not address here recent reports that some patients diagnosed as being in a persistent vegetative state demonstrate deep brain activity in response to stimuli using advanced imaging techniques. Such studies do not prove that the patient is aware of the stimulus.) Apart from the possibility of error in the diagnosis, it is unclear whether such a patient has any interests, positive or negative.

Even a patient who is awake and alert may be suffering so extremely and have so little prospect of improvement, that treatment that is effective in prolonging life may not be in the patient's interest. A parent's insistence on treatment may be so clearly contrary to the child's interests that it should be challenged and in some cases overruled. A familiar example might be a child with multiple relapses of leukemia, not responsive to bone marrow or stem cell transplantation, who experiences severe graft versus host disease, multi-organ system failure, drug-resistant infection, no plausible prospect of survival beyond the ICU, and a parent insisting on hemodialysis to treat renal failure.

Physicians in such cases are often tempted to say that such treatment would be medically futile, but the problem is really the opposite; namely, a concern that the treatment will be effective, and the consequence of effective treatment would be continued suffering with little benefit to the child. Physicians might more accurately say that they believe the treatment is futile in the social sense of not being in the child's interests, but there is little advantage in invoking futility. The more candid course would be to explain to the parent that further treatment will not be offered, because the physician strongly believes it is not serving the child's interests.

Third, expensive treatment could be refused based on consideration of costs with little or no prospect of benefit. If there is no benefit that the patient can experience, then the cost/benefit ratio for the patient is infinity (the denominator is "zero"). Even if there is a remote but infinitesimally small chance of benefit, the cost/benefit ratio might be far beyond what any society would support. No one is entitled to all the goods and services s/he desires, whether it be food, shelter, education, or health care, nor can any society afford to provide it. Rationing is unavoidable in all societies and cost per quality-adjusted life-year is one generally accepted basis for deciding which services are owed to persons.

A physician who unilaterally refuses to provide medically effective treatment for any of these reasons should strongly consider seeking support for his/her position from an institutional ethics committee. There are ethical and legal reasons for this, beyond the scope of this chapter.

Regardless of whether ethics consultation is obtained, the physician considering unilateral withholding or withdrawal of treatment owes it to the patient/parents to be open and candid about his/her intentions, the reasons for that position, and a display a willingness to actively listen to the parents' views. This duty derives from the obligation to be truthful and respectful with patients. Invoking futility, particularly medical futility, risks concealing the physician's real reasons for wanting to withhold or withdraw treatment.

Other issues

This discussion has focused on situations in which the physician wishes to discontinue life-sustaining treatment unilaterally, since these are the cases that evoke the most disagreement and uncertainty. It is important to recognize, however, that the term can be used inappropriately in collaborative decisions if the physician uses "futility," as if it is a medical judgment, to short-circuit or avoid what is really a value judgment.

Two important points should be made about the legal aspects of unilateral withholding or withdrawing of life-sustaining treatment. First, the legal risks are generally over rated, as ultimate liability for withholding or withdrawing life-sustaining treatment is virtually unknown unless "the provider's conduct is outrageous" (Pope, 2008). The risks of inciting a lawsuit, or even criminal prosecution, are not zero, and the personal and financial costs of such an experience are not trivial, but if decisions are being heavily influenced by legal considerations, estimates of the actual risks should be based on data.

Some states have passed statutes to support unilateral refusal to provide life-sustaining treatment. The highly publicized Texas law (Texas statutes, 1999), passed in 1999, was the first. Part of its advance directive statute, it is commonly referred to as a "futility" statute, though it does not use that word, substituting the equally ambiguous phrase, "inappropriate treatment." Whether or not it provides a satisfactory solution to relevant cases has been widely debated (Fine, 2009; Truog, 2009).

Finally, Truog (2010) has argued that physicians may have a duty to provide treatment that the physician believes is futile to advance the interests of family members. He cites a case in which he provided what he considered to be medically futile CPR (a sham resuscitation) to assure the parents that their child was receiving the maximal treatment they desired. This position was criticized on various grounds, including violation of the physician's primary duty to promote the patient's interests; using the patient as an means to an end; inadequate concern for possible suffering of the patient; participating in an intentional deception; contributing to popular misconceptions; and inadequate consideration of costs to providers and other patients (Hanto et al., 2010).

Case resolution

Carlos has no plausible prospect of a meaningful life. If he does survive, he is virtually certain to require permanent residence in the ICU, unconscious and ventilator dependent, and will become increasingly susceptible to infection and probable death in the ICU.

Reducing or withdrawing the drugs needed to suppress his seizures will also result in his death, due to uncontrolled status epilepticus. Watching him die this way would be an extraordinarily difficult course for the medical team as well as his mother. On the other hand, withdrawing the ventilator and maintaining suppression of seizures would require such high doses of medications as to raise questions of whether the cause of death was the medications, rather than his illness, raising concerns about violation of restrictions on active euthanasia (see Chapters 22 and 24).

Assuming extensive and skilled efforts to persuade the mother to agree to a palliative care plan have failed, there is a temptation for the physician to unilaterally decide to discontinue life-sustaining treatment by invoking futility. A claim of medical futility cannot yet be made, as the treatment has obviously been effective in maintaining the child's life. A claim of qualitative futility would be plausible; i.e., that the child's quality of life will be so poor that continued treatment is not serving his interests. But using the "F" word risks confusion with claims of medical ineffectiveness, and risks avoiding candid discussion of the real reasons for wanting to discontinue life support.

Because the case has unusual legal risks, related to the high doses of suppressive medications that will probably be needed to ensure a peaceful death, it would be especially prudent for the physician to seek consultation from the hospital ethics committee, and if the hospital attorney is not typically involved in that process, s/he should be consulted.

In summary, if parental agreement cannot be obtained, unilateral cessation of treatment can be justified in this case, but the reasons for such a decision should be stated directly and candidly, without appeal to claims of futility.

References

Fine, R.L. (2009). Point: the Texas Advance Directives Act effectively and ethically resolves disputes about medical futility. *Chest*, **136**(4), 963–967.

Fost, N., Chudwin, D., & Wikler, D. (1980). The limited moral significance of 'fetal viability'. *Hastings Center Report*, **10**(6), 10–13.

Hanto, D.W., Fine, R.L., Sadovnikoff, N., et al. (2010). Is it always wrong to perform futile CPR? *New England Journal of Medicine*, **362**(21), 2034–2037.

Helft, P.R., Siegler, M., & Lantos, J. (2000). The rise and fall of the futility movement. *New England Journal of Medicine*, **343**, 293–296.

Jecker, N.S. & Schneiderman, L.J. (1993). Medical futility: the duty not to treat. *Cambridge Quarterly of Healthcare Ethics*, **2**, 151–159.

Mercurio, M. (2005). Physicians' refusal to resuscitate at borderline gestational age. *Journal of Perinatology*, **25**, 685–689.

Moreno, S. (2007). Case puts Texas futile-treatment law under a microscope. *Washington Post*, Apr 11, **2007**, A03.

Pope, T. (2008). Involuntary passive euthanasia in YS Courts: reassessing the judicial treatment of medical futility cases. *Marquette Elders Advisor*, **9**(2), 229.

Texas statutes (Added 1999; Amended 2003). Advanced Directives Act. Health and Safety Code, Title 2, Subtitle H, Chapter 166.046. Available at www.statutes.legis.state.tx.us/docs/Hs/htm/HS.166.htm. Last accessed January 24, 2011.

Truog, R.D. (2009). Counterpoint: the Texas Advance Directives Act is ethically flawed: medical futility disputes must be resolved by a fair process. *Chest*, **136**(4), 968–971.

Truog, R.D. (2010). Is it always wrong to perform futile CPR? *New England Journal of Medicine*, **362**, 477–479.

Wilkinson, D. (2009). The self-fulfilling prophecy in intensive care. *Theoretical Medicine and Bioethics*, **30**(6), 401–410.

Willoughby, Jr., R.E., Tieves, K.S., Hoffman, G.M., et al. (2005). Survival after treatment of rabies with induction of coma. *New England Journal of Medicine*, **352**, 2508–2514.

Further reading

Fost, N. (1995). Medical futility: commentary. In *Ethics and Perinatology*, ed. A. Goldworth, W. Silverman, D.K. Stevenson, E.W.D. Young, & R. Rovers. New York: Oxford University Press.

Chapter 20

Advance directives and DNR orders

Jeffrey P. Burns and Christine Mitchell

Case narrative

A 16-year-old female with advanced cystic fibrosis is admitted to the pediatric intensive care unit in severe respiratory distress. She is being supported by non-invasive ventilation, but her respiratory failure is progressing and she will likely need to be intubated in the next several hours. She has adamantly refused her pulmonologist's request that she be listed for lung transplant, stating "I have thought about this for years, I have talked with other CF patients who did and did not get a lung transplant, and I would rather die than go through that." Her parents want her to be listed for lung transplant. A short time later, while in severe respiratory distress, the patient asks to speak to her attending physician without her parents present. In this conversation she tells her physician, "I know I will not be able to communicate much longer, but no matter what happens do not let my parents list me for a lung transplant. I would rather die than go through all that transplant stuff." Should the patient's physician honor the adolescent's wishes or those of her parents?

Introduction

In August 1976 the *New England Journal of Medicine* published the first descriptions of do-not-resuscitate (DNR) policies. The issue contained two separate articles from two Harvard teaching hospitals describing their policies on the framework for decision-making about the resuscitation status of patients at their hospital (Clinical Care Committee, 1976; Rabkin et al., 1976). A third article on the subject in that issue was a commentary by a Harvard law professor, and later Solicitor General of the United States, arguing that orders not to resuscitate were likely consistent and legal under the United States constitution (Fried, 1976).

There was even a fourth article on these polices in that issue – written by philosopher Sissela Bok (1976). She noted that the DNR order focused on *what would not* be done for the patient, and only addressed decisions at the very end of life, instead of promoting in advance what *would* be done for the patient regarding a range of decisions, not solely resuscitation decisions, across the trajectory of illness. Bok's article was one of the first to prominently call for advance directives to ensure that patients have the opportunity to identify and clarify their personal values about medical treatment decisions. What are advance directives, how do DNR orders fit into advance directives, and do these concepts even have meaning for the pediatric patient?

Advance directives

Advance care planning is the process of planning for future medical care in the event that the patient is unable to make his or her own decisions. In its ideal form, the process helps patients clarify their personal values and goals about medical treatment, articulate what they would like or not like to receive in various situations, and name the person whom they want to make health care decisions on their behalf in the event they cannot do so for themselves. Importantly, advance care planning is ideally not an event, but an ongoing process as life circumstances and personal values evolve over time (President's Commission, 1983).

Types of advance directives

Advance directives fall into two basic categories: those concerning instructions for medical care and those concerning designation of a proxy for the patient. Instructional directives for care can be recorded in a number of types of documents. The most common, a "living will," directs clinicians and loved ones as to

Clinical Ethics in Pediatrics: A Case-Based Textbook, ed. Douglas S. Diekema, Mark R. Mercurio and Mary B. Adam. Published by Cambridge University Press. © Cambridge University Press 2011.

the wishes of the now incapacitated patient regarding medical treatments at the end of life. Other types of instructional directive include a "values history," which describes overarching values regarding health care in life-threatening illness situations, and more specific "medical directives" which specify choices based on likely scenarios of illness. Many of these include a proxy designation section.

A person who is empowered to make decisions in place of the patient may be called a health care proxy, a durable power of attorney for health care, a legal guardian, or a surrogate decision-maker. Depending on the state, a durable power of attorney for health care will typically be the incapacitated patient's "agent," "proxy," or "attorney-in-fact." The typical legally recognized prerogatives of this health care proxy include participating in medical decisions that are not covered in an instructional directive, having full access to the medical record, and granting or refusing consent for all treatments. Clinicians should familiarize themselves with the specific advance directive authority and requirements of their state (IOM, 1997). In some states either an instructional directive or a health care proxy are recognized as legally valid surrogates for the incapacitated patient. A few states, such as Massachusetts, do not legally recognize instructional directives in medical decision-making, and only recognize a duly appointed health care proxy.

"My wishes" and other tools to guide planning

Guidance in advance care planning is often facilitated by going through various scenarios as outlined in a worksheet or a validated tool. This provides a structure to more comprehensively elucidate and capture the patient's personal values and threshold for use of potential medical interventions. One of the most widely used tools for advance care planning is a process entitled "Five Wishes" and, more recently, a version for children, entitled "My Wishes." Five Wishes was introduced in 1997 and originally distributed with support from a grant by the Robert Wood Johnson Foundation. It has now been broadly implemented, currently exists in 26 languages, and is legally valid under the advance directive statutes in most states. It is designed to be an advance directive/living will that addresses the full range of a person's concerns, not just the medical and legal ones. For example, matters of comfort, dignity, pain management, personal and spiritual issues, family

reconciliation, and memorial matters are all addressed (Aging with Dignity, 2010).

No matter how thorough they are, however, as a practical matter advance directives cannot anticipate all possible circumstances. The legally authorized surrogate and the physician must often extrapolate from the advance directive to the current situation, and apply this as the basis for substituted reasoning about what the patient would want.

Principles for surrogate decision-making

What is the hierarchy of guidance in the advance planning process? The generally accepted order is that a legally developed instructional directive should guide decision-making and be followed as the most authoritative indication of the patient's wishes when they exist. Next in the hierarchy of guidance is substituted judgment, which should be utilized when there is no instructional directive, but a duly appointed surrogate possesses sufficient relevant knowledge of the patient values. Third would be the "best interest" standard, which applies when there is no advance directive and no surrogate with knowledge of the patient's relevant preferences and values. Actual circumstances often do not present themselves as neatly as this ranking suggests, and it is often necessary to utilize a combined approach. For example, even if an instructional directive exists it may not clearly address the circumstances at hand and thus it may be necessary to rely more heavily on substituted judgment reasoning by the surrogate (Appelbaum & Grisso, 1988; Meisel & Cerminara, 2010).

Equally important, clinicians must understand the proper role of surrogates. This is necessary both to provide the surrogate with guidance, as well as to recognize that there are limits to the surrogate's decision-making authority and to ensure that these limits are not exceeded. Typical durable powers of attorney for health care, for example, explicitly deny to the surrogate any authority to make decisions in conflict with the patient's known wishes or, if the patient's wishes are not known, that conflict with the patient's fundamental interests. When there is a serious question about the appropriateness of the surrogate's decision, the physician should explore the decision with the surrogate and other family members. If that does not resolve the issue, consultation with a clinical ethics committee or, if necessary, appeal to the courts for the purpose of appointing a different surrogate to protect the patient's interests may be necessary, although the latter is fortunately rare in actual practice (Meisel & Cerminara, 2010).

Advance directives for the pediatric patient

The process of advance care planning for the pediatric patient works in much the same way for young children as for the adult patient. The patient's parents, as the legal surrogate decision-makers, are ideally provided with the information and guidance they need to reflect on their child's prognosis and potential treatment options, enabling them to select treatment options they believe to be in the child's best interests. Deference to parents' decisions for their children is based, not merely on their legal status, but as well on the recognition that a child's parents are almost always in the best position to determine the best interests of their child (AAP, 1995). One notable exception to this general rule is children in the custody of the state, for whom parents are no longer the child's legal surrogate decision-makers. Depending on state law, decisions about whether to limit life-sustaining treatments such as CPR (cardiopulmonary resuscitation) for a child who is a ward of the state may be made by responsible persons in the state Department of Health and Human Services, by the court, or by a court-appointed guardian.

Advance directives for the adolescent patient

Advance care planning for the adolescent patient requires special considerations. More than 3000 adolescents in the United States die annually from the effects of chronic illness, and while adolescents lack the strict legal authority to make binding medical decisions for themselves (including decisions to discontinue life-sustaining treatment), many, if not most, will meet all of the necessary cognitive and emotional criteria for having the capability to do so. In such situations, a broad ethical and medical consensus supports respecting the decisional authority of the mature minor patient. For example, the American Academy of Pediatrics and the Institute of Medicine both support advance care planning as determined by the input of the adolescent patient (AAP, 1995; IOM, 1997; Field & Behrman, 2002).

Legally, certain minors under the age of 18 are deemed "emancipated" and treated as adults for all purposes. Definitions of the emancipated minor may include those who are: (1) self-supporting and/or not living at home; (2) married; (3) pregnant or a parent; (4) in the military; or (5) declared to be emancipated by a court. Second, many states give decision-making authority (without the need for parental involvement) to some minors who are otherwise unemancipated but who have decision-making capacity ("mature minors") or who are seeking treatment for certain medical conditions, such as sexually transmitted diseases, pregnancy, and drug or alcohol abuse. Recent legislation in a number of states grants mature minors the right to initiate advance directives and make independent end-of-life decisions.

Strong moral arguments exist for taking serious account of the adolescent's treatment preferences, even when full decisional authority is not appropriate. This sentiment is well supported by the Committee on Bioethics of the American Academy of Pediatrics in a policy statement entitled "Informed Consent, Parental Permission, and Assent in Pediatrics" where they write, "Decision-making involving the health care of older children and adolescents should include, to the greatest extent feasible, the assent of the patient as well as the participation of the parents and the physician. Pediatricians should not necessarily treat children as rational, autonomous decision makers, but they should give serious consideration to each patient's developing capacities for participating in decision-making … If physicians recognize the importance of assent, they empower children to the extent of their capacity" (AAP, 1995).

DNR orders: the first advance directive?

The DNR order can be seen as among the first examples of advance directives. Even today it retains special symbolism in the care of the patient, but why did this form of advance directive emerge in the first place?

The absence of an established and transparent framework for resuscitation decisions in the event of cardiac arrest was an increasing concern to many health care professionals in the late 1960s and early 1970s (Burns et al., 2003). First reported in the medical literature by Kouwenhoven and colleagues in 1960, CPR as originally described was intended only for patients experiencing a witnessed cardiac arrest from an etiology thought to be easily reversible. The first description of CPR reflected precisely this context by presenting a case series of 20 patients who experienced a witnessed cardiac arrest either upon the induction of anesthesia, or upon emergence from anesthesia, at Johns Hopkins Hospital in the late 1950s. The simplicity of the technique and its application in many respects were the source of the problems that soon emerged in hospitals across the world. As there was no framework for decision-making about which patients would receive a resuscitation attempt, decisions by medical staff became increasing ad hoc, in the absence of conversations about it with the patient and family. Terms such as "chemical code," "show code," "Hollywood code," and "slow code," describing situations where the staff employed less than a full resuscitation attempt in the belief that CPR was not "beneficial," became commonplace in hospitals. Reports in the medical literature described repeated resuscitation attempts on terminally ill patients that appeared only to prolong suffering and delay death.

In 1974 the American Heart Association first proposed that decisions not to resuscitate be formally documented in progress notes and communicated to all clinical staff. This movement toward explicit DNR policies rapidly spread, with the result that medical staff now had a framework to deliberate with the patient or patient's surrogate on the rationale for attempting or withholding CPR in the event of cardiac arrest, and could have these discussions well before the event.

DNR order as threshold for discussion of the goals of therapy

As Bok noted in 1976, discussion about DNR, an order that focuses strictly on what will not be done in the specific circumstances of cardiopulmonary arrest at the very end of life, would seem to be an illogical starting point for the inherently important discussion of "what is important to you in the last few months of your child's life." Yet, in a culture that assiduously avoids contemplating death, the DNR discussion is usually an inducement for even the most reluctant parent, guardian, or clinician to articulate, in some fashion, what is important to them. Discussions with parents about resuscitation sometimes become misdirected to a focus on specific medical procedures that might be performed in the event of cardiac arrest; yet, by incorporating the principles of advance care planning, such discussions become an opportunity to elucidate the full range of possible medical treatments and comfort measures as they relate to the patient's goals. Reframing the DNR discussion away from a checklist

about specific therapies (procedure-directed/specific DNR orders), and toward a more focused discussion of the patient's goals and values (goal-directed DNR orders), appropriately reorients the role of the physician in these discussions as the medical expert about treatment alternatives, recommending treatment plans that align with the expressed goals and values of the patient. This results in a decision-making framework that focuses on learning what the patient or their surrogate values most and what goals they are trying to achieve in selecting whether CPR or a DNR order is best for their child.

The goal-directed approach to thinking about DNR decisions allows for more comprehensive treatment plans to be entertained as needed, such as in the care of patients with a DNR order who may benefit from an operative or interventional procedure. For example, the parents of a child with a terminal disorder may decide to temporarily suspend a DNR order during a surgical procedure intended to make the child more comfortable. They may agree to certain resuscitation interventions in the event that their child develops a readily reversible cardiopulmonary complication in the operating room as a result of the anesthetic or surgical procedure. This suspension of the DNR may only apply to a brief and defined period around the anesthetic for the procedure, with resumption of the DNR status immediately after an agreed upon perioperative period. For this reason, both the American Society of Anesthesiologists and the American College of Surgeons have adopted formal positions that automatic suspension of DNR orders is not appropriate and that all decisions about resuscitation status should be based on the goals of the informed patient undergoing surgery or a procedure requiring anesthesia (or their surrogate decision-maker), using the goal-directed approach outlined above (Burns et al., 2003).

DNR in the home and school

Emergency medical services (EMS) personnel were traditionally expected to initiate CPR on all persons found in cardiopulmonary arrest. As it became clear that CPR is not always a beneficial intervention in every case of cardiac arrest, and as policies permitting decisions not to resuscitate have become more widespread, all states have procedures allowing EMS personnel to be guided by out-of-hospital DNR orders. As directed by some unique identification procedure to certify the authenticity of the DNR order, most policies still allow EMS personnel to provide transport to a medical facility and care directed toward comfort only. Similarly, the validity of DNR orders in the school setting is also increasingly established. The Americans with Disabilities Act of 1990, the Education for All Handicapped Children Act of 1975, and advances in health care have allowed minors with disabilities greater access to public education. As a result, some chronically ill or technology-dependent children are at risk for having a cardiopulmonary arrest while at school. The American Academy of Pediatrics, the National Education Association, and the National Association of School Nurses all have statements affirming the inclusion of students with DNR orders in the school setting (Burns et al., 2003). Despite this, only a few state protocols for emergency medical service personnel explicitly extend out-of-hospital DNR orders to cover minors, and even fewer encompass the school setting.

Summary and case resolution

How should medical decisions for the adolescent patient described here be made? What framework for reasoning about this dilemma should be applied to guide decisions? Standard types of normative ethical theories, typically grouped as utilitarian or ends-based theories, as compared with formalist, Kantian, or duty-based theories, point to forms of reasoning about the good to be achieved (such as living longer or dying well) or the duties to be considered (such as duties to avoid harm, and duties to the patient or duties to the parents). Rules and reasoning drawn from such theoretical frameworks when applied to the case and facts at hand are referred to as "applied ethics."

Appealing directly to abstract normative theories provides little concrete guidance in specific cases; however, general ethical principles drawn from such theories emphasize common moral duties that have evolved from collective moral experience over centuries. These core principles include duties to: (1) respect the capacity of individuals to make their own decisions, choose their own vision of the good life, and act accordingly; (2) foster the interests and happiness of other persons and of society at large; (3) refrain from harming other persons; and (4) act fairly – distributing benefits and burdens in an equitable fashion, and resolving disputes by means of fair procedures (Arras & Steinbock, 1995). These principles are often identified, respectively, as the principles of autonomy, beneficence, nonmaleficence, and justice. But how are we

to weigh and balance the various principles against one another in this case? Does our duty to respect the decisions of others, especially those who most directly bear the consequences of the decision, apply to the patient or her parents? Critics of principlism argue that in actual clinical dilemmas a principle-based approach can only take us so far.

A casuist approach to moral decision-making is based on the idea that moral wisdom resides and moral reasoning emerges in our responses to paradigmatic cases, rather than in abstractions of theory or principle. By this framework, one can learn how to proceed in new cases by reflecting on the reasoning of similar past cases and the emerging consensus about end-of-life decisions over the past 40 years as part of the advance planning movement; i.e., that competent patients have a well-established moral and legal right to make their own decisions about health care. This includes the informed refusal of life-sustaining treatments. Moreover, this consensus denies the patient's surrogate any authority to make decisions in conflict with the patient's known wishes or, if they are not known, in conflict with the patient's fundamental interests. By extension of this evolved consensus, pediatric patients have the same rights, though they must be exercised by a surrogate decision-maker, usually their parents, who are presumed to be responsible for determining either what their child would want if the child could choose for herself (substituted judgment) or what would be best for the child (best interests). Health care professionals too – especially those in pediatrics and those caring for adults who cannot make their own decisions – also have a responsibility to consider and advocate for what they believe to be in the best medical interests of their pediatric patients.

Whether proceeding from a principle of autonomy or the casuistic reasoning pattern of similar cases, both approaches require assessment of this 16-year-old patient's decisional capacity at the time she made these statements. Was she adversely affected by her advanced illness or medications or some combination of the two? Was there any known or suspected psychiatric illness at the time? If the answer to these questions is affirmative, then the weight we attach to her statements is less because she would be less cognitively capable of reasoning about the various alternatives for care and the benefits and risks associated with each, of applying her own values and vision of a good life and death, or of arriving at an enduring decision. On the other hand, if her statements reflect a well-informed understanding of the risks and benefits of lung transplant and beliefs about the value of various treatments as her illness has evolved (preferably, as corroborated by clinicians with a longstanding relationship), then her decision should be respected, despite the possibility that she may die without a lung transplant. An adolescent who has weighed the burdens of illness, especially in the case of those with a life-shortening illness such as cystic fibrosis, should be given great deference if their articulated advance directive about medical decisions is based on accurate information about the risks and benefits of potential therapies, unclouded by acute illnesses or medications.

If possible, a joint discussion with the patient, her parents, and the relevant clinicians should take place immediately before this patient loses effective decisional capacity from illness progression and intubation for mechanical ventilation (AAP, 1994). If this is not possible, or if such a discussion does not resolve the issue, the physician should discuss the patient's expressed advance directive with her parents and all longstanding clinicians in an attempt to reach consensus about honoring the treatment decisions expressed by the adolescent. If that does not resolve the issue, the next step would involve consultation with a medical ethics committee or, if necessary, appeal to the courts to either seek a determination that the adolescent is a mature minor or to seek the appointment of a different surrogate decision-maker to work with the physician to protect the patient's interest.

References

Aging with Dignity (2010). Five wishes. Available at www.agingwithdignity.org. Last accessed February 1, 2011.

American Academy of Pediatrics (AAP), Committee on Bioethics (1994). Guidelines on foregoing life-sustaining medical treatment. *Pediatrics*, **93**(3), 532–536.

American Academy of Pediatrics (AAP), Committee on Bioethics (1995). Informed consent, parental permission, and assent in pediatric practice. *Pediatrics*, **95**(2), 314–317.

American Heart Association (1974). Standards and guidelines for cardiopulmonary resuscitation (CPR) and emergency cardiac care (ECC): medicolegal considerations and recommendations. *JAMA*, **227**(Suppl), 864–866.

Appelbaum, P. & Grisso, T. (1988). Assessing patients' capacity to consent to treatment. *New England Journal of Medicine*, **319**, 1635–1638.

Arras, J.D. & Steinbock, B. (1995). Moral reasoning in the medical context. In *Ethical Issues in Modern Medicine*, ed. J.D. Arras & B. Steinbock. Mountain View: Mayfield Publishing Co., 1–39.

Bok, S. (1976). Personal directives for care at the end of life. *New England Journal of Medicine*, **295**, 367–369.

Burns, J.P., Edwards, J., Johnson, J., Cassem, N.H., & Truog, R.D. (2003). Do-not-resuscitate order after 25 years. *Critical Care Medicine*, **31**, 1543–1550.

Clinical Care Committee of the Massachusetts General Hospital (1976). Optimum care for hopelessly ill patients: a report of the Clinical Care Committee of the Massachusetts General Hospital. *New England Journal of Medicine*, **295**, 362–364.

Field, M.J. & Behrman, R.E. (eds.), Committee on Palliative and End-of-Life Care for Children and Their Families, Board on Health Sciences Policy (2002). *When Children Die: Improving Palliative and End-of-Life Care for Children and their Families*. Washington, DC: National Academies Press.

Fried, C. (1976). Terminating life support: out of the closet! *New England Journal of Medicine*, **295**, 390–391.

Institute of Medicine (IOM), Committee on Care at the End of Life (Field, M.J. & Cassel, C.K., eds.) (1997). *Approaching Death: Improving Care at the End of Life*. Washington, DC: National Academy Press.

Kouwenhoven, W.B., Jude, J.R., & Knickerbocker, G.G. (1960). Closed-chest cardiac massage. *JAMA*, **173**, 1064–1067.

Meisel, A. & Cerminara, K.L. (2010). Decisionmaking standards for incompetent patients. In *The Right to Die*, 3rd edn. Frederick, MD: Aspen.

President's Commission for the Study of Ethical Problems in Medicine and Biomedical and Behavioral Research (1983). *Deciding to Forego Life-Sustaining Treatment*. Washington, DC: US Government Printing Office. Available at http://bioethics.georgetown.edu/pcbe/reports/past_commissions/deciding_to_forego_tx.pdf. Last accessed February 1, 2011.

Rabkin, M.T., Gillerman, G., & Rice N.R. (1976). Orders not to resuscitate. *New England Journal of Medicine*, **295**, 364–366.

Chapter

21

The determination of death

Geoffrey Miller

Case narrative

She had planned to leave him; take her 3-year-old son somewhere safe. Her husband (the child's father) returned to the apartment in the early evening in the full throes of a paranoid psychosis, fueled by a prolonged binge on alcohol and methamphetamine. The mother and child were found the following morning. She was in a coma, suffering from hemorrhage of her liver and spleen after blows to her head had caused loss of consciousness and kicks to her abdomen had ruptured organs. The boy was also comatose. He had struck the side of his head on the edge of a wall, thrown there by his father after trying to intervene. His extradural hemorrhage had plenty of time to expand, and his brain to shift, herniate, and infarct. The diagnosis was not difficult for the neurosurgery or emergency room teams, but following surgery, the boy arrested in the recovery room and, although eventually resuscitated, was asystolic for at least 30 minutes. He was now intubated, ventilated and receiving full vasopressor support. Twelve hours later, a rigorous examination showed no signs of brain activity, and a repeat examination 30 hours later was unchanged. The boy's next of kin was the father, the violent offender, recently arrested and placed in jail. The paternal grandparents were constantly present at the child's bedside, often praying together. They did not believe the child was dead as he was clearly warm, breathing with a ventilator, and had a heartbeat.

Introduction of issues and historical context

The question that is raised in this chapter is whether we can and ought to declare death when we reliably recognize the existence of brain death, or total brain failure that is irreversible. It is not the concept and consequences of death which are in question. Death is existential, an inevitable part of living. Its consequences may be viewed differently, but its existence is certain. These consequences may be interpreted as biological by medical scientists, or simply as a transition in religious traditions (Miller & Ashwal, 2009). Philosophers might state that it is the loss of a person's interests and obligations owed them as these depend on qualities possessed only by the living, and the anthropologist will appreciate the customs, norms, rituals, and prohibitions that surround death, as well as the initiation of a social event and a ceremonial process (Kaufmann, 2003). Legally its determination is required to allow burial or cremation, an autopsy, organ transplantation, inheritance, and when a spouse may remarry. It may also trigger an investigation as to whether the death was criminal or accidental, natural or suicide.

Historically death was recognized when the heart stopped beating, breathing ceased, and the individual was unconscious and unresponsive. When a person was found in this state, a state resembling death, the passage of time would confirm the situation and a physician was not necessarily involved. As medical expertise and understanding increased, the cardiopulmonary criteria for death became easier to confirm. However, as medical technology improved it became possible to maintain respiratory and cardiac function where previously this would not have been possible (Miller & Ashwal, 2009). Medical intervention was often able to maintain respiration and circulation in the unconscious, brain-damaged patient, and by the 1950s there was an acknowledgment that absence of brain function – particularly when the pathological state of the brain was such that life could be maintained only by artificial means – might signify death (Mollard & Goulon, 1995). During the next decade an Ad Hoc Committee of the Harvard Medical School (1968) described this pathological state of irreversible

Clinical Ethics in Pediatrics: A Case-Based Textbook, ed. Douglas D. Diekema, Mark R. Mercurio and Mary B. Adam. Published by Cambridge University Press. (c) Cambridge University Press 2011.

coma and proposed a definition of brain death. Loss of somatic integration underpinned the reasons for describing brain death as an acceptable way to recognize death. Brain death was the irreversible loss of total brain function and was equivalent to a cardiopulmonary death as there was loss of integrative unity of the organism (Truog, 2007; Shewmon, 2009). It was believed that once brain death had occurred it was a matter of limited time before the rest of the body would stop functioning. But as Shewmon reported (2009), some patients with total loss of brain function who were maintained on ventilators and other supports can continue to physiologically function and were not the same as "non-heart-beating corpses." Furthermore, several critical brain structures may remain viable and continue integrative neurological functioning after clinically determined brain death. These include, among others, electroencephalogram activity, brainstem auditory and somatosensory-evoked potentials, and hypothalamic function (Verheijde et al., 2009). Despite this, the two standards for determining death – the cardiopulmonary standard and the brain death standard – were readily accepted. More recently there has been renewed criticism of the brain death standard (Verheijde et al., 2009). Agreed upon criteria for the determination of death are not required when death is obvious, as occurs when one is confronted with a decapitated or decomposed body or when a body demonstrates the signs that occur after death such as *algor mortis, livor mortis, rigor mortis*, and putrefaction. We do want to know when death occurs, but in particular we want to know when we are able to declare that it has occurred. It is this ability that has been affected by time and technology. I will argue for the continued use of the concept of brain death as equivalent to cardiopulmonary death based on its operational usefulness and its moral rightness in that it can provide good in the absence of harm and, for most, there is no offense to intuition or moral sense (Miller & Ashwal, 2009).

Diagnosis of death

To diagnose death requires that it be understood as a biological phenomenon that can be reliably and repeatedly determined. There should be standards, a cardiopulmonary standard and a brain death standard, and criteria for these standards. The cardiopulmonary standard requires the irreversible cessation of cardiac and respiratory function and will ultimately lead to brain death. Brain death is the irreversible cessation of whole brain function, which would be followed by the cessation of cardiopulmonary function provided artificial measures are not instituted. In the United Kingdom brain death is viewed as equivalent to brainstem death because whole brain function cannot be sustained when there is complete absence of brainstem function. The finding of some non-functional activity in the heart or the brain following a diagnosis, using standardized methods, that death has occurred does not negate the diagnosis of death. The point at which we can reliably, reasonably, and acceptably recognize and declare death is the point at which the functional cessation of all organs is unpreventable and inevitable. Accepting two means of recognizing death does not imply that there are two forms of biological death, only that there are two forms of recognition (Bernat, 2002).

Some believe that irreversible neocortical death, even with functional brainstem activity, is equivalent to a biological cardiopulmonary death (Laureys, 2005; Veatch, 1975). It is understood as a philosophical or social death. But the recognition of neocortical death is neither reliable nor generally accepted. Because the determination of death serves a social function as well as a medical one, it requires that the methods we choose are reliable, repeatable and predictable, and involve criteria that are accepted by the wider community as representative of death and being dead. A higher (neocortical) brain standard would most likely not be acceptable to the wider community, since it would potentially allow burial of bodies that were warm with still-beating hearts. While spiritual, cultural, legal, and philosophical concepts of death are important in their own contexts, they are not necessarily relevant to the biological concept of death, which should be unambiguous and rest on the determination of irreversibility (Bernat, 2002). Necessary criteria for determining death include reaching a point of no return; that the point of no return is associated with a loss of function of the human organism as a whole (President's Council on Bioethics, 2008); irreversible loss of consciousness and irreversible apnea; and that this point is one at which no one has ever been revived. Death is the point at which those criteria are met. It is not the process leading up to that point – that is dying – nor is it the biological changes which follow that point.

The clinical criteria used to determine brain death can be reliable and repeatable. As a means for determining death, these criteria have proven to be acceptable to the general public and political bodies, although there is variability in their performance (American

119

Academy of Neurology, 1995; Canadian Neurocritical Care Group, 1999; Haupt & Rudolf, 1999; Wijdicks, 2007). The core features of the clinical determination of brain death are similar worldwide but there are variations (Miller & Ashwal, 2009). These variations include the need for and type of ancillary testing; performance recommendations for tests such as the apnea test; the required numbers of physicians involved; and differing hospital policies. Variability has also been found in brain death determinations in children (Mejia & Pollack, 1995; Joffe & Anton, 2006; Greer et al., 2008; Mathur et al., 2008). This variability is poorly explained and does not have a firm empirical explanation or scientific basis (Baron et al., 2006; Wijdicks, 2006). It is important ethically that the practice is standardized and rests on sound empirical grounds. Recently the Society of Critical Care Medicine and the American Academy of Pediatrics published amended guidelines for the determination of brain death in children (Nakagawa et al., 2011). They endorsed the view that brain death is a clinical diagnosis characterized by the absence of brain function that has resulted in irreversible coma and the following six necessary requirements: (1) establish an irreversible and proximate cause of coma; (2) normal core temperature; (3) normal blood pressure for age of child; (4) normal metabolic parameters; (5) examination unaffected by medication; (6) a neurological examination which should establish coma, absence of brainstem reflexes, and apnea. The details of how these requirements are achieved are described in the guidelines. Two examinations plus apnea testing with each are required. The examinations should be performed by different attending physicians, but the apnea tests can be performed by the same physician. The observation periods are 24 hours for term newborns up to 30 days old, and 12 hours for older infants and children. Assessment of neurologic function following cardiopulmonary resuscitation or severe acute brain injury should be deferred for 24 hours. Apnea testing must be performed safely and requires adequate oxygenation (techniques for this are described) and an arterial pCO_2 20 mmHg above baseline and equal to or greater than 60 mmHg. A positive test occurs when there is no respiratory effort. If an apnea test cannot be completed safely, an ancillary test such as cerebral blood flow estimation using angiography or radionuclide scanning, or an electroencephalogram should be performed. Ancillary tests are not required to establish brain death and should only be used if the apnea test cannot be completed or there is uncertainty about the neurological examination. The purpose of the first examination is to establish brain death; the purpose of the second examination is to show that the findings are unchanging. There are no reports of infants or children recovering neurological function after meeting brain death criteria when the present accepted medical standards for its diagnosis were met (Ashwal, 2001).

In many international jurisdictions the law sets the general legal standard for determining death, but not the medical criteria (Miller & Ashwal, 2009). In the United States the Uniform Determination of Death Act states that, "An individual who has satisfied either (1) irreversible cessation of circulatory and respiratory function, or (2) irreversible cessation of all functions of the entire brain, including the brain stem, is dead. A determination of death must be made in accordance with acceptable medical standards." Thus, medical science is left to determine the criteria by which the legal standard is met. In the United States, all states recognize that brain death is legal death, but in New York State and New Jersey a religious exemption is allowed. In these states if a family does not accept the concept of brain death, they can demand that cardiopulmonary criteria be met before a declaration of death.

The cultural and societal importance of the diagnosis of death

When death occurs or someone is declared dead, it initiates many actions of social and legal importance to the family and the community in which the deceased lived. Arguments about whether death is a process or an event (Morrison, 1971), while of interest, operationally "miss the point," failing to recognize what is important about the general use of the term death: it initiates a cascade of events related to mourning and remembrance rituals, burial and funeral arrangements, legal recognition of a person's death and the concomitant implications for inheritance, public benefits, and transfers of power or role. Precision in the timing of death may be important legally or in clinical situations, but for the general public, recognizing the time of death is more a matter of consensus than mathematical certitude and rests upon acceptability of the methods used to determine death and the belief that the findings are irreversible. Put another way, whether physicians use a cardiopulmonary standard or a neurological standard to declare death, the accepted criteria must be followed unfailingly and must irreversibly be associated with death in order for trust to be maintained. This is particularly important if organ donation will be considered, since most communities will not find organ donation acceptable unless it is preceded by death and living people are not killed for their organs (Robertson, 1999; Huddle et al., 2008).

Not every society has recognized that brain death is equivalent to death. In the 1990s the Danish Council of Ethics declared that the irreversible loss of cardiac function was necessary to declare death and that when brain death occurs while a patient is on a ventilator, death cannot be declared until the ventilator is removed and cardiac function has ceased irreversibly (Rix, 1990). Under those circumstances, cardiac transplantation would not be possible. A similar situation existed in Japan during the same time period (Miller & Ashwal, 2009). However, a recent Japanese organ transplant law acknowledges brain death in a person of any age to constitute human death, but only when a transplant is to be performed, the family agrees to the transplant, and the potential donor had not objected to becoming a donor previously. While this approach may not quite be coherent, it is certainly pragmatic and reasonable, and seeks to accommodate different acceptable ethical views.

The concept of brain death and its equivalence to human death is widely accepted, but there are detractors (Seifert, 1993; Shewmon, 2001; Laureys, 2005). Their objections are based upon reports of artificially maintained cardiopulmonary function for prolonged periods in individuals who met the criteria for brain death, as well as the maintenance of pregnancy in and the delivery of an infant from a woman who was brain dead (Loewy, 1987; Kantor & Hoskins, 1993; Feldman et al., 2000). Shewmon (1998) reports that, given the right circumstances, brain death is not the same as the complete cessation of functioning of the organism, and he provocatively uses the term "chronic brain death." Taylor (1997) supports this argument and states that brain death is really only "near death" and is a legal fiction that allows for organ procurement and transplant. Shewmon (1998) persuasively argues that the continuation of integrative bodily functions after brain death is not an irreversible loss of integrative unity of the organism. Because of this, a recent President's Council on Bioethics report (2008) suggested the use of the term total brain failure instead of brain death. The concept of the loss of integrated somatic functioning was also rejected. However, the report stated that irreversible total brain failure could "serve as a criterion for declaring death" because "it is a sign that the organism can

no longer engage in the essential work that defines living things" which includes the ability to breathe and to be conscious. Irreversible loss of both of these constitutes loss of the organism as a whole (Shewmon, 2009). The meaning of the term "as a whole" could be argued, but these arguments become specious and irrelevant. The irreversible loss of consciousness with no ability to breathe independently sets in motion a process that is readily recognized biologically, philosophically, anthropologically, and socially as that which occurs after death.

Conclusion

Irreversible brain death or total brain failure may not be recognized by everyone as equivalent to cardiopulmonary death, and this should be respected. While some argue that technological support can forestall death, others argue that technology simply masks it (President's Council on Bioethics, 2008; Shewmon, 2009). The important question is whether we allow death to be declared in circumstances where there is irreversible total brain failure with absence of consciousness and irreversible apnea, provided certain provisions are met and accepted clinical procedures are followed. The declaration of death is not necessarily the time when there is total cessation of all physiological processes that occur in the living body. The precise moment when this happens is difficult, if not impossible, to identify easily. However, we can identify the point at which this will inevitably occur. Brain death criteria reliably identify that point, and represent an ethically appropriate means to determine death.

References

Ad Hoc Committee of the Harvard Medical School (1968). A definition of irreversible coma; report of the Ad Hoc Committee of the Harvard Medical School to examine the definition of brain death. *JAMA*, **205**, 337–340.

American Academy of Neurology, Quality Standards Subcommittee (1995). Practical parameters for determining brain death in adults. *Neurology*, **45**, 1012–1014.

Ashwal, S. (2001). Clinical diagnosis and confirmatory testing of brain death in children. In *Brain Death*, ed. E.F.M. Wijdick. Philadelphia, PA: Lippincott, Williams & Wilkins, 91–114.

Baron, L., Shemie, S.O., Teitelbaum, J., & Doig, C.J. (2006). Brief review: history, concept and controversies in the neurological determination of death. *Canadian Journal of Anaesthesia*, **53**, 602–608.

Bernat, J.L. (2002). The biophilosophical basis of whole-brain death. *Social Philosophy and Policy Foundation*, **12**, 324–342.

Canadian Neurocritical Care Group (1999). Guidelines for the diagnosis of brain death. *Canadian Journal of Neurological Sciences*, **26**, 64–66.

Feldman, D.M., Borgida, A.F., Rodis, J.F., & Campbell, W.A. (2000). Irreversible maternal brain injury during pregnancy: a case report and review of the literature. *Obstetrical and Gynecological Survey*, **55**, 708–714.

Greer, D.M., Varelas, P.N., Haque, S., & Wijdicks, E.F.M. (2008). Variability of brain death determination guidelines in leading US neurologic institutions. *Neurology*, **70**, 284–289.

Haupt, W.F. & Rudolf, J. (1999). European brain death codes: a comparison of national guidelines. *Journal of Neurology*, **246**, 432–437.

Huddle, T.S., Schwartz, M.A., Bailey, F.A., & Bos, M.A. (2008). Death, organ transplantation and medical practice. *Philosophy, Ethics and Humanities in Medicine*, **3**, 1–5.

Joffe, A.R. & Anton, N. (2006). Brain death: understanding of the conceptual basis by pediatric intensivists in Canada. *Archives of Pediatrics and Adolescent Medicine*, **160**, 747–751.

Kantor, J.E. & Hoskins, I. (1993). Brain death in pregnant women. *Journal of Clinical Ethics*, **4**, 308–314.

Kaufmann, S.R. (2003). Dying and death. In *Encyclopedia of Medical Anthropology*, ed. C.R. Ember & M. Ember. New York: Kluwer Academic, 245.

Laureys, S. (2005). Death, unconsciousness and the brain. *Nature Reviews Neuroscience*, **6**, 899–909.

Loewy, E.H. (1987). The pregnant brain dead and the fetus: must we always try to wrest life from death? *American Journal of Obstetrics and Gynecology*, **157**, 1097–1101.

Mathur, M., Petersen, L., Stadfler, M., et al. (2008). Variability in pediatric brain death determination and documentation in Southern California. *Pediatrics*, **121**, 988–993.

Mejia, R.E. & Pollack, M.M. (1995). Variability in brain death determination practices in children. *JAMA*, **274**, 550–553.

Miller, G. & Ashwal, S. (2009). Brain death, minimal consciousness, and vegetative states in children. In *Pediatric Bioethics*, ed. G. Miller. New York: Cambridge University Press, 247–261.

Mollard, P. & Goulon, M. (1995). Le coma depasse [in French]. *Revue Neurologique*, **101**, 3–15.

Morrison, R.S. (1971). Death: process or event? *Science*, **173**, 694–698.

Nakagawa, T.A., Ashwal, S., Mathur, M., & Mysore, M. and the Committee for Determination of Brain Death in Infants and Children, Society of Critical Care Medicine and the American Academy of Pediatrics (2011). Guidelines for determination of brain death in infants and children: an update of the 1987 Task Force recommendations. *Critical Care Medicine*, 2011; in press.

President's Council on Bioethics (2008). *Controversies in the Determination of Death*. Washington, DC: Government Publishing Office.

Rix, B.A. (1990). Danish ethics council rejects brain death as the criterion of death. *Journal of Medical Ethics*, **16**, 5–7.

Robertson, J.A. (1999). The dead donor rule. *Hastings Center Report*, **6**, 6–14.

Seifert, J. (1993). Is "brain death" actually death? *Monis*, **76**, 175–202.

Shewmon, D.A. (1998). Chronic "brain death": meta-analysis and conceptual consequences. *Neurology*, **51**, 1538–1545.

Shewmon, D.A. (2001). The brain and somatic integration: insights into the standard biological rationale for equating "brain death" with death. *Journal of Medicine and Philosophy*, **26**, 457–478.

Shewmon, D.A. (2009). Brain death. Can it be resuscitated? *Issues in Law & Medicine*, **25**, 3–14.

Taylor, R.M. (1997). Re-examining the definition and criterion of death. *Seminars in Neurology*, **17**, 265–270.

Truog, R. (2007). Brain death – too flawed to endure, too ingrained to abandon. *Journal of Law, Medicine and Ethics*, **35**, 273–281.

Veatch, R.M. (1975). The whole-brain oriented concept of death: an outmoded philosophical formulation. *Journal of Thanatology*, **3**, 13–30.

Verheijde, J.L., Rady, M.Y., & McGregor, J.L. (2009). Brain death states of impaired consciousness, and physician-assisted death for end-of-life organ donation and transplantation. *Medicine, Health Care and Philosophy*, **12**, 409–421.

Wijdicks, E.F.M. (2006). The clinical criteria of brain death throughout the world: why has it come to this? *Canadian Journal of Anaesthesia*, **53**, 540–543.

Wijdicks, E.F.M. (2007). The diagnosis of brain death. *New England Journal of Medicine*, **344**, 1215–1221.

Chapter

22

Physician-assisted dying in children

Alexander A. Kon

Case narrative

Zak was a happy, healthy 3-year-old boy. One morning, Zak's parents had difficulty waking him. They noted some spots on Zak's chest and face, and thought that he had a mild viral infection. As the day progressed, Zak became increasingly lethargic and the spots increased, so his mother brought him to the doctor. The pediatrician was very concerned and activated the emergency medical services. Zak was taken to a local emergency department where he was quickly diagnosed with meningococcal septic shock. Appropriate therapies were initiated and Zak was transported to the regional pediatric intensive care unit (PICU).

In the PICU, Zak continued to receive appropriate treatment. His parents remained at his bedside and were clearly loving and very concerned for their child's welfare. After several days, it was apparent that the septic emboli (which are the hallmark of meningococcal sepsis) had blocked blood flow in many of Zak's capillary beds. In addition to renal and hepatic impairment, Zak's hands and feet had obvious signs of necrosis, and it was assumed that there were infarcted areas in his brain (although this could not be confirmed because he was not stable enough to move to the scanner).

Zak's condition stabilized and the clinicians were able to wean him off vasoactive medications and the ventilator. Because Zak had been on analgesic and anxiolytic medications for some time, his medications were gradually weaned to avoid opiate and benzodiazepine withdrawal. As the narcotic doses were decreased, Zak appeared uncomfortable. He moaned and writhed on his bed.

Additionally, the necrosis on his extremities placed him at risk for developing secondary infections. Because the dead tissue would never regenerate, it was recommended that one foot be amputated at the ankle,

the other foot amputated at mid-calf, his right hand amputated at the elbow, and three fingers amputated from his left hand.

Zak's parents agonized over his condition. They loved their son, and wanted him to recover and live a long and healthy life, but what kind of a life would he have? A life with such severe amputations. A life with potential long-lasting renal and hepatic impairment. A life with uncertain neurological sequelae. As they watched Zak suffer in the PICU bed, moaning constantly, thrashing wildly, they wept. How they hated to watch him suffer so.

After many hours of discussion, the parents finally decided that letting Zak continue to suffer in this way was inhumane. Together, they asked the PICU attending physician to help end Zak's suffering. Since his body no longer required vasoactive medications or mechanical ventilation, there was no life support to withdraw. The only option that they felt would end Zak's suffering was to administer a lethal injection. They wanted to hold their beloved child during this process so that they could be with him and love him during his death. They made this request out of love and compassion for their son; no one in the PICU believed otherwise.

When a child suffers unbearably

Unfortunately, Zak's story is not unique. Many infants and children suffer tremendously in neonatal intensive care units (NICUs) and PICUs. In some units, almost every day there is at least one patient for whom parents and/or staff wonder whether ongoing life-prolonging measures are justified. Statements like "we're torturing him" and "keeping him on the ventilator is just cruel" are not uncommon. For many of these children, parents and health care providers decide that withdrawing life-prolonging interventions is

Clinical Ethics in Pediatrics: A Case-Based Textbook, ed. Douglas S. Diekema, Mark R. Mercurio and Mary B. Adam. Published by Cambridge University Press. © Cambridge University Press 2011.

appropriate. It is now well accepted that withdrawing vasoactive medications or extubating a child's trachea when doing so will certainly lead to death can be ethically justifiable (Mercurio et al., 2008). Infants and children can generally be made comfortable throughout the dying process using state-of-the-art palliative treatment interventions (Catlin & Carter, 2002; Kon & Ablin, 2009, 2010). Some children die quickly after life-prolonging interventions are withdrawn; others live hours or days.

Other children, however, do not require medical technology to survive. Like Zak, some children who are able to maintain circulation, oxygenation, and ventilation without medical intervention also suffer greatly. For these children, there is often no "good" option. Although discontinuation of medically administered nutrition and hydration is ethically permissible in many cases (Diekema et al., 2009), children can often survive for weeks without nutrition and hydration. Although palliative sedation (sometimes referred to as terminal sedation) can be used to minimize suffering during the dying process, there is reason to believe that a significant minority (perhaps as many as 20% of patients) may suffer considerably in spite of such medication (Davis, 2009).

Because the dying process may be quite prolonged, and children may suffer during this process, some have advocated for actively hastening the child's death in order to alleviate suffering. This option has been proposed for children who remain in the hospital setting as well as for children cared for at home or in chronic care facilities.

Forms of physician-assisted dying

Methods of physician-assisted dying (PAD) may be separated into two categories based on who administers the lethal compound. In self-administered physician-assisted dying (SAPAD), it is the patient who performs the final act of administering the lethal dose. This may be accomplished in several ways. The patient's physician may write a prescription for a lethal dose of an approved medication, and the patient then fills the prescription and self-administers the lethal dose. Alternatively, the physician may set up an intravenous line with a lethal compound that is administered when the patient presses a button. This category has also been referred to as physician-assisted suicide; however, due to the pejorative connotations of that term many who advocate for legalization of this option prefer the term SAPAD.

The term euthanasia (or active euthanasia) is used to indicate the other category of PAD in which the lethal compound is administered by someone other than the patient. Under the umbrella of euthanasia, there are three sub-categories: voluntary active euthanasia (VAE), non-voluntary euthanasia (NVE), and involuntary euthanasia (Brock, 1992). In VAE the physician and patient discuss the available options, they agree that VAE is the best alternative, and the physician administers a lethal compound with the informed consent of the patient. When the patient is incompetent, the surrogate decision-maker(s) discusses the options with the patient's physician and they decide that euthanasia is the best option for the patient. The physician (or someone else) then administers a lethal compound with the informed permission of the surrogate(s). Because the patient does not consent to the euthanasia, this option is termed NVE. When the patient does not wish to be euthanized and is euthanized against his/her will it is termed involuntary euthanasia.

It should be noted, however, that the ethical distinction between SAPAD and VAE is tenuous. Brock (1992) argued that the individual who actually administers the lethal compound has little moral importance. Indeed, if one accepts SAPAD as ethically permissible, significant ethical concerns arise if patients who are unable to self-administer medications are denied access to PAD (e.g., if a patient who is quadriplegic would otherwise meet criteria for SAPAD but is unable to self-administer the lethal compound, to deny him/her appropriate intervention based solely on their physical disability would be untenable). As such, Brock (1992) argued that if one accepts SAPAD as ethically permissible, VAE must also be deemed permissible.

This chapter will focus solely on PAD in children. There is a tremendous body of literature on PAD in adult patients; however, a recitation of those writings is beyond the scope of this chapter. For the sake of brevity and clarity, this chapter will focus on the ethical issues of PAD in children in the context of ethically permissible PAD in competent adult patients who have decisional capacity. Clearly, there remains significant debate and disagreement regarding the permissibility of PAD in the care of competent adults; however, this chapter is written under the assumption that PAD may be permissible in some cases because if PAD is considered impermissible in competent adult patients who have decisional capacity, then it would seem unreasonable to ever consider PAD permissible in the care of children.

Ethical arguments in support of physician-assisted dying

Much of the ethical literature in support of PAD focuses on two basic values: individual self-determination (related to the principle of respect for patient autonomy) and individual well-being (related to the principle of beneficence) (Brock, 1992; Emanuel, 1994). In the case of a competent adult patient who, when fully informed, wishes to hasten their death, PAD may be ethically permissible based on the argument that the physician's participation in PAD supports the patient's ability to decide what happens to their body (i.e., individual self-determination). PAD may also be seen as enhancing individual well-being if the patient and physician agree that the patient's suffering outweighs the benefits of living. In such cases, it may be in the patient's best interest to hasten death.

PAD may be viewed as therapeutic (and therefore as medically indicated) in a small group of cases. If (1) a patient is suffering unbearably (Dees et al., 2010; Kon & Ablin, 2010), (2) the agreed upon goal of treatment is alleviating that suffering, (3) all attempts to alleviate suffering have failed to reduce it to a tolerable level, and (4) suffering will end only upon death, then the only medical intervention that will further the stated goal of treatment is PAD (Kon & Ablin, 2010).

PAD for minors with decisional capacity

Although patients under the age of majority are generally incompetent by law (i.e., they lack the legal authority to consent for medical procedures), many have decisional capacity. Older adolescents may have already developed adult levels of comprehension and decision-making ability, and even younger children who live with chronic illness often have an ability to understand medical information and appreciate the ramifications of medical decision-making well beyond "healthy" children of similar age.

Decisional capacity encompasses four elements: the ability to understand the relevant information, an appreciation of the current situation and the consequences of choice-making, the ability to manipulate information rationally, and the ability to make a choice and state it clearly (Applebaum & Grisso, 1988; Grisso et al., 1997). If a minor meets criteria for decisional capacity, it can be argued that they have a right to autonomous decision-making. Because minors lack capacity, however, their right to have their autonomy respected is limited.

Although lacking competence, a minor with decisional capacity may actively participate in the shared decision-making process. If PAD is chosen and if that choice is fully informed and voluntary, then PAD would be ethically similar to SAPAD or VAE for an adult patient. Certainly, there are other factors of great importance when considering SAPAD or VAE in a minor. The patient's guardian(s) must ensure that the decisions made are appropriate and consistent with the child's best interest. When a child is in favor of PAD and the parents are opposed to such intervention, PAD may be unjustifiable (Ross, 2009). However, if the competent minor and parents are in agreement that PAD is preferable to other medical interventions, then SAPAD or VAE may be ethically permissible. Indeed, VAE has been available to adolescents in the Netherlands since 2002. The Termination of Life on Request and Assisted Suicide (Review Procedures) Act 2002 specifies that children as young as 12 years of age qualify for VAE if the child asks for it and the parents agree.

PAD for children who lack decisional capacity and who are terminally ill

Children who are terminally ill and near death may suffer tremendously. Data suggest that many terminally ill children suffer from untreatable pain, dyspnea, fatigue, and other distressful symptoms (Wolfe et al., 2008; Heath et al., 2010). Some centers have protocols for the use of palliative sedation in children, and data suggest that when used in patients near the end of life, palliative sedation itself does not hasten death (Maltoni et al., 2009), However, even this form of treatment may fail to adequately alleviate the suffering of a substantial percentage of patients (Davis, 2009).

Because many terminally ill children derive no benefit from interventions aimed at prolonging life, it can be appropriate to withhold such interventions (Mercurio et al., 2008). Indeed, withholding medically administered nutrition and hydration may be appropriate when parents and physicians concur that such interventions do not provide a net benefit to the child (Diekema et al., 2009). When nutrition, hydration, and other life-prolonging medical interventions are discontinued, however, it may take days to weeks for a child to die. During this time, many children experience ongoing suffering in spite of excellent care (Wolfe et al., 2008; Maltoni et al., 2009; Heath et al., 2010).

If one accepts that there are cases in which an adult patient near the end of life is suffering unbearably and considers hastening death as being in their best interest, and the physician concurs that PAD is appropriate (or even medically indicated) for this patient at this time, then it would be reasonable to postulate that there are pediatric cases in which parents and physicians believe that a terminally ill child's suffering is unbearable, that hastening death is in the child's best interest, and that therefore PAD might be appropriate (and potentially medically indicated).

The question at hand is whether it is in the child's best interest to either have that life terminated quickly to alleviate suffering or to continue the dying process through its natural course. The primary argument in favor of NVE in such a case is based on a desire to minimize the child's suffering. If death is inevitable and the patient is suffering unbearably in spite of best medical treatment, then it may be permissible to hasten death in order to relieve suffering. Alternatively, the primary argument against NVE in such a case is that without knowing the child's experience of suffering, we can never be certain whether that suffering is unbearable. While we may make assumptions about the child's level of comfort based on external signs (e.g., facial expression, body position, vital signs), without knowing what they are actually feeling we run the risk of euthanizing the child when in fact their suffering is bearable. The answer to this question depends on which one believes to be the lesser of the two evils: Is it better to hasten the death of a dying child knowing that in fact his/her suffering may be bearable, or is it better to allow a child to continue through the natural dying process even when that suffering may be unbearable? There are significant data demonstrating that SAPAD and VAE for adult patients is not uncommon (Kuhse & Singer, 1988; Brahams, 1992; Meier et al., 1998; Maitra et al., 2005), and some physicians participate in NVE for incompetent adult patients (van der Maas et al., 1996); however, few data have been published regarding PAD practices in pediatric setting. Data suggest, however, that many parents consider requesting PAD for their terminally ill child (Dussel et al., 2010).

PAD for children who lack decisional capacity and who are in a persistent vegetative state

The rationale for PAD in the case of a child in a persistent vegetative state (PVS) rests on the question of best interests. When parents and physician agree that a child in PVS derives no net benefit from life-prolonging medical interventions, it may be permissible to withhold all such interventions (including medically administered nutrition and hydration) (Diekema et al., 2009). The question of whether it is in the child's best interest to die from dehydration after the discontinuation of medically administered nutrition and hydration, which may take days to weeks, or to have death occur more rapidly through NVE depends on whether the child in PVS can suffer and whether they have any interests.

PVS and suffering

If the child in PVS cannot suffer, then there appears to be no justification for NVE. Because the ethical basis for NVE is to relieve unbearable suffering, NVE cannot be justified in a patient who is not suffering. If, however, the child in PVS can suffer and can experience unbearable suffering, then once nutrition and hydration have been removed this would be considered terminal, and the same arguments discussed above would be applicable.

PVS and interests

If the child in PVS has interests, those interests must be considered and should guide decision-making. If, however, the child in PVS is considered to have no interests whatsoever, then he/she can have no "best interest." If there are no interests, it makes no difference to the child whether death occurs from dehydration or from NVE. Because there remains disagreement regarding whether adults in PVS can have interests, we cannot at this time definitively answer the question of whether children in PVS have interests.

If we believe that the child in PVS has no interests, then whose interests should guide decision-making? One could consider the preferences of the parents. Parents may prefer to allow death to occur more slowly so that they and other family members have time to say goodbye, because they have personal moral objections to hastening death, or for other personal reasons. Alternatively, they may prefer to hasten their child's death so that they feel there can be no suffering, so that they can plan better for their child's final hours, or because ongoing medical care represents a financial or emotional burden for the family. Alternatively, one could consider the interests of society, balancing the desire to minimize health care costs and facility utilization against the desire to protect the most vulnerable members of our society.

PAD for incompetent children who are not terminally ill and are not in PVS

Much of the debate regarding PAD has focused on terminally ill patients. If, however, the ethical justification for PAD is based on the values of individual self-determination and individual well-being (Brock, 1992; Emanuel, 1994), there seems no requirement that PAD be restricted to terminally ill patients. Many focus on PAD in terminally ill patients because hastening death that is imminent is more palatable than is hastening death that is otherwise unlikely to occur in the near future. It may be argued, however, that due to the mortal nature of human existence and the inevitability of death inherent in all human life, we are all terminal. If we are all terminal, then the distinction between terminally ill patients and the rest of society is arbitrary and has little ethical basis. Indeed, if a non-terminally ill person suffers unbearably (e.g., a patient with severe chronic pain that is refractory to aggressive palliative treatment, a person who is unable to perform even the most basic tasks of self-care due to permanent spinal injury, a person with an untreatable progressive neurodegenerative disease who currently has decisional capacity but who will soon become severely demented), the same values of self-determination and well-being apply. If there are cases of non-terminally ill competent adult patients who have decisional capacity for whom PAD is permissible, then one must consider whether there are non-terminally ill children for whom PAD is permissible as well.

This section analyzes the ethical implications of PAD in non-terminally ill children with the assumption that PAD may be permissible for a non-terminally ill competent adult patient who has decisional capacity. This assumption is made not because the permissibility of PAD in non-terminally ill adults has been established (indeed, it has not), rather this assumption is made because if PAD is impermissible in non-terminally ill competent adult patients who have decisional capacity, then there can be no justification for PAD in non-terminally ill children.

Because the value of self-determination has minimal impact in the care of children who lack decisional capacity, the justification for PAD must rest on the child's well-being. PAD would therefore be permissible in a child only if: (1) the child is suffering unbearably, (2) the agreed upon goal of treatment is alleviating that suffering, (3) all attempts to alleviate suffering have failed to reduce it to a tolerable level, and (4) the suffering will end only upon her death (Kon & Ablin, 2010). To meet these criteria, it is necessary to know whether the child's suffering is unbearable. If continued existence represents a fate worse than death, then PAD may be seen as supporting the child's well-being.

Like Zak, many non-terminally ill children are felt to suffer unbearably. In response to the suffering of infants whose current and future quality of life is dismal, the University Hospital in Groningen developed what has been termed the Groningen Protocol (Verhagen & Sauer, 2005). This protocol was designed for use with infants who do not require life support and are not terminally ill but whose current and future quality of life is considered unacceptably low. While the Groningen Protocol was designed solely for use in the NICU, there is no reason that it could not also be implemented for older children. This author and others have written on the ethical quagmire raised by this practice (Chervenak et al., 2006; Kon, 2007, 2009; Kodish, 2008); however, others have argued that, based on Dutch culture and values, the Groningen Protocol is justifiable in the Netherlands even if the protocol is ethically impermissible outside of the Netherlands (Lindemann & Verkerk, 2008).

The rationale for allowing NVE for non-terminally ill infants and children is based on a realization that some children suffer unbearably and a belief that NVE can be permissible if this is the only option that will alleviate the child's suffering. By allowing NVE in such cases, we can support the well-being of those children whose suffering is unbearable. However, because suffering is necessarily a first-person subjective experience, it is impossible for any person other than the patient to assess their level of suffering with certainty. Care providers and parents may use clues to assist is assessing suffering (e.g., facial expressions, etc.); however, they can never judge with certainty whether the child's suffering is unbearable. Children who have decisional capacity may be capable of informing others whether their suffering is unbearable, and even those without decisional capacity may be able to judge whether their suffering is unbearable and may be able to clearly communicate their assessment to others; however, younger children and those with more limited cognitive abilities are unable to provide this first-person subjective information to providers and parents.

When parents and providers lack the first-person report of the child, the judgment of the *unbearableness* of the suffering is inexact and unreliable. If we allow NVE in such cases, physicians will necessarily hasten the death of some children whose suffering is real but not unbearable. In those cases, death does not further the child's well-being, and therefore hastening death cannot be considered permissible. Alternatively, if we forbid NVE, there will necessarily be some children who are condemned to ongoing unbearable suffering. As such, either alternative is suboptimal. Is it better to hasten the death of some children whose suffering is not unbearable in order to provide NVE to those who suffer unbearably, or is it better to condemn some to a life of unbearable suffering in order to ensure that we never hasten the death of a child for whom the benefits of life are greater than the burdens? This author has argued that we should not allow NVE in non-terminally ill children without the child's first-person report because we must ensure that we never hasten the death of a child who is not suffering unbearably (Kon, 2007, 2008). Others, however, believe that it may be reasonable under some value systems to inadvertently hasten the death of some infants whose suffering is real but not unbearable in order to make PAD available to the widest range of patients (Lindemann & Verkerk, 2008).

Summary

As noted above, this discussion of PAD in the pediatric setting is predicated on the ethical permissibility of PAD in the care of competent adult patients. Clearly, PAD in the care of competent adult patients it not universally accepted. Indeed, governments who have legalized such a practice are in the minority, and there remains significant debate within medicine, health care, bioethics, and society in general regarding the permissibility of PAD for competent adults. The states (and health care professionals) are obligated to afford greater protection to children than to competent adults because of the dependency of children on others to protect their interests. Where PAD for competent adults is prohibited, any discussion of PAD in the care of children is moot.

Some states (the Netherlands, Oregon, etc.) provide legal access to PAD for some adults. Under such systems, the question of whether to allow similar access for some children must be considered, and, as discussed above, there may be reasonable arguments made for either position. In general, providers should be cognizant of the laws governing PAD where they

practice, and any consideration of PAD in pediatric settings should be discussed openly with input not only from health care providers and ethicists, but also from the broader society (such discussions should also include representatives from the disabled community to ensure the broadest range of input).

Case resolution

The entire PICU staff were distraught about Zak's moaning and thrashing, and many agreed with the parents that he should be "put out of his misery." The PICU physician agreed that Zak was suffering unbearably and that his future quality of life was unreasonably low. The physician ordered a lethal dose of potassium chloride (a medication that if given in high doses can cause cardiac arrest); however, the patient's nurse refused to administer the medication for fear of losing her nursing license. The PICU nurse manager obtained the medication from the locked medication area (the physicians did not have access to this area), and she gave the medication to the physician. The physician then administered the medication to Zak. Within seconds, Zak's heart ceased to beat and he was declared dead. The parents were appropriately upset; however, they were grateful for the care that Zak had received and thanked the physician for ending Zak's suffering. The PICU staff generally agreed that this was the most humane course of action, but there was great surprise that the physician had carried out this NVE.

The hospital administration was less supportive of this action and investigated the incident. Because the nursing administration and the medical staff administration were wholly separate, each independently reviewed the case and determined appropriate actions for those under their supervision. Both administrations focused primarily on state law, risk of legal action, and public perception; neither asked for an ethics consultation to assist in case review.

The nursing administration determined that the nurse manager acted inappropriately when she obtained the potassium chloride and gave it to the doctor because she knew that the doctor was planning to use it to euthanize the child. The nurse manager was fired for her actions; however, no action was taken against her nursing license. The medical staff administration also determined that the physician's actions were inappropriate and therefore restricted her hospital privileges. The physician was no longer allowed to attend in the PICU; however, she continued to care for patients in other areas of the hospital.

Unfortunately, neither the nursing administration nor the medical staff administration discussed the most salient ethical question in this case: Was Zak better off dead than alive? It was clear that Zak was suffering, but was his suffering *unbearable*? There is no question that life with significant amputations is burdensome; however, if Zak had been supported through his illness, if he had had access to high-quality prosthetics, if his family had helped him overcome his handicaps, would he have felt that he would have been better off dead or would he have savored his life and lived it as fully as possible? There is a wealth of data demonstrating that medical professionals over estimate the burdens associated with disabilities and underestimate the quality of life of children living with handicaps (Sprangers & Aaronson, 1992; Saigal et al., 1996, 1999, 2006; Janse et al., 2004); therefore allowing physicians to determine whether a child's presumed future quality of life is sufficiently low to justify NVE is unwise. It is likely that a clinical ethics consultation could have assisted the clinicians in understanding these issues more fully.

Disclaimer

The view expressed are solely those of the author and do not represent the official opinion of the United States government, the Department of Defense, or the Department of the Navy.

References

Appelbaum, P.S. & Grisso, T. (1988). Assessing patients' capacities to consent to treatment. *New England Journal of Medicine*, **319**(25), 1635–1638.

Brahams, D. (1992). Euthanasia: doctor convicted of attempted murder. *Lancet*, **340**(8822), 782–783.

Brock, D.W. (1992). Voluntary active euthanasia. *Hastings Center Report*, **22**(2), 10–22.

Catlin, A. & Carter, B. (2002). Creation of a neonatal end-of-life palliative care protocol. *Journal of Perinatology*, **22**(3), 184–195.

Chervenak, F.A., McCullough, L.B., & Arabin, B. (2006). Why the Groningen Protocol should be rejected. *Hastings Center Report*, **36**(5), 30–33.

Davis, M.P. (2009). Does palliative sedation always relieve symptoms? *Journal of Palliative Medicine*, **12**(10), 875–877.

Dees, M., Vernooij-Dassen, M., Dekkers, W., & van Weel, C. (2010). Unbearable suffering of patients with a request for euthanasia or physician-assisted suicide: an integrative review. *Psychooncology*, **19**(4), 339–352.

Diekema, D.S., Botkin, J.R. & the Committee on Bioethics, American Academy of Pediatrics (2009). Clinical report – forgoing medically provided nutrition and hydration in children. *Pediatrics*, **124**(2), 813–822.

Dussel, V., Joffe, S., Hilden, J.M., et al. (2010). Considerations about hastening death among parents of children who die of cancer. *Archives of Pediatrics and Adolescent Medicine*, **164**(3), 231–237.

Emanuel, E.J. (1994). Euthanasia. Historical, ethical, and empiric perspectives. *Archives of Internal Medicine*, **154**(17), 1890–1901.

Grisso, T., Appelbaum, P.S., & Hill-Fotouhi, C. (1997). The MacCAT-T: a clinical tool to assess patients' capacities to make treatment decisions. *Psychiatric Services*, **48**(11), 1415–1419.

Heath, J.A., Clarke, N.E., Donath, S.M., et al. (2010). Symptoms and suffering at the end of life in children with cancer: an Australian perspective. *Medical Journal of Australia*, **192**(2), 71–75.

Janse, A.J., Gemke, R.J., Uiterwaal, C.S., et al. (2004). Quality of life: patients and doctors don't always agree: a meta-analysis. *Journal of Clinical Epidemiology*, **57**(7), 653–661.

Kodish, E. (2008). Paediatric ethics: a repudiation of the Groningen protocol. *Lancet*, **371**(9616), 892–893.

Kon, A.A. (2007). Neonatal euthanasia is unsupportable: the Groningen protocol should be abandoned. *Theoretical Medicine and Bioethics*, **28**(5), 453–463.

Kon, A.A. (2008). We cannot accurately predict the extent of an infant's future suffering: the Groningen Protocol is too dangerous to support. *American Journal of Bioethics*, **8**(11), 27–29.

Kon, A.A. (2009). Neonatal euthanasia. *Seminars in Perinatology*, **33**(6), 377–383.

Kon, A.A. & Ablin, A.R. (2009). It's not palliative care, it's palliative treatment. *Lancet Oncology*, **10**(2), 106–107.

Kon, A.A. & Ablin, A.R. (2010). Palliative treatment: redefining interventions to treat suffering near the end of life. *Journal of Palliative Medicine*, **13**(6), 643–646.

Kuhse, H. & Singer, P. (1988). Doctors' practices and attitudes regarding voluntary euthanasia. *Medical Journal of Australia*, **148**(12), 623–627.

Lindemann, H. & Verkerk, M. (2008). Ending the life of a newborn: the Groningen Protocol. *Hastings Center Report*, **38**(1), 42–51.

Maitra, R., Harfst, A., Bjerre, L., Kochen, M., & Becker, A. (2005). Do German general practitioners support euthanasia? Results of a nation-wide questionnaire survey. *European Journal of General Practice*, **11**(3–4), 94–100.

Maltoni, M., Pittureri, C., Scarpi, E., et al. (2009). Palliative sedation therapy does not hasten death: results from a prospective multicenter study. *Annals of Oncology*, **20**(7), 1163–1169.

Meier, D.E., Emmons, C.A., Wallenstein, S., et al. (1998). A national survey of physician-assisted suicide and euthanasia in the United States. *New England Journal of Medicine*, **338**(17), 1193–1201.

Mercurio, M.R., Maxwell, M.A., Mears, B.J., Ross, L.F., & Silber, T.J. (2008). American Academy of Pediatrics policy statements on bioethics: summaries and commentaries: part 2. *Pediatrics in Review/American Academy of Pediatrics*, **29**(3), e15–e22.

Ross, L.F. (2009). Against the tide: arguments against respecting a minor's refusal of efficacious life-saving treatment. *Cambridge Quarterly of Healthcare Ethics*, **18**(3), 302–315; discussion 315–322.

Saigal, S., Feeny, D., Rosenbaum, P., et al. (1996). Self-perceived health status and health-related quality of life of extremely low-birth-weight infants at adolescence. *Journal of the American Medical Association*, **276**(6), 453–459.

Saigal, S., Stoskopf, B.L., Feeny, D., et al. (1999). Differences in preferences for neonatal outcomes among health care professionals, parents, and adolescents. *Journal of the American Medical Association*, **281**(21), 1991–1997.

Saigal, S., Stoskopf, B., Pinelli, J., et al. (2006). Self-perceived health-related quality of life of former extremely low birth weight infants at young adulthood. *Pediatrics*, **118**(3), 1140–1148.

Sprangers, M. & Aaronson, N. (1992). The role of health care providers and significant others in evaluating the quality of life of patients with chronic disease: a review. *Journal of Clinical Epidemiology*, **45**(7), 743–760.

van der Maas, P.J., van der Wal, G., Haverkate, I., et al. (1996). Euthanasia, physician-assisted suicide, and other medical practices involving the end of life in the Netherlands, 1990–1995. *New England Journal of Medicine*, **335**(22), 1699–1705.

Verhagen, E. & Sauer, P.J. (2005). The Groningen protocol – euthanasia in severely ill newborns. *New England Journal of Medicine*, **352**(10), 959–962.

Wolfe, J., Hammel, J.F., Edwards, K.E., et al. (2008). Easing of suffering in children with cancer at the end of life: is care changing? *Journal of Clinical Oncology*, **26**(10), 1717–1723.

Chapter 23

The Groningen Protocol

A.A. Eduard Verhagen and John D. Lantos

Case narrative

When Marieke was born, her pediatrician noticed skin erosions and blistering of the skin on all extremities. The lips and skin of her face showed raw red areas but otherwise she was vigorous and appeared healthy. She was transferred to a university hospital on the second day of life. Skin tests and biopsy revealed the diagnosis of severe dystrophic epidermolysis bullosa.

Epidermolysis bullosa (EB) is a rare skin disorder that manifests itself with an exceptional liability of the skin to blister after minor mechanical trauma. Because of a genetic abnormality, the different skin layers do not stick together adequately, so that the skin surface can easily break down after cuddling, rubbing, scratching, or swallowing. Marieke suffered from the most severe form in which permanent scarring leads to deformities, and involvement of various organs results in early postnatal death or chronic progression. There is no cure for EB.

The physicians discussed the diagnosis and outlook with her parents who were determined to take their child home in anticipation of an early death. They were taught how to take care of the skin and change the bandages. Home-care nurses administered strong analgesics (opioids) and sedatives to help alleviate the pain. Feeding was problematic because of the oral lesions and strictures in the esophagus. Intravenous access was very difficult to obtain or maintain as the tape holding the catheters in place caused blistering and skin sloughing.

Marieke's parents managed to care for her at home for 2 months. Over this time, she was in constant pain despite high doses of medications. She had not gained any weight in 2 months. She was brought back to the hospital for re-evaluation.

On re-admission to the hospital, the parents and the medical team decided to intensify analgesic

medications as much as possible without sedating her so heavily that she would be unable to interact with her parents. They tried to continue oral feeds since Marieke seemed to be comforted by drinking. The parents and the medical team had decided not to add any additional medical treatments, including evaluations for sepsis or treatment of respiratory distress. Marieke was expected to die soon from infection, medication side effects, and/or dehydration and malnutrition.

This, however, didn't happen. Instead, she drank just enough milk to stay alive while the pain and suffering increased. Nobody could bring themselves to withhold her oral feedings. Her parents considered the dying process inhumane and Marieke's suffering unnecessary. They requested the physicians to consider actively ending her life as soon as possible. The medical team understood the parents' arguments and agreed. The pediatrician followed the Groningen Protocol and ended Marieke's life with lethal medication.

Marieke's case illustrates three sources of ethical tension in the care of a baby who is dying of an incurable chronic disease. First, sometimes a newborn's suffering from an incurable disease is considered intractable and unbearable for the child. Even expert pain management cannot always relieve pain and suffering. Second, withholding potentially supportive treatments does not always result in the anticipated death. Third, parents may ask for termination of life if they consider the suffering unnecessary and inhumane. The dilemma for physicians is whether or not they should comply with such a parental request.

Although several interesting ethical issues are raised, the focus of this chapter will be the ethical and legal aspects of the physicians' decision to terminate life in newborns. A special emphasis will be given to the

Clinical Ethics in Pediatrics: A Case-Based Textbook, ed. Douglas S. Diekema, Mark R. Mercurio and Mary B. Adam. Published by Cambridge University Press. © Cambridge University Press 2011.

developments in the Netherlands where termination of life of severely defective newborn babies has become legal under very narrowly defined circumstances.

End-of-life decisions in different categories of newborns

Many medical decisions can have the effect of hastening death. Decisions to write do-not-resuscitate orders, to withdraw mechanical ventilation, to withhold fluid and nutrition, or to give high doses of opioid analgesics fall into this category. So do decisions to deliberately terminate a newborn's life with lethal drugs. We refer to all of these as end-of-life decisions (EoLDs).

Newborns in whom an EoLD is being considered can be classified in three groups along the dimensions of their dependency on intensive care for physiologic stability (stable/unstable) and prognosis (Verhagen & Sauer, 2005a; Verhagen et al., 2010).

Group I encompasses physiologically unstable infants whose death is imminent. These newborns are actually dying (heart rate falling, blood pressure dropping, and oxygen saturation dropping). In most countries, it is ethically acceptable and legal to withhold or withdraw interventions for such babies. Furthermore, in most countries, withholding and withdrawing interventions are seen as morally equivalent. The legal status of these EoLDs in many, but not all, countries is that they are considered "normal medical practice" and the resulting death subject to no specific control through criminal law (McHaffie et al., 1999). Sometimes, cases that fall into group I are considered to be cases of medical futility.

Group II consists of infants who are dependent upon intensive care and who have a very poor prognosis for survival or neurocognitive outcome but who are physiologically stable and not actively dying. In such infants, a decision to withhold or withdraw life support is sometimes made because of their poor prognosis, even though, unlike infants in group I, they could be kept alive.

Withholding or withdrawing mechanical ventilation for quality of life reasons is more controversial than withholding or withdrawing life support in a moribund infant. Medical practice in group II newborns appears to vary between units. A recent international comparison has shown no extubations in stable newborns in one unit, while in three other units 19–35% of extubations were performed in stable infants for quality of life reasons (Verhagen et al., 2010).

In many countries, doctors and professional societies develop criteria to help doctors decide when it is appropriate or acceptable to withhold or withdraw treatment. In the Netherlands, by contrast, influential reports by the medical profession have recognized that the medical behavior that needs legitimation is not the artificial shortening of life but the prolongation. These reports invoke the ethical principle of "in dubio abstine." Quality of life considerations can give rise to doubt about whether the potential life to be won from continued treatment will ultimately benefit the patient. In such cases, Dutch doctors think that it would be wrong for the doctors to give or continue the treatment (Griffiths et al., 2008). Thus, in the Netherlands, physicians are not required to give treatment that they view as "not in the child's best interest" and they determine what constitutes this.

A third group of infants is even more controversial. Group III encompasses stable newborns with a very poor prognosis and intractable suffering who are not dependent on intensive care. Because these newborns are stable without life support, withdrawal of the ventilator is simply not an option. We will explore the decision-making in these newborns in more depth below.

Decision-making in newborns with intractable suffering (group III)

There are four possible strategies for parents and physicians caring for these newborns.

The first is to not make an EoLD. With unrestricted medical treatment, many such infants can live for years or decades.

The second is to withhold medical treatment, including medically provided fluid and nutrition, or other treatments such as antibiotics, because these interventions can be considered not to be in the interest of the child. Most infants will not be able to take sufficient oral nutrition and will eventually die. This strategy may be acceptable and justifiable for a number of physicians and parents. It has been endorsed by the American Academy of Pediatrics (Diekema & Botkin, 2009). It remains controversial, however, in part because of the emotional and social symbolism associated with feeding children.

A third approach, sometimes combined with the second, is to gradually increase the dose of sedatives and analgesics in group III infants. This has been referred to as "palliative sedation" or "terminal sedation." It is frequently accompanied by the withdrawal or withholding of life-sustaining interventions, such as medically provided fluids and nutrition. It is typically a measure of last resort to be considered in situations where all other measures to reduce pain and suffering have failed (Jansen & Sulmasy, 2002).

Some people argue that palliative sedation is an appropriate EoLD in group III infants because this effectively alleviates the pain and discomfort. Palliative sedation is controversial in newborns. Standards for this type of sedation at the end of life are not available and guidelines for practice vary considerably (de Graeff & Dean, 2007). The goals of palliative sedation are often ambiguous. Is the true goal the relief of suffering, with the shortening of life being a foreseeable but not desired side effect? Or is the true goal to hasten death, but to do so in way that is not obviously euthanasia? In addition, the timing of newborn deaths on palliative sedation protocols is often difficult to predict.

A fourth approach to group III infants is to deliberately end their lives using lethal drugs. This approach is sometimes used in the Netherlands. It is illegal in most other countries.

It is widely known that the Netherlands was the first country in the world to legalize euthanasia in adults. An adult with a hopeless prognosis and unbearable suffering would be permitted euthanasia on his/her request under the 2002 Euthanasia Law, which is a manifestation of the commitment to patient autonomy in Dutch medical law. A newborn, however, cannot make a euthanasia request, and parents are not accepted as their legal representatives in such a matter. Does that mean that these children cannot be afforded the same considerations?

The justification of euthanasia in Dutch law has never rested only on the voluntary request of the patient. Trial verdicts have consistently referred specifically to the norms of the medical profession as defining the boundaries of euthanasia. These norms require both respect for autonomy and a situation of necessity that the doctor finds himself in because of the patient's hopeless and unbearable suffering. In the 1990s, these norms were tested in court in the context of newborns. Two doctors were prosecuted for murder after having reported their cases of neonatal termination of life – as required by the 1992 reporting guidelines. One baby suffered from complicated spina bifida and the other from trisomy 13. Based on the verdicts in these cases, known as the Prins and Kadijk cases, it is now accepted that if the parents agreed and under certain circumstances the physician can claim impunity,

i.e., the defense of necessity. In such circumstances the newborn's suffering should be extreme, thus compelling the physician to choose between the duty to save lives, on the one hand, and to do everything possible to prevent unbearable suffering, on the other hand. If the physician exercises due care, termination of life may be justified. The requirements of due medical care were formulated for the first time in the Prins and Kadijk cases.

The creation of the Groningen Protocol

In 2002, in response to these legal cases and to other cases in the neonatal intensive care unit, a group of physicians of the University Medical Center in Groningen started a discussion with the local prosecutor regarding termination of life in newborns. They were aware of recent publications about Dutch end-of-life practice suggesting the existence of covert termination of life in an estimated 20 newborns per year (Vrakking et al., 2005). Anonymous interviews in a nationwide survey had indicated that fear of prosecution and uncertainties about the reporting procedure were the main reasons for physician non-reporting of these cases (van der Wal & van der Maas, 1996). Moreover, the Groningen group had recently dealt with a case like the Marieke case, in which parents asked for the termination of life of their 2-month-old baby with lethal EB. Although the parents' request was understandable for the medical team, and the ethical committee and medico-legal experts agreed that termination of the baby's life would be appropriate, no doctor was prepared to be the responsible physician terminating the baby's life. Despite the verdicts in the Prins and Kadijk cases, termination of life was (and still is) a criminal offense (murder) for which the responsible physician risked being prosecuted. The child was discharged and died after 3 months of intense suffering in a local hospital. This course of events caused very negative emotions in the Groningen medical team.

The aim of the discussion with the prosecutor was twofold: first, to try to prevent police investigations and formal prosecution by agreeing which information the prosecution authorities needed for the decision whether or not to prosecute, and second, to publish the outcomes to guide the behavior of doctors in termination of life and to promote reporting. The "Groningen Protocol" was the result of this discussion, enriched with the main findings of the analysis of 22 previously

Table 23.1. The main requirements for termination of life in newborns in the Groningen Protocol*

The diagnosis and prognosis must be certain
Hopeless and unbearable suffering must be present
Both parents must give informed consent
The diagnosis, prognosis, and unbearable suffering must be confirmed by at least one independent doctor
The procedure must be performed in accordance with the accepted medical standard

* Additional information needed to support and clarify the decision is published in Verhagen and Sauer (2005a).

unpublished cases of termination of life in newborns and a review of the legal issues. The cases occurred nationwide over a 10-year period and concerned newborns with severe congenital malformations, mostly complex neural tube defects. None of these cases had been prosecuted. The main requirements set in the protocol, which became a national guideline in 2005, are given in Table 23.1. In 2007, a multidisciplinary review committee for termination of life in newborns, consisting of lawyers, ethicists, and neonatologists, was installed. The committee's duty was to advise the prosecuting authorities on the carefulness of the decision-making in each reported case. The medical profession had asked for such a committee for a long time because it was expected to facilitate reporting and review.

The doctors who developed the protocol published it in peer-reviewed medical journals, and invited scrutiny and feedback (Verhagen & Sauer, 2005a, 2005b; Verhagen, 2006).

International response to the Protocol

The Groningen Protocol has received intense criticism, and the international debate is still ongoing. One argument that is often raised against the Groningen Protocol and acceptance of deliberate ending of life in newborns is the "slippery-slope" argument (Kon, 2008). It is argued that accepting this practice will lead to a failure of safeguards and erosion of norms so that forms of termination of life that are currently considered undesirable will be practiced without discussion. Interestingly, similar arguments had once been made against legalizing do-not-resuscitate orders, or allowing the withdrawal of life support (Arras, 1982). The dilemma in responding to such arguments is that they are theoretical. It is hard to know, in advance, which slopes will be slippery or which practices will lead to stable, definable, and defensible new norms.

Furthermore, it is clear that, at least in the Netherlands, the practice of deliberately ending lives

of newborns existed long before the publication of the Protocol. It probably does in other countries as well. It was going on, at least partly, "under the table." The Protocol's main goal was to regulate and control that practice, to make it transparent and subject to public review. The Protocol allows doctors to be openly accountable for their decisions to all members of society. An opposing view might be that there are many bad things going on "under the table" in all societies, things so evil that we would not want to make them transparent and accept them. In Dutch society, however, there is a shared understanding that hastening death is not always the worst thing that can happen to a human being and that death is not synonymous with "evil." Where the Dutch go further than other countries is in their shared belief that even newborns have a fundamental interest in not prolonging a life that is or soon will become an intolerable burden to them.

Some critics of the Protocol worry that the required criterion for lethal injection – "sustained suffering that cannot be relieved" – was far too subjective to be applied consistently or fairly. Others have argued in support of the Protocol, confirming that babies can certainly suffer pain to excruciating degrees, other kinds of serious and unrelievable conditions like total lifelong dependency, or lack of any capacity for communication (Lindemann & Verkerk, 2008).

There have been many misunderstandings about the Protocol, including that it is aimed at babies with spina bifida. In fact, nowhere in the Protocol is spina bifida represented as a condition associated with hopeless and sustained suffering. Other misunderstandings concern the role of parents, and the claim that they could be tempted to kill their baby so they do not have to look after it. Publications describing the parents' role in end-of-life decisions in the Netherlands do not at all support that assumption (van der Heide et al., 1998; Verhagen et al., 2009a). These sorts of concerns should not be limited to the interventions described in the Groningen Protocol. They are equally concerning in every decision to withhold or withdraw life-sustaining treatment from a newborn. In the Groningen Protocol, as in other EoLDs, parental requests for termination of a baby's life are not automatically implemented. The medical team always makes the final decision.

The Groningen Protocol 5 years later

Was the Groningen Protocol really a first step down a slippery slope that would lead to widely increased use of neonatal euthanasia? In the years between 2005 and 2010, only two cases of termination of life in newborns were reported and both involved patients with EB. Did physicians still terminate lives without reporting or had the number of cases indeed dropped considerably? A chart review of all newborns who died in the ten Dutch NICUs during a 12-month period between 2005 and 2006 and interviews with the responsible physicians following the publication of the Groningen Protocol revealed only one case of intentional ending of life (Verhagen et al., 2009b). Interestingly, in these years, there has been a sharp increase in the prenatal diagnosis of congenital anomalies after the decision was made to offer structural ultrasound examination to every pregnant woman in the Netherlands at 20 weeks, and late abortions have doubled. Until that decision, routine screening policy for the detection of fetal structural abnormalities had not been an integral part of antenatal care. Many people, including the Health Inspectorate, think the increase in abortions and decrease in termination of life after birth are related to the introduction of the ultrasound examination. From that perspective, the effects of the Groningen Protocol were different from those predicted by either its supporters or critics.

Resolution of Marieke's case

The responsible pediatrician reported the medical team's actions to the review committee and to the local prosecutor, who gave permission for the child's funeral. The committee examined the case thoroughly and reported to the prosecuting authority that the termination of life was careful and consistent with currently accepted medical and ethical considerations and protocols dealing with this topic. The prosecuting authority decided to refrain from prosecution. The pediatrician, who was notified about the decision about 3 months after Marieke's death, supported the parents in their grieving during several follow-up consultations. Because the gene mutation that caused EB was identified, prenatal screening became available for Marieke's parents. In the following years, the mother delivered one healthy boy and had one miscarriage of a healthy fetus as a complication of villous biopsy at 16 weeks. She also had an abortion at 20 weeks after the results of another biopsy showed that the fetus had EB. Despite all emotions, she never expressed regret about the decision-making in Marieke's case nor in the pregnancies that followed.

References

Arras, J.D. (1982). The right to die on the slippery slope. *Social Theory and Practice*, **8**, 285–328.

de Graeff, A. & Dean, M. (2007). Palliative sedation therapy in the last weeks of life: a literature review and recommendations for standards. *Journal of Palliative Medicine*, **10**, 67–85.

Diekema, D.S. & Botkin, J.R. (2009). Clinical report – forgoing medically provided nutrition and hydration in children. *Pediatrics*, **124**, 813–822.

Griffiths, J., Weyers, H., & Adams, M. (2008). Termination of life in neonatology. In *Euthanasia and Law in Europe*. Oxford and Portland, OR: Hart Publishing.

Jansen, L.A. & Sulmasy, D.P. (2002). Sedation, alimentation, hydration, and equivocation: careful conversation about care at the end of life. *Annals of Internal Medicine*, **136**, 845–849.

Kon, A.A. (2008). We cannot accurately predict the extent of an infant's future suffering: the Groningen Protocol is too dangerous to support. *American Journal of Bioethics*, **8**, 27–29.

Lindemann, H. & Verkerk, M. (2008). Ending the life of a newborn: the Groningen Protocol. *Hastings Center Report*, **38**, 42–51.

McHaffie, H.E., Cuttini, M., Brolz-Voit, G., et al. (1999). Withholding/withdrawing treatment from neonates: legislation and official guidelines across Europe. *Journal of Medical Ethics*, **25**, 440–446.

van der Heide, A., van der Maas, P.J., van der Wal, G., et al. (1998). The role of parents in end-of-life decisions in neonatology: physicians' views and practices. *Pediatrics*, **101**, 413–418.

van der Wal, G. & van der Maas, P.J. (1996). *Euthanasie en andere medische beslissingen rond het levenseinde: de praktijk en de meldingsprocedure [Euthanasia and other medical end-of-life decisions: practice and the reporting procedure]*. The Hague: SDU Uitgevers.

Verhagen, A.A.E. (2006). End of life decisions in newborns in The Netherlands: medical and legal aspects of the Groningen protocol. *Medicine and Law*, **25**, 399–407.

Verhagen, A.A.E. & Sauer, P.J. (2005a). End-of-life decisions in newborns: an approach from The Netherlands. *Pediatrics*, **116**, 736–739.

Verhagen, A.A.E. & Sauer, P.J. (2005b). The Groningen proto-col – euthanasia in severely ill newborns. *New England Journal of Medicine*, **352**, 959–962.

Verhagen, A.A.E., de Vos, M., Dorscheidt, J.H., et al. (2009a). Conflicts about end-of-life decisions in NICUs in the Netherlands. *Pediatrics*, **124**, e112–e119.

Verhagen, A.A.E., Dorscheidt, J.H., Engels, B., Hubben, J.H., & Sauer, P.J. (2009b). End-of-life decisions in Dutch neonatal intensive care units. *Archives of Pediatrics and Adolescent Medicine*, **163**, 895–901.

Verhagen, A.A.E., Janvier, A., Leuthner, S.R., et al. (2010). Categorizing neonatal deaths: a cross-cultural study in the United States, Canada, and the Netherlands. *Journal of Pediatrics*, **156**, 33–37.

Vrakking, A.M., van der Heide, A., Onwuteaka-Philipsen, B.D., et al. (2005). Medical end-of-life decisions made for neonates and infants in the Netherlands, 1995–2001. *Lancet*, **365**, 1329–1331.

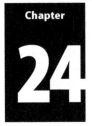

Defining beneficence in the face of death: symptom management in dying children

Marcia Levetown

Case narrative

Cole is an 8-month-old first-born child, diagnosed at 4 months of age with Werdnig–Hoffmann disease (spinal muscular atrophy, SMA 1), a severe form of autosomal recessive muscular dystrophy. SMA 1 has historically led to death from respiratory insufficiency before age 2 and is incurable. Cole's parents are aware of the nature and prognosis of his condition and have been apprised of all potential measures to prolong Cole's life and enhance his comfort.

Cole presents to the palliative care team with a 2-week history of irritability, frequent night-time awakenings, and increasingly frequent and brief daytime naps. He is afebrile and has no new symptoms. His respiratory rate is 60 per minute and shallow; a full physical examination is otherwise unremarkable. Cole's parents report that shortly after commencing sleep, his breathing becomes shallower and then he awakens, never getting adequate rest. Though not in severe distress, it is very likely that the etiology of his irritability is borderline respiratory insufficiency when awake, resulting in sleep disruption and deprivation, which is further exacerbated by the decreased conscious control of breathing when asleep. No soporifics are approved for this age group. Further, any lessening of his consciousness risks respiratory failure and even respiratory arrest. Cole's parents remain adamant that they wish no form of mechanical respiratory support.

Exploring ethically appropriate options and "best interests"

As with adults, our obligation to pediatric patients of all ages and diagnoses is to promote their well-being in the health care context (beneficence), such as diagnosing and managing distressing symptoms; to avoid maleficence (not to ignore the distress, nor do additional harm); to honor the autonomy of the patient (or surrogate's representation of the patient's preferences and priorities, such as goals of care); and to be just. However, in cases such as Cole's, there is tension between the ideal of improving symptom distress and the potential of hastening death. In all health care decision-making, one must weigh the known and potential benefits of the proposed choices versus the known and potential burdens and risks. Most often, the benefit–burden calculus is a subjective one. In the case of immature children, such as Cole, parents are then left to weigh options on behalf of their child, within the context of the family. Many bioethicists will argue that the child has an independent "best interest" to be honored and may assert that an independent agent should represent the child. Who is qualified to do so and by whose authority, as well as whether this person or entity is able to judge "independently" or fairly, to the benefit of the child, is rarely addressed. Children who will die in the near future certainly should have the opportunity to live as long and as comfortably as possible, given the realities of their conditions. Most children prefer to live with their families in their home environment (Hammes et al., 2005; Hinds et al., 2005a; Surkan et al., 2006). This should be kept in mind when deciding what is in his/her best interests. The psychosocial and spiritual well-being of a child are at least of equal importance to their physical well-being when death is inevitable, and is of particular significance when death is imminent (Hinds et al., 2005a; Weiner et al., 2008; Lyon et al., 2009).

Cole's parents feel that mechanical ventilation (MV) is not in their child's best interests, while recognizing it would likely extend his life duration; nevertheless, they feel that lying encased in an immobile body, dependent on machines to breathe, with no potential for reversal of the underlying condition, is unfair to an infant who should be exploring the world with his eyes,

Clinical Ethics in Pediatrics: A Case-Based Textbook, ed. Douglas S. Diekema, Mark R. Mercurio and Mary B. Adam. Published by Cambridge University Press. © Cambridge University Press 2011.

hands, feet, and mouth. Another individual may vehemently disagree with this view. In the United States, as of this writing, parents have the legal right as guardians to make this choice. His parents' view is one of several legitimate interpretations of Cole's best interests. Further, from a practical standpoint, it would be difficult to force parents to maintain a child on a ventilator at home against their wishes. It would also be difficult to wrest the child from the parents' loving arms to institutionalize him for the purpose of mechanical ventilation for his remaining months, based on the arguable claim that this action would serve the child's best interests.

The shifting balance of symptom control versus risk of death

For a child with an acute reversible illness, the decision to allow a death in exchange for more effective symptom control would almost always be considered inappropriate. However, in the case of a child who is certainly going to die from his disease in the near future, the prevention and relief of suffering is at least as pressing a priority as the prevention of premature death. It is clear that, as death approaches, the intensity of symptom distress often escalates dramatically (Kenny & Frager, 1996; Houlahan et al., 2006; Friedrichsdorf & Kang, 2007). Prior to that time, clinicians with expertise in palliative care (the interdisciplinary art and science of preventing and relieving physical, psychosocial, emotional, and spiritual suffering of a patient and his or her self-defined family throughout the trajectory of a serious illness) are able to manage symptoms with minimal risk in the vast majority of cases. Thus, the need to balance the risk of death with the benefit of symptom control rarely arises until death is near.

In caring for terminally ill children, it is critical to honor the principles of patient- and family-centered care. Parents, siblings, other family members, and friends have indelible memories of the dying child's final moments of life (Hinds et al., 2005b). Thus, mitigating the suffering of the child also mitigates the suffering of the family. Families witness to severe symptom distress struggle with feelings of having been inadequate to protect their child, leading to difficulties in their bereavement adaptation (Kreicbergs et al., 2005; Mack et al., 2009).

In the case presented here, Cole's parents do not wish their child to be subjected to suffering. Mechanical ventilation represents suffering to them, so they wish to avoid it. At the same time, they want his symptoms to be effectively managed. As a consequence of severe muscular weakness, Cole has the potential for dyspnea (feeling short of breath), as well as aspiration of mouth and stomach contents into his pharynx (causing choking) and lungs (with the potential for pneumonitis/pneumonia and increased dyspnea). It also appears that he is experiencing sleep deprivation due to hypoventilation. Opioids, including morphine, are the only class of agents demonstrated to manage dyspnea, irrespective of underlying cause (Bruera et al., 1990; Cohen et al., 1991; Campbell, 1996; Kenny & Frager, 1996; Houlahan et al., 2006).

Given the lack of lung or circulatory pathology, "standard" treatments such as bronchodilators and oxygen will not make Cole more comfortable, so opioids are the most likely medications to be effective. But there are risks in using opioids to relieve Cole's symptom distress, since opioids can slow respirations and suppress respiratory drive when he is already teetering on the edge of respiratory failure.

Theoretical and practical support for prioritizing symptom control at the end of life

The principle of double effect (PDE) is often used in the context of the care of terminally ill patients to justify attempts to control symptoms that may be associated with the risk of hastening the death itself. PDE derives from the Catholic Church, which recognized that in some instances it may be justifiable to proceed with an action that intends good, even when there is the risk that a bad outcome may arise as an unintended but foreseeable result of the action. The *New Catholic Encyclopedia* provides four conditions for the application of the principle of double effect (McCormick, 1978):

1. The act itself must be morally good or at least indifferent.
2. The agent does not intend the bad effect, but may permit it. If he could attain the good effect without the bad effect he should do so.
3. The good effect must flow directly from the action and not from the bad effect. Otherwise the agent would be using a bad means to a good end, which is never allowed.
4. The good effect must be sufficiently desirable to compensate for the allowing of the bad effect.

Returning to the case of Cole and the prospect of using opioids for his sleep disturbance and dyspnea, and noting these conditions point by point, the act of giving medicine with the goal of relieving symptom distress is a moral good. The intent is not to cause harm or hasten death by the use of this agent, while recognizing that there is a risk of that outcome. The good effect (relief of pain and symptoms) is achieved directly through the action of the medication, and not through the potential of a hastened death. In fact, doses will be started at the lowest possible effective dose and his responses will be meticulously monitored. At the time of any adverse effect, the decision regarding whether to continue to use the medication or not will be revisited and discussed with the parents, based on the effectiveness of relief of distress and re-evaluation of the risks. The relief of severe symptom distress offsets the potential for hastened death in the eyes of many, though not all.

Realities of symptom control and the end of life: is the principle of double effect needed?

Now that the theoretical justification for using opioids in the management of severe dyspnea (and other symptoms, particularly pain) has been proffered, is it needed? In the few papers researching the risk of hastened death with the use of opioids to manage severe distress at the end of life, the conclusion is that the resolution of the symptoms, even by means of opioids, actually prolongs the life of the individual in a statistically though not always clinically meaningful way (Partridge & Wall, 1997; Quill et al., 1997; Bengoechea et al., 2010). Thus, a clinician's fear of hastening death and the resultant willingness to allow a child to suffer from inadequate treatment of symptoms is not justified by the evidence and represents a violation of the principle of beneficence. Lack of knowledge is insufficient justification for this persistent and pervasive problem; clinicians must either become more evidence-based in their management of symptom distress at the end of life, or they should consult others with greater expertise to assist them.

Intractable symptoms and "options of last resort"

Very rarely, symptoms cannot be adequately controlled while simultaneously maintaining the patient's consciousness, even by clinicians who are very knowledgeable and highly skilled in palliative care. Thus, in these uncommon situations, unusual measures may be required to relieve escalating symptoms as death approaches (Kenny & Frager, 1996). Symptom distress is thought to be a conscious experience; therefore, one approach to severe and intractable symptom distress management is to render the patient unconscious, even knowing the fact that many parents wish to interact with the child to the last possible moment (Pritchard et al., 2008). Patients with severe dyspnea, pain, or other symptom distress are generally not capable of such affirming communication in a way their parents desire.

Variably referred to in the literature as "terminal" (out of favor), "total," or "palliative" sedation (PS), this option is only considered when there has been expert consultation and all other treatment options have been tried and proven to be unsuccessful. Issues that must be considered when using PS include (Kirke et al., 2010):

1. Is there any justification for lightening or forgoing the sedation?
    *   If the symptom is likely to come under control in the future, the answer is yes.
    *   If the symptom is expected to last for the remainder of the child's life (most likely worsening over time), the answer is generally no.
2. Who will be responsible to turn the child every 2 hours or more often, day and night, to prevent pressure ulcers? Who will do the frequent mouth care?
    *   Even if parents are willing and able to provide such care at home, they most likely will need assistance, either through the use of trained volunteers, paid caregivers, or hospice care. An alternative is to admit the child to a nursing home or hospital for nursing care.
3. What are the pros and cons of the medical provision of nutrition and/or hydration during PS?
    *   If the symptoms are anticipated to resolve with time, and a trial of awakening is planned, maintenance of nutritional support is appropriate.
    *   If the symptoms are unlikely to resolve, and death is anticipated in hours, days or a few weeks, then forgoing artificial nutrition and hydration may be considered (Diekema et al., 2009).

Case resolution

After thoroughly reviewing both invasive and non-invasive ventilation options, Cole's parents again requested symptom management without MV. Thus, to address his dyspnea and sleep deprivation, Cole was given a trial of low dose oral morphine (half the usual starting dose for an opioid-naïve patient of his age and weight) via his gastrostomy tube (G-tube). No effect was noted after 1 hour, when the medication would have achieved its peak effect. Using the principle of titration to effect, a second dose (this time the usual starting dose) was administered. Cole slept though the night and was restored to his usual pleasant demeanor, smiling at his parents, with full resolution of his irritability. He remained on that dose of morphine, given one to two times daily, which effectively addressed his symptoms, for 5 months. He required a laxative to manage the constipation associated with opioids, but otherwise had no adverse effects. Cole then developed pneumonitis associated with aspiration at age 13 months. He was treated with antipyretics to lower his fever and a slightly increased and more frequent dose of morphine to address his increased dyspnea. He died at his home, while being held by his parents, 1 week later. The primary cause of his death was SMA 1, with the anticipated complication of aspiration pneumonitis. By bravely being willing to use opioids in his care, his clinicians enabled Cole to live comfortably for his last 5 months and allowed his parents the ability to enjoy his company. Their bereavement will be enhanced due to the fact that their values were honored, their child was comfortable until his death, and he remained at home in their care for his entire life.

The hastening of a child's death, even in the face of symptom distress, by giving an older child the means to commit suicide, by directly providing a treatment with the intent to end life or in anticipation of the parents or someone else administering the medication with the explicit goal of hastening death (euthanasia), is not legally permitted in the United States, and many feel that it is ethically inappropriate. In almost all cases, there are ethically acceptable means to address symptom distress without resorting to these options.

Summary and key points

Beneficence and nonmaleficence are honored in the care of children with life-threatening conditions by:

- recognizing the primacy of family-centered care, including giving parents and children wide discretion in evaluating the benefits and burdens of treatments, even at the risk of a potentially hastened death, rather than assuming the medical community knows the child's best interests;
- being knowledgeable about symptom distress management and the evidence regarding the associated risks or lack thereof;
- prioritizing symptom distress as a goal of care, even in the face of the theoretical potential of a hastened death;
- being knowledgeable about and open to considering technically and ethically challenging options, such as palliative sedation.

References

Bengoechea, I., Gutiérrez, S.G., Vrotsou, K., Onaindia, M.J., & Quintana Lopez, J.M. (2010). Opioid use at the end of life and survival in a hospital at home unit. *Journal of Palliative Medicine*, **13**(9), 1079–1083.

Bruera, E., Macmillan, K., Pither, J., et al. (1990). Effects of morphine on the dyspnea of terminal cancer patients. *Journal of Pain and Symptom Management*, **5**, 341–344.

Campbell, M.L. (1996). Managing terminal dyspnea: caring for the patient who refuses intubation or ventilation. *Dimensions in Critical Care Nursing*, **15**, 4–11.

Cohen, M.H., Anderson, A.J., Krasnow, S.H., et al. (1991). Continuous intravenous infusion of morphine for severe dyspnea. *Southern Medical Journal*, **84**, 229–234.

Diekema, D.S., Botkin, J.R., & Committee on Bioethics, American Academy of Pediatrics (2009). Forgoing medically provided nutrition and hydration in children. *Pediatrics*, **124**, 813–822.

Friedrichsdorf, S.J. & Kang, T.I. (2007). The management of pain in children with life-limiting illnesses. *Pediatric Clinics of North America*, **54**, 645–672.

Hammes, B.J., Klevan, J., Kempf, M., & Williams, M.S. (2005). Pediatric advance care planning. *Journal of Palliative Medicine*, **8**, 766–773.

Hinds, P.S., Drew, D., Oakes, L.L., et al. (2005a). End-of-life care preferences of pediatric patients with cancer. *Journal of Clinical Oncology*, **23**, 9146–9154.

Hinds, P.S., Schum, L., Baker, J.N., & Wolfe, J. (2005b). Key factors affecting dying children and their families. *Journal of Palliative Medicine*, **8**(Suppl 1), S70–S78.

Houlahan, K.E., Branowicki, P.A., Mack, J.W., Dinning, C., & McCabe, M. (2006). Can end of life care for the pediatric patient suffering with escalating and intractable symptoms be improved? *Journal of Pediatric Oncology Nursing*, **23**(1), 45–51.

Kenny, N.P. & Frager, G. (1996). Refractory symptoms and terminal sedation of children: ethical and practical management. *Journal of Palliative Care*, **12**, 40–45.

Kirk, T.W. & Mahon, M.M. For the Palliative Sedation Task Force of the NHPCO Ethics Committee. (2010). National hospice and palliative care organization (NHPCO) position statement and commentary on the use of palliative sedation in imminently dying terminally ill patients. *Journal of Pain and Symptom Management*, **39**, (5), 914–923.

Kreicbergs, U., Valdimarsdóttir, U., Onelöv, E., et al. (2005). Care-related distress: a nationwide study of parents who lost their child to cancer. *Journal of Clinical Oncology*, **23**, 9162–9171.

Lyon, M.E., Garvie, P.A., McCarter, R., et al. (2009). Who will speak for me? Improving end-of-life decision-making for adolescents with HIV and their families. *Pediatrics*, **123**(2), e199–e206.

Mack, J.W., Wolfe, J., Cook, E.F., et al. (2009). Peace of mind and sense of purpose as core existential issues among parents of children with cancer. *Archives of Pediatrics and Adolescent Medicine*, **163**(6), 519–524.

McCormick, R.A. (1978). Ambiguity in moral choice. In *Doing Evil to Achieve Good: Moral Choice in Conflict Situations*, ed. R.A. McCormick & P. Ramsey. Chicago: Loyola University Press, 7–53.

Partridge, J.C. & Wall, S.N. (1997). Analgesia for dying infants whose life support is withdrawn or withheld. *Pediatrics*, **99**, 76–79.

Pritchard, M., Burghen, E., Srivastava, D.K., et al. (2008). Cancer-related symptoms most concerning to parents during the last week and last day of their child's life. *Pediatrics*, **121**(5), e1301–1309.

Quill, T.E., Dresser, R., & Brock, D.W. (1997). The rule of double effect – a critique of its role in end-of-life decision making. *New England Journal of Medicine*, **37**, 1768–1771.

Surkan, P.J., Dickman, P.W., Steineck, G., et al. (2006). Home care of a child dying of a malignancy and parental awareness of a child's impending death. *Palliative Medicine*, **20**(3), 161–169.

Weiner, L., Ballard, E., Brennan, T., et al. (2008). How I wish to be remembered: the use of an advance care planning document in adolescent and young adult populations. *Journal of Palliative Medicine*, **11**(10), 1309–1313.

Minors as recipients and donors in solid organ transplantation

Aviva M. Goldberg and Joel Frader

Case narrative 1: a minor as solid organ donor

A 15-year-old girl with end-stage kidney disease due to Wegener's granulomatosis has been on dialysis since her diagnosis 18 months before. Her lung disease is quiescent. The transplant team has determined that she is ready for transplant and has identified no psychological or medical issues to delay the procedure. Each parent volunteered to be a living kidney donor, but both were blood type incompatible (they were both type A and she was a type O). The patient is highly sensitized due to transfusions received early in her illness, suggesting a long wait on the deceased-donor kidney list, even with some priority accorded children awaiting a kidney. Her fraternal twin accompanied her to a clinic visit and stated, "I want to give my sister my kidney. I'm blood type O, I know what I'm getting myself into, and I understand the risks. How do we make this happen?"

Should the transplant team accept the twin's offer and proceed with a donor evaluation? Would the situation be different if the girls were identical twins? What if the twins were 8 years old?

Discussion of ethical issues in case 1

Live organ donation is common for kidneys, and is now possible for liver, lung, and even small bowel transplants. Live donation does not benefit the donor medically, but may provide some psychological reward. Donors do incur risks, including death (approximately 3/1000 for kidney donors), medical complications (the quantification of these varies widely among reports), and negative psychological sequelae, including low self-esteem or feelings of guilt if the transplant fails. Proponents of living donation justify donor risks by appealing to the

psychological benefits that donors may accrue, as well as benefits to family functioning arising from reduced family burdens associated with the sick relative. Kidney recipients generally experience substantial benefits, including the increased quality and quantity of life that a successful transplant offers over dialysis. In the case of identical twins, the medical benefits to the recipient are even greater, given the reduced need for immunosuppression and the resultant avoidance of the significant side effects of immunoregulatory medications. Some also argue that the psychological benefit to an identical twin donor may exceed the rewards experienced by other siblings, given the strong bond that many identical twins share.

While data from the United Network for Organ Sharing (UNOS) show that minors do sometimes act as organ donors, they comprise less than 0.1% of living kidney donors to date (49 donors as of December 2010). American courts have repeatedly authorized minors to serve as organ donors with parental permission as long as there is some perceived benefit to the potential donor (usually psychological). However, some ethicists feel that courts have too readily accepted the donor benefit argument, stating that it is "a speculative rationalization that allowed courts sympathetic to patients with renal failure to feel more comfortable about imposing a nephrectomy on vulnerable people unable to defend themselves" (Steinberg, 2004)

As with adult donors, some argue that minor donors who undergo a procedure primarily for the benefit of another person should have to provide a higher level of informed consent than would be necessary for a typical medical procedure. Some express concern that a minor may be especially vulnerable to feeling compelled to donate in order to preserve family peace or to please his or her parents (a theme that is played to dramatic

Clinical Ethics in Pediatrics: A Case-Based Textbook, ed. Douglas S. Diekema, Mark R. Mercurio and Mary B. Adam. Published by Cambridge University Press. © Cambridge University Press 2011.

effect in the novel and movie *My Sister's Keeper*; Picoult, 2004).

The Amsterdam Consensus Panel (an international panel of experts) does not endorse minor donations under any circumstances, but the American Academy of Pediatrics (AAP) Committee on Bioethics (Ross et al., 2008) state that "minors can morally serve as living organ donors but only in exceptional circumstances." The AAP delineates five conditions for a minor to be considered a solid organ donor:

1. The potential donor and recipient must each have a high likelihood of benefit (and the donations should generally be restricted to intimate family members to improve the likelihood of benefit).
2. Surgical risks to the donor must be extremely low.
3. All other opportunities for transplantation must have been exhausted, with no potential adult living donor available, and low likelihood of timely and/or effective transplantation from a deceased donor. The AAP makes no exception for identical twins, stating "if it is ethically impermissible for a minor to serve as a living donor to a sibling because of the risks or because the child cannot make a voluntary and informed decision, the same standards should hold if the potential child donor is an identical twin."
4. The minor must freely agree to donate without coercion as established by an independent donor advocate.
5. Emotional and psychological risks to the child must be minimized (by preparing donors through role playing, allowing them to ask questions, including them in the decision-making process, etc.).

Crouch and Elliott (1999), among others, have argued that family life offers special privileges and obligations and one may sometimes justify family member organ donation based on the implicit obligations arising from family relationships. Others disagree, stating that an act is not necessarily morally justified simply because it takes place within a family (Steinberg, 2004). In reality, many adult donors report that they made an "automatic" decision to donate when given the opportunity. They admit that their consent was not truly "informed" because they could not adequately understand the risks of the procedure given their emotional situation. Despite this, few regret the decision (Glannon & Ross, 2002, Papachristou et al., 2004). This suggests the relational importance of many donation decisions made within families. From this perspective, an adolescent could legitimately donate even when recognizing some influence by his or her parents, siblings, or other close relatives. The challenge faced by clinicians lies in ascertaining whether a potential family donor has been provided the opportunity to adequately consider the decision, voice reservations about his or her role, and express a desire not to donate without undue pressure or coercion. The appointment of an independent donor advocate for the teen and ample opportunities to meet privately with the donor evaluation team can provide important protections for a possible donor.

Not all adolescents will be suitable organ donors, just as many adults do not qualify for medical or psychological reasons. Once other alternatives have been exhausted and proper protective procedures have been followed, however, we believe adolescents with adequate capacity and strong ties to the intended recipient may ethically serve as donors.

Summary

- All donors should be medically and psychologically healthy, regardless of the donor's age and the impact that a decision not to donate might have on the intended recipient.
- Potential donors from within a family cannot make donation decisions completely free from emotional pressure or "auto-coercion," but that fact does not, in and of itself, undermine the validity of the donation.
- Minors wishing to serve as donors may be evaluated if appropriate conditions are met (benefit to the donor, minimization of surgical and psychological risks, lack of other donors, and a process to assure free agreement), though these situations should remain exceptional.

Resolution of case 1

The transplant team sat down with the potential donor (both with her parents and on her own) to further investigate her wishes and motivations. An independent donor advocate (a social worker at the hospital not involved in the care of the sister with kidney disease) was appointed to protect the potential donor. After an extensive evaluation, the fraternal twin was approved to be a donor and underwent a successful transplant nephrectomy.

This decision could not be similarly justified for an 8-year-old potential donor. Such a young child is unlikely to understand the risks and benefits of donation in sufficient depth. Identical twins should have protections similar to those for fraternal twins or other minor siblings; the risks to twin donors do not differ from risks to other donors. The key issue involves establishing the minor's capacity to understand the risks and consider the decision in light of those risks.

Case narrative 2: transplantation of solid organs with limited proof of clinical superiority

A 7-month-old boy presented to the emergency room of a small community hospital with vomiting and dehydration. He had previously experienced episodes of intermittent vomiting which resolved without intervention. This time the vomiting had persisted and telephone management by the primary care physician did not succeed. At presentation the child was tachycardic, with poor peripheral perfusion and marginal blood pressure. His abdomen was distended and firm. After fluid resuscitation, he was taken to the operating room (OR) where the surgeon reduced a volvulus with only slight improvement in the dusky appearance of the bowel. Emergency transport to a regional pediatric center was arranged.

After a short stop in the children's hospital pediatric intensive care unit for stabilization, the boy was taken to the OR. Surgeons found extensive necrosis of the bowel and resected all but 20–25 centimeters of the small intestine. Following surgery, the boy experienced slow growth on parenteral nutrition (PN), and efforts to provide enteral nutrition resulted in vomiting and/or large fluid losses through his stoma. The pediatric surgeons advised the family to take their child to another center for small bowel transplantation. When the parents asked about alternatives to transplantation, the physicians responded that without a transplant the boy would succumb because of repeated central venous catheter complications or liver failure from toxic effects of PN, or both.

Discussion of ethical issues in case 2

Though transplant teams have made considerable progress in understanding the challenges associated with small bowel transplantation (SBTx), many serious problems remain. In this case, the patient's surgeons tell the parents the child should undergo SBTx in order

to save the boy's life. However, the doctrine of informed consent requires a more comprehensive discussion of the risks, benefits, and reasonable alternatives to the recommended intervention. (Nothing about a good informed consent process precludes a medical recommendation.) Especially in situations like this one, where the suggested intervention itself involves substantial risks and difficulties (recurrent or chronic graft rejection, graft versus host disease, a higher risk of post-transplant lymphoproliferative disease [PTLD] and/or aggressive malignancy than occurs with other solid organ transplants, and poor neurodevelopmental outcomes), referral for transplantation without a thorough discussion of the risks of transplantation and alternatives to transplantation violates even minimal notions of informed consent (Committee on Bioethics, 1995).

In the twenty-first century, the approach to short bowel syndrome (SBS) ideally involves multidisciplinary and multimodal interventions. Continuous enteral feeding with elemental formulas and bowel surgeries, such as serial transverse enteroplasty, to lengthen the residual bowel and increase absorptive capacity, have enabled many patients to come off PN, avoiding the vascular and hepatic complications of PN (Mazariegos, 2009; Avitzur & Grant, 2010). A consensus seems to have emerged that many patients previously felt to have no chance for survival without transplant may actually experience successful bowel rehabilitation and thrive on oral nutritional intake alone. Non-transplant approaches may succeed in some patients with as little as 10–15 cm of residual bowel (Avitzur & Grant, 2010).

In addition, the risks of transplantation have become somewhat clearer. While fatal Epstein–Barr virus-associated PTLD no longer poses the threat it did in the early years of SBTx, due to improved immunosuppression regimens and various antiviral strategies, the risk of PTLD following SBTx remains substantially higher than that seen after other solid organ transplants (Abu-Elmagd et al., 2009). The large amount of lymphoid tissue in the graft makes SBTx patients more vulnerable to developing graft versus host disease than is seen with other solid organ transplants. Rejection of the transplanted bowel, whether occurring as intermittent acute episodes or chronic rejection, poses both diagnostic and treatment difficulties. Physicians may have trouble distinguishing symptoms and signs of rejection from those associated with viral and other infections of the graft. Children typically require frequent biopsies of their grafts, as often as twice a week, accomplished by endoscopy through a stoma. These procedures may require sedation and/or produce psychological distress for the child. Uncertainty about the diagnosis of rejection may delay closure of stomas which, in turn, may have an impact on the child's quality of life.

Finally, the SBTx group at the University of Miami has found persistent and troubling neurocognitive deficits in children who have had SBTx. They found severe motor delay in more than 95% of those transplanted before 3 years of age, compared with ~70% of similarly aged liver transplant patients with serious delays. They also documented cognitive delay in 74% of SBTx survivors compared with 54% of those following liver transplantation (Thevenin et al., 2006).

Despite substantial improvements in SBTx outcomes, 5-year survival remains somewhere around 50% with considerable concern about poor developmental status, risk of acute and chronic rejection and recurrent infection, risk of cancer, and the need for repeated hospitalizations and procedures. Under these circumstances thoughtful and concerned parents might well see non-transplant treatment as preferable. At what point a family might reasonably refuse non-transplant therapies, such as repeated surgical procedures to increase bowel surface area or artificial feedings, seems somewhat less clear. Ross and Frader (2009) argued that risk-averse parents looking at the likelihood of bad outcomes could well choose palliative care over surgery in hypoplastic left heart syndrome. At the very least, under similar circumstances physicians have a duty to disclose the option of non-intervention, even if the professionals feel they could not support such a decision by the parents.

The lack of clarity about when patients with SBS might benefit from transplantation versus non-transplant approaches continues to suggest the need for head-on comparative trials of the alternative approaches, something that has changed little since a similar examination of the ethics of SBTx in 1998 (Frader & Caniano, 1998). Over the past 10–15 years, controlled clinical trials involving different surgical techniques or comparing surgery with other interventions have established the feasibility and acceptance of such research. SBS seems a good candidate for an attempt to examine the comprehensive advantages and disadvantages of transplantation compared with other management strategies.

Summary

- Informed consent for complex procedures must involve a thorough discussion of the risks, benefits, and reasonable alternatives to the procedure.
- Small bowel transplantation, given its high rate of complications and the availability of alternative treatments, is a good example of a situation where deciding not to consent to the proposed treatment may be a reasonable choice for informed parents.

Resolution of case 2

The boy's parents used resources at the children's hospital to investigate the outcomes of and alternatives to SBTx. The father flew to a transplant center with extensive pediatric SBTx experience and met with representatives of the gastroenterology service, pediatric surgery, transplantation surgery, and nutrition services. After a two hour meeting he tentatively agreed to bring his son for a trial of intestinal rehabilitation. In a later family meeting, the boy's mother agreed. Over 6 months the child had serial enteroplasties and appeared to make some progress in weaning from PN. However, he continued to refuse oral feedings and options for vascular access were eventually exhausted. The boy lost weight despite vigorous attempts at enteral nutrition. His parents declined SBTx and returned home with their son. With support from a regional pediatric hospice program, the family decided to withdraw the boy's feeding tube. He died several days after medically provided nutrition and hydration were stopped.

The parents of the boy in this case made independent efforts to obtain adequate information before giving their permission for one of the alternative treatments for SBS. After examining and understanding information about the results of SBTx, they took the relatively unusual step of refusing the physician-preferred treatment. These parents felt that the burdens of transplantation outweighed a potential survival benefit for their son. Given the state of knowledge about competing approaches to this clinical problem, they applied their own values to a very difficult choice. This is the way parental decision-making is supposed to happen, despite the discomfort and opposition of some of the professionals involved.

References

Abu-Elmagd, K.M., Mazariegos, G., Costa, G., et al. (2009). Lymphoproliferative disorders and de novo malignancies in intestinal and multivisceral recipients: improved outcomes with new outlooks. *Transplantation*, **88**, 926–934.

Avitzur, Y. & Grant, D. (2010). Intestine transplantation in children: update 2010. *Pediatric Clinics of North America*, **57**, 415–431.

Committee on Bioethics, American Academic of Pediatrics (1995). Informed consent, parental permission, and assent in pediatric practice. *Pediatrics*, **95**, 314–317.

Crouch, R.A. & Elliott C. (1999). Moral agency and the family: the case of living related organ transplantation. *Cambridge Quarterly of Healthcare Ethics*, **8**, 275–287.

Frader, J.E. & Caniano, D.A. (1998). Research and innovation in surgery. In *Surgical Ethics*, ed. L.B. McCullough, J.W. Jones, & B.A. Brody. New York: Oxford University Press, 216–241.

Glannon, W. & Ross, L.F. (2002). Do genetic relationships create moral obligations in organ transplantation? *Cambridge Quarterly of Healthcare Ethics*, **11**, 153–159.

Mazariegos, G. (2009). Intestinal transplantation: current outcomes and opportunities. *Current Opinion in Organ Transplantation*, **14**, 515–521.

Papachristou, C., Walter, M., Dietrich. K., et al. (2004). Motivation for living-donor liver transplantation from the donor's perspective: an in-depth qualitative research study. *Transplantation*, **78**, 1506–1514.

Picoult, J. (2004). *My Sister's Keeper*. New York: Atria Books.

Ross, L.F. & Frader, J. (2009). Hypoplastic left heart syndrome: a paradigm case for examining conscientious objection in pediatric practice. *Journal of Pediatrics*, **155**, 12–15.

Ross, L.F., Thistlethwaite, J.R., Jr., & Committee on Bioethics, American Academy of Pediatrics (2008). Minors as living solid-organ donors. *Pediatrics*, **122**, 454–461.

Steinberg, D. (2004). Kidney transplant from young children and the mentally retarded. *Theoretical Medicine*, **25**, 229–241.

Thevenin, D.M., Baker, A., Kato, T., et al. (2006). Neurodevelopmental outcomes for children transplanted under the age of 3 years. *Transplantation Proceedings*, **38**, 1692–1693.

Chapter 26

Enhancement technologies and children

Jennifer C. Kesselheim

Case narrative

Kyle is a 4-year-old patient in your primary care practice. He is the third son born to Dara and Max, a couple you know well because you have been their family's pediatrician for 12 years. Dara and Max are both highly educated professionals who consistently emphasize dedication to school work and scholastic achievement in their parenting. Kyle's parents raise no concerns about Kyle's physical health but they express frustration about his behavior. As compared with their other sons, Dara and Max feel that Kyle is less able to focus on "educational activities" such as puzzles and books; he seems to favor more active play and prefers activities where he can run and climb. He can be "very oppositional" when they try to redirect him towards "educational activities." Dara and Max worry that Kyle's behavior may indicate attention-deficit/hyperactivity disorder (ADHD). Although his preschool teachers do not suspect ADHD and express no concerns about Kyle's behavior at school, Kyle's parents request a trial of Ritalin. Dara says "Kyle is so unlike our other sons. I just want to see if the medicine can help him focus and behave differently." You respond by asking what she means by "differently," to which Max replies "We would like him to behave ... better."

The quest for "better": defining enhancement

The desires of Dara and Max may resonate with many parents. Many large and small decisions of parenthood are usually guided by the parents' desire to help their children live better lives. Parents are expected to maximize their children's opportunities for success by making thoughtful choices for their children in the home, in the classroom, in the pediatrician's office, and in all domains of life.

At times, it can be difficult to identify the limits of this intrinsic parental duty. When does the parental quest for "better" grow beyond the bounds of good parenting to become ethically problematic? Ethical dilemmas can stem from discrepant definitions of "better." For Dara and Max, their son could behave "better" by engaging in activities that they feel would benefit his cognitive development and place him on a path towards academic excellence. But to different parents, the meaning of "better" may also differ. Better may entail athletic talents for some, while others might favor creative expression, an ear for music, or demonstration of particular character traits such as sense of humor, optimism, or empathy. The moral ambiguity of these decisions is further intensified when one considers the meaning of childhood. By definition, a child is in the midst of a journey, on the way to something, in the process of realizing a mature self. There is a unique openness to the existence of a child that is related to having an unwritten future. But this definition of childhood can be difficult to reconcile with the parent's role in shaping the future of their child. In their report entitled "Beyond Therapy: Biotechnology and the Pursuit of Happiness," the President's Council on Bioethics (2003) notes "the notorious paradox of parenthood: we love our children unconditionally ... yet we are constantly doing everything in our power to get them to be different, to *change*."

The Council goes on to note that new technologies, some available in the present and others imagined for the future, will bring renewed attention to the quest for "better." As technology gives us new ways to improve upon the natural state of our children, it will become increasingly essential for pediatricians to be able to distinguish where proposed interventions sit on the spectrum between medical therapy and enhancement. The former improves the biological functioning of the

Clinical Ethics in Pediatrics: A Case-Based Textbook, ed. Douglas S. Diekema, Mark R. Mercurio and Mary B. Adam. Published by Cambridge University Press. © Cambridge University Press 2011.

body by preventing, alleviating, or reversing a disease state (Daniels, 2000). On the other hand, *enhancement aims to improve function that is already within the normal range*. In so doing, enhancement technologies can raise ethical dilemmas for parents and pediatricians who struggle with the quest for "better."

"Better" minds

In the 1990s, psychotropic medication revolutionized the disciplines of pediatrics, child neurology, and child psychiatry by introducing new drugs to the pediatric population. Several classes of drugs, including stimulants, antidepressants, anxiolytics, and antipsychotics were used to treat an array of disorders including attention-deficit disorder (ADD), attention-deficit/hyperactivity disorder (ADHD), conduct disorder, depression, schizophrenia, and various other disorders of behavior, mood, and learning (Conrad, 2004). Each of these disorders takes a serious toll on children and families. Kyle's parents fear ADHD, which can certainly cause suffering in children who experience both failure in school and disruptive conflict at home. While the advent of these new medications for children has sparked certain controversies, these medicines can alleviate symptoms for children with genuine psychiatric diagnoses. For example, in children with true ADD or ADHD, the use of stimulants like methylphenidate (Ritalin) or amphetamine (Adderall) can be life changing. Medication, usually in conjunction with extra support from parents, services from the child's school, and competent counseling, can help a struggling child adjust socially, succeed academically, and gain self-esteem (President's Council on Bioethics, 2003).

But what role should psychotropic medications play for a child like Kyle? Does Kyle have a true diagnosis of ADHD that justifies treatment with methylphenidate? Making a diagnosis such as ADHD, for which there is no objective medical test, is inherently more subjective than for a disease with an easily identifiable biological marker. From his parents' point of view, he does not focus on the activities they prefer him to pursue and is oppositional when they try to guide his play. However, his preschool teachers remain unconcerned about his behavior and his pediatrician believes these "symptoms" are less consistent with ADHD than with normal, albeit sometimes frustrating, behaviors inherent to childhood. In all likelihood, Kyle is a normal 4-year-old boy. Nonetheless, parents like Dara and Max may desire their normal children to behave

"better," by which they may mean more attentive, more flexible, more sociable, or more tranquil. This desire may lead to a request for stimulants, or other psychotropic medications, even in the absence of true disease. Such requests represent enhancement because they involve psychopharmacologic strategies to "improve" upon the normal.

Ethical analysis

Responding to Dara and Max's request for a trial of stimulant therapy must involve a delineation of the risks and potential benefits of the medication. First, while stimulants and other psychotropic medications have a low incidence of toxicity overall when used properly, they are nonetheless associated with short-term side effects such as insomnia and weight loss due to appetite suppression (Diller, 1996). In addition, the effect that multiple years of stimulant use in childhood may have on the mid-life or elderly adult is entirely unknown (President's Council on Bioethics, 2002). Moreover, certain psychotropic medications are prescribed for children in an off-label manner, indicating that the Food and Drug Administration (FDA) has not yet found sufficient evidence for the drugs' safety and efficacy in the pediatric population (Cooper et al., 2004). While off-label prescribing is common in pediatrics, it is still a source of risk to patients that should contribute to ethical reasoning.

Second, the President's Council on Bioethics (2003) notes that "the use of such drugs to shape behavior raises serious questions concerning the liberty of children." To the extent that children are owed an open and unwritten future, the use of psychotropic medications in the absence of psychiatric disease may constitute an excess of adult control.

Third, the drug may be difficult to discontinue once initiated. Ritalin can enhance the performance of anyone, whether or not ADD or ADHD is present, by decreasing distractibility and increasing concentration and alertness. If Kyle has such a response while taking methylphenidate, his parents may misconstrue this response as a benefit of the drug, thereby reinforcing the drug's utility and possibly committing Kyle to many more years of stimulant use in the absence of true disease. This ongoing use of stimulants may cause future teachers and peers to make assumptions about his abilities and wrongly consider him to have a disorder. In addition, the continuing "need" for this medication can undermine Kyle's self-esteem by leading to his own erroneous conclusion that he has a disorder.

Lastly, the use of stimulants may unfairly deprive Kyle of the opportunity to experience other interventions. Kyle may experience greater benefit from other therapies to address his parents' concerns, such as play therapy. Stimulant use for Kyle may distract his parents and pediatrician from pursuing these non-pharmacologic avenues that may, in the end, be more useful to him.

Parents and physicians alike must sometimes confront the risks of medications in order to ameliorate disease. However, the risks of methylphenidate or other psychotropic medications are less acceptable when no true psychiatric disorder is present. In those cases, the medications do not yield the benefit of alleviating disease, and the risks accompanying their use are therefore difficult to justify without concomitant medical benefits.

"Better" bodies

The quest for "better" can also lead patients and families to try to improve a child's body. Many believe that particular physical traits and abilities can optimally position children to live happy and successful lives. This belief has manifested itself in the debate about human growth hormone supplementation for children with short stature.

Recombinant DNA technology has allowed human growth hormone (hGH) to be produced in abundance. Therapy with hGH has therefore expanded beyond its traditional use for growth hormone-deficient children. Human growth hormone has been approved by the FDA for the treatment of short stature due to numerous organic causes, several of which, such as chronic renal insufficiency and Turner syndrome, do not involve hGH deficiency. The unifying feature of the various indications for hGH supplementation is *disability*; the intention behind hGH therapy is to ameliorate the disability introduced by extreme short stature (Allen & Fost, 2004). But defining disability can be subjective, and as technologic advances made hGH supplementation more prevalent, pediatricians and pediatric endocrinologists have been confronted with an increasing array of requests for hGH.

Consensus is emerging that short stature causes significant disability for patients below the 5th percentile for height, such that hGH supplementation for this population of patients constitutes medical therapy (Drug and Therapeutics Committee, 1995; Allen & Fost, 2004). Patients whose height is at or above the 5th

percentile are unlikely to experience disability from their short stature; the use of hGH supplementation for this cohort, who enjoy normal function, should be considered enhancement (Drug and Therapeutics Committee, 1995).

Ethical analysis

How should a physician respond to a parent's request for hGH supplementation for a child whose stature is not likely to cause disability? Are physicians ethically justified in refusing such a request?

While human growth hormone supplementation has been shown to be non-toxic overall, physicians may still refuse to prescribe hGH for reasons of safety. Supplementing hGH is associated with intracranial hypertension as well as with slipped capital femoral epiphysis (Wyatt, 2004). As in the case of stimulants, hGH is sometimes prescribed for children in an off-label manner, which can raise further doubts about the safety of supplementation.

In addition, physician refusal could arise from justice considerations, for enhancement of vertical growth using hGH carries a hefty price tag. One child's (30 kg) supplementation can yield an annual cost as high as US$15 000–20 000 (Allen & Fost, 2004). Although cost is certainly not the only morally relevant consideration, the expense of this technology used for the purposes of enhancement, not treatment, should prompt prescribers to exercise caution, as the benefits of the hormone may not justify the expense.

What benefits might come from hGH supplementation for children at or above the 5th percentile of height? While it has been widely assumed that short stature yields psychological strain while being taller leads to better psychological health, research may not substantiate these claims. Data do *not* reveal a relationship between the adult height of hGH-supplemented individuals and their quality of life (Allen & Fost, 2004). Therefore, children who are already at or above the 5th percentile, who experience no disability from their short stature, may not truly benefit from more vertical growth. In fact, such children may be harmed by this intervention, because inherent in the request for hGH supplementation is the message that the child has failed to meet parental expectations (Diekema, 1990). Concerns over the psychological welfare of the child may therefore provide ethical justification for refusing parental requests for hGH supplementation.

How should pediatric endocrinologists address parents who feel their child is *entitled* to an intervention that will help him or her to become as tall as possible? Although parents and patients may experience disappointment or frustration that the child will not grow to his or her full potential height, the pediatrician should remember that the patient is not morally entitled to the added height. Patient and family members' expectations should not oblige physicians to provide hGH supplementation for enhancement purposes (Daniels, 2000; Allen & Fost, 2004).

"Better" genes

Enhancement technologies can also be applied to "improve" children before they are even born. As the use of assisted reproductive technologies becomes more prevalent, and as we increasingly learn the links between particular human traits (phenotypes) and certain combinations of genes (genotypes), medical technology is opening the door for the enhancement of future children by manipulation of sperm, eggs, and embryos. To explore the ethical issues raised by these technologies, we must first define the various strategies proposed for enhancing genes and distinguish between those already in use and those which are not *yet* feasible, but are theoretically plausible.

- Prenatal diagnosis: Illnesses for which genetic testing is available may be diagnosed during an established pregnancy (with amniocentesis or chorionic villus sampling). For example, a fetus whose parents are known carriers of Tay–Sachs disease can be diagnosed with the disease early so that the couple could consider termination of the pregnancy. This technology allows parents to avoid the birth of a child with certain undesired traits, but the potential for this technology to be used to select for a "better" baby, rather than select against a diseased one, is low.
- Preimplantation genetic screening and selection: Testing of sperm, eggs, or embryos newly conceived through in vitro fertilization (IVF) allows selective implantation of embryos that are known to express desirable genotypes. This technology is far more expensive than prenatal diagnosis and must include IVF. While this approach usually aims to optimize the future child's health, it can also be applied to select for the sex of the baby or to ensure that the baby will be compatible with an ill family member in need of a

stem cell transplant. The use of this technology is currently limited as it can only select for a limited number of genes and traits at a time. That said, this technology will likely become increasingly applicable with the identification of more genes that control traits of interest to parents.
- Directed genetic change (genetic engineering): This technology warrants consideration since it exists as a theoretical possibility for the future, even though it is not feasible currently and poses numerous safety concerns. This strategy would seek to directly improve embryos by introducing more desirable genes.

To make clear the distinctions between these three approaches, the President's Council on Bioethics wrote that the first represents "eliminating the bad (screening out)," the second represents "selecting the good (choosing in)," while the third represents "redesigning for the better (fixing up)" (President's Council on Bioethics, 2003).

Ethical analysis

The President's Council on Bioethics clearly expresses concern about all three of these technologies due to safety (President's Council on Bioethics, 2003). The methods of making a prenatal diagnosis can increase the chances for infection, miscarriage, or fetal demise. Preimplanatation genetic diagnosis involves gamete manipulation and IVF, which are known to carry risks of congenital malformations and preterm labor. Directed genetic change can also be risky as the intervention may disrupt the function of other genes, beyond the gene of interest. The risk of harm to the fetus or future child may be justified if the intention is medical therapy. For example, a risk of miscarriage may be justified by the benefits of knowing the fetus is not affected by a devastating condition like Tay–Sachs disease. In such a case, the decision to accept these risks can justifiably be left to parental discretion. But if the intention is enhancement, if the intervention neither treats nor prevents suffering from true medical illness, the risks of detrimental outcomes for the fetus or future child are more difficult to accept.

Enhancing the genes of the next generation raises ethical concerns about justice because these expensive technologies are not equally accessible to all couples. Therefore, couples with economic riches will also be more likely to have children with "genetic riches," thereby widening the already vast disparity between rich and poor families (President's Council on Bioethics, 2003).

As it is currently applied, prenatal diagnosis seeks to prevent medical disease and is therefore rarely used as an enhancement technology. That said, this technology raises ethical questions by giving parents a new form of adult control over their future child and by sending a message that every child may not be welcome, that parental acceptance may be conditional (President's Council on Bioethics, 2003). In addition, prenatal diagnosis may blur the line between medical therapy and enhancement when the traits being selected against are deemed negative for reasons other than health. In this way, prenatal diagnosis importantly opens the door to enhancement by optimizing a parent's choice about the qualities of his or her offspring (President's Council on Bioethics, 2003) Preimplantation genetic screening and directed genetic change can each be used to prevent or treat medical disease, but both have the potential to serve enhancement purposes as well. Using these technologies for enhancement would raise ethical questions by interfering with the open future of children. When parents choose positive traits for their children, they set up *a priori* expectations for how their children will excel. Children's talents would be chosen for them, depriving them of the unscripted discovery of their own passions. As the President's Council on Bioethics wrote, these technologies were "designed to free us from the tyranny of our genes" but may in turn "narrow our freedom as individuals" in a new way.

Conclusions

Enhancement technologies may well lead to an unprecedented change in pediatric practice and could redefine the relationship between parents and their children. As advances continue to emerge, it will become increasingly essential for pediatricians to feel confident responding to requests for enhancement. A critical first step is developing an understanding of enhancement, in order to recognize the true nature of a patient's or parent's request. Unlike medical treatment, which improves the biological functioning of the body by preventing, alleviating, or reversing a disease state, enhancement aims to improve function that is already within the normal range. Therefore, enhancement interventions do not have the potential to yield the same appreciable benefits as have medical therapies; this essential distinction must remain at the forefront of ethical reasoning about enhancement.

Once a pediatrician becomes aware that a proposed intervention actually constitutes enhancement, careful consideration should follow. Some of the salient ethical questions to ask include:
- What safety concerns accompany this intervention and are these risks ethically justifiable in light of the limited benefits?
- Would acquiescing to the request for enhancement possibly prevent the patient from enjoying the benefits of other therapeutic interventions?
- Does the enhancing intervention represent an excess of adult control over the pediatric patient? Could the proposed enhancement inappropriately interfere with the child's access to an open and unscripted future?
- Would the enhancement technology, if adopted more widely, create concerns about justice or fairness due to a high price or unequal access to the technology?

These questions can help guide ethical reasoning about a request for enhancement. In many cases, proposed enhancement technologies will fare poorly in the face of these considerations. Such is the case for Kyle's parents, whose plea for methylphenidate certainly constitutes a request for enhancement. Due to the potential for short-term side effects, the risks of long-term use (both physical and emotional), the missed opportunity for other more beneficial interventions, and the excess of adult control, methylphenidate use for Kyle should be avoided. Under circumstances similar to Kyle's, and in the setting of other pleas for enhancement technologies, the pediatrician is ethically justified in refusing such requests. As experts in protecting and restoring the health of children, pediatricians are optimally positioned to help define the limits of the quest for "better."

References

Allen, D.B. & Fost, N. (2004). hGH for short stature: ethical issues raised by expanded access. *Journal of Pediatrics*, **144**, 648–652.

Conrad, P. (2004). Prescribing more psychotropic medications for children: what does the increase mean? *Archives of Pediatrics and Adolescent Medicine*, **158**, 829–830.

Cooper, W.O., Hickson, G.B., Fuchs, C., Arbogast, P.G., & Ray, W.A. (2004). New users of antipsychotic medications among children enrolled in TennCare. *Archives of Pediatrics and Adolescent Medicine*, **158**, 753–759.

Daniels, N. (2000). Normal functioning and the treatment-enhancement distinction. *Cambridge Quarterly of Healthcare Ethics*, **9**, 309–322.

Diekema, D.S. (1990). Is taller really better? Growth hormone therapy in short children. *Perspectives in Biology and Medicine*, **34**, 109–123.

Diller, L.H. (1996). The run on Ritalin. Attention deficit disorder and stimulant treatment in the 1990s. *Hastings Center Report*, **26**, 12–18.

Drug and Therapeutics Committee, Lawson Wilkins Pediatric Endocrine Society (1995). Guidelines for the use of growth hormone in children with short stature. A report by the Drug and Therapeutics Committee of the Lawson Wilkins Pediatric Endocrine Society. *Journal of Pediatrics*, **127**, 857–867.

President's Council on Bioethics (2002). Staff Background Paper: Human flourishing, performance enhancement, and Ritalin. December 2002. Available at http://bioethics.georgetown.edu/pcbe/background/humanflourish.html. Last accessed December 29, 2010.

President's Council on Bioethics (2003). Beyond Therapy: Biotechnology and the Pursuit of Happiness. A report by the President's Council on Bioethics. Washington, DC: Government Printing Office. Available at http://bioethics.georgetown.edu/pcbe/reports/beyondtherapy/beyond_therapy_final_webcorrected.pdf. Last accessed December 29, 2010.

Wyatt, D. (2004). Lessons from the national cooperative growth study. *European Journal of Endocrinology*, **151**(Suppl. 1), S55–S59.

Chapter

27

Cochlear implants and deaf children

Halle Showalter Salas

Case narrative

After an uneventful pregnancy, a woman delivers a healthy baby boy. Prior to discharge from the hospital, the infant undergoes newborn screening and is found to be prelingually deaf with complete sensorineural hearing loss. The family is referred to an audiologist who recommends a cochlear implant for the child. He is physically an ideal candidate and an implant would give him the best chance at spoken communication.

The parents, who are both culturally Deaf, oppose the cochlear implant. They view his deafness as a part of who he is rather than as a deficit or a disability requiring medical intervention. They desire for their son to fully share in their family's culture and communicate fluently with them in ASL, their native language. They worry that an implant could potentially inhibit his full participation in their community. They also express fears that an implant would signal to their child and society that something was wrong with him by viewing his deafness as pathological rather than an integral piece of his identity.

When asked to further clarify their concerns, the parents state that at the very least, the decision to implant should be made by their son when he is at an age to appropriately weigh the pros and cons of the procedure, the risks/benefits of the device, and the resulting impact of an implant on his life.

Introduction to cochlear implants

Understanding cochlear implants from a variety of perspectives is critical to defining and understanding the ethical issues inherent in the case. I will first present a basic explanation of cochlear implants followed by a short description of the device from a Deaf perspective. Finally, I will briefly describe how cochlear implants fit in to a much larger debate that has existed for over a

century about deaf children, their education, and the notion of a Deaf community. This background information will provide a factual foundation on which to discuss the ethical issues of beneficence, nonmaleficence, and respect for persons as they present themselves in this case.

A cochlear implant is a small electronic device that bypasses damaged portions of the ear and directly stimulates the auditory nerve. Signals generated by the implant are transmitted via the auditory nerve to the brain, which then recognizes these signals as sound (NIDCD, 2009). Approximately one month after implantation, the device is "turned on" and, ideally, a number of professionals provide long-term support to assist the implantee to utilize the device and develop aural speech (D'Silva et al., 2004, p. 113). The device includes two major components: an internal portion that is surgically implanted and an exterior portion that can be seen on the user's head that connects to a device that sits behind the ear (Figure 27.1). Rather than restoring normal hearing, the implant allows a person to experience a representation of sound, the ultimate goal of which is to aid an individual in understanding speech (NIDCD, 2009).

Cochlear implants were first approved by the Food and Drug Administration (FDA) in 1990 for children 2–17 years of age, and are now approved for use in certain children as young as 12 months of age (Kim et al., 2010, p. 11). According to the FDA, as of April 2009, approximately 188 000 people worldwide have received implants. Of those, roughly 41 500 adults and 25 500 children have been implanted in the United States (www.nidcd.nih.gov/health/hearing/coch.asp). The use of cochlear implants has increased in recent years (Kim et al., 2010). Several factors contribute to this change, including newborn screening programs, which promote earlier identification of children with

Clinical Ethics in Pediatrics: A Case-Based Textbook, ed. Douglas S. Diekema, Mark R. Mercurio and Mary B. Adam. Published by Cambridge University Press. © Cambridge University Press 2011.

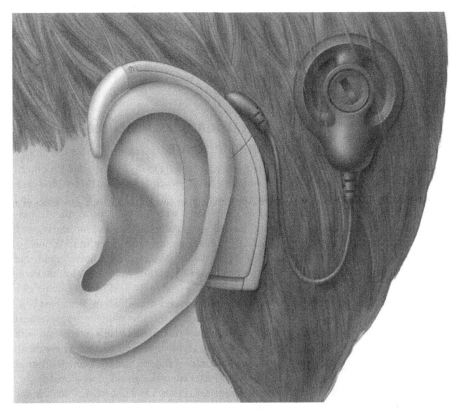

Figure 27.1. Cochlear implant. Photo courtesy of Cochlear Americas, ©2010.

hearing issues, allowing for earlier intervention and ever broadening criteria for implant candidates (Hyde et al., 2010; Kim et al., 2010).

Discussion of the issues

Unlike the case presented above, nearly 90% of deaf children are born to hearing parents (Berg et al., 2007, p. 13). Most hearing parents see deafness as a deficit and as a barrier to communicating with their child in the way that is most comfortable to them and commonly used by their family. Few of these parents know a deaf adult, and most have little contact with the Deaf community (Christiansen & Leigh, 2002).

In contrast, the parents in our case identify as culturally Deaf and consider themselves members of the Deaf community. The term "Deaf," with an uppercase "D," emphasizes a language and cultural affiliation. Typically this includes deaf people in the United States and Canada whose everyday means of communication is American Sign Language (ASL). The term "deaf" (lowercase "d") refers to people with a medical condition that does not allow them to hear (Padden & Humphries, 1988). Not all deaf people or hard of hearing individuals belong to the Deaf community or desire to be part of it. Some prefer to be part of the mainstream hearing culture.

As with all discrete communities, there exists a great deal of diversity within the Deaf community, and its response to cochlear implants also varies. Initially, organizations like the National Association of the Deaf (NAD) were staunchly opposed to implants, as evidenced in their 1991 position paper on cochlear implants. Some advocates used terms like "genocide" or "child abuse" when referring to implants. As technology has improved and more deaf children are receiving and living with cochlear implants, the opinions and positions of many have softened (Christiansen & Leigh, 2002; Drolsbaugh, 2008), due in part to the recognition that every child is different and requires a variety of means to accomplish his or her potential. Nonetheless, many people in the Deaf community are still opposed to or struggle with the idea of implants for children that are prelingually deafened (Drolsbaugh, 2008).

Another concern surrounding cochlear implantation commonly discussed in Deaf publications is the preferential focus on aural or spoken language rather than concentrating on language acquisition (Christiansen & Leigh, 2002). Many in the Deaf community are concerned that the focus on spoken language, which accompanies a cochlear implant, constitutes a major disservice to deaf children, especially if sign language is not part of that education. People who are deaf obtain information primarily through visual means, making sign language one of the most accessible media for immediate communication and as such, many believe signed language should have a prominent place in the education of all deaf children. The NAD supports and endorses innovative educational programming for all deaf children that includes auditory and speech skills in a "dynamic and interactive visual environment that utilizes sign language and English" (NAD, 2000).

The education of deaf children and selection of the best communication methods have created tension in the United States for over a century. Understanding the historical background provides context for discussing the ethical implications surrounding cochlear implants. The nineteenth century was rife with debate between the manualists who advocated for deaf children to be educated using mainly sign methods, and the oralists who promoted a speech-only environment and the prohibition of sign language. One thing these two groups had in common was paternalism. Baynton (1996) comments that "Both saw deafness through their own cultural biases and sought to shape deaf people accordingly. Both forged metaphors of deaf people as fundamentally flawed, incomplete, isolated and dependent. And both used that imagery to justify the authority of the hearing over the deaf." Some would argue that not much has changed. Many years of such a paternalistic approach eventually led to protests and other acts of advocacy, which evolved out of deeply held beliefs of Deaf individuals who wanted some control over their education and lives and their voices heard by the leadership that represented who they were (Deaf President Now Protest, 2010).

Today, with the advances of cochlear implant technology and improved access to such treatment, many of these questions persist. What is normal? How should hearing differences be treated? What is best for an individual living in this culture? Who decides the notion of "best" for a deaf child? On one hand, many in society support the notion that differences should be not only tolerated but embraced. On the other hand, the social majority highly values science and technology, and holds a worldview informed by the fact that they perceive much of the world through auditory means. Several ethical issues emerge from these differing values and views.

Ethical principles: beneficence and nonmaleficence

Beneficence, or seeking to do what is good for others, is a major ethical principle with bearing in this case. Medical teams seek the good of their patients, and many individuals with medical backgrounds perceive deafness as a pathology – a lack of hearing as a medical problem requiring intervention (Weinberg, 2005). Many within the medical culture argue that the principle of beneficence would require intervening on behalf of a deaf individual because living in a world of sound benefits deaf children. Perceived benefits of implantation include auditory improvement and speech production which enable interaction with hearing society, ability to respond to the environment, and a reduction of social stigma, all of which presumably lead to better educational and professional opportunities for deaf children (Okubo et al., 2008). Many in the Deaf community, however, do not perceive that these benefits are superior to the lives they lead in the absence of implants, lives full of communication, rich relationships, and fulfilling careers. They worry that irreparable harm is being done to children who may never feel comfortable being deaf and will continually strive to become hearing – something that will always elude them. Rather than promoting good, implants can lead to great harm.

The parents in the case at the opening of the chapter seek to do what is best for their child by promoting his sense of self through a focus on capability. From their perspective, their child will "fit" better in the family without the ability to hear. "Being very rational about it, hearing adults can no more become deaf than deaf adults can become hearing. Neither culture considers it normal for members to have had a childhood in the other culture" (Tuchler, 2009). Christiansen and Leigh (2002) point out that for a deaf child born to a hearing family, "enabling the profoundly deaf child to participate in the culture of the parents contributes to the principle of beneficence, or doing good for the child." However, in the case of a deaf child born to Deaf parents, Christiansen and Leigh emphasize the potential for harm in the event the child feels estranged from his family of origin. This concern invokes the principle of nonmaleficence, the principle that we should not cause unnecessary harm to others. What harm can be done to the child by requiring a cochlear implant and what harm can be done by refusing? Lane and Bahan (1998) describe prelingually deaf children as visual, and rather than viewing deafness as a disability to conquer, the focus should be on deafness as a way of life defined by social values and relationships. They assert that allowing a deaf child to be deaf does not by definition exclude them from connection with the hearing community.

The Deaf family in this case argues that their child would potentially be more estranged from the family's community by virtue of receiving a cochlear implant. After all, a child's environment and family support are very important to the implant's success (Kim et al., 2010). Depending on the child's family situation, an implant may result in great benefit or may do harm. The harm/benefit calculation should be made for each individual child to assure to the greatest extent possible that the potential benefits outweigh the potential harms. From the perspective of the parents in our case, however, the implant offers little benefit. Despite the relative safety of the surgery, repeat surgery may be required if the device fails. Effectiveness of the implant is variable and dependent on many things including non-modifiable factors such as IQ, socioeconomic status, gender, family size, and educational programs available (Berg et al., 2005). For these reasons, it is difficult to predict outcomes with implants as they do not guarantee the ability to hear or to acquire spoken language. From the perspective of the medical staff, however, the potential benefits may outweigh the harms. The surgery is considered medically safe with a very small number of patients experiencing medical complications (Christiansen & Leigh, 2002). And, with proper support, this child will likely develop aural speech, granting him better access to the hearing majority culture.

Is it possible that placement of a cochlear implant could *interfere* with the good the parents or the medical team seek for the child? Cochlear implants can present what seems like a "quick fix" that makes it possible for the deaf child to participate in the hearing family and culture. Some suggest that the idea of a quick solution could lead hearing parents to unrealistic expectations of their child's social, developmental, and linguistic future (Berg et al., 2005). This would not seem to be

the case with Deaf parents and a deaf child. However, the necessary support for the child to achieve the benefit of spoken communication may be a greater burden to the Deaf family given that spoken communication is not used in the household. Looking at it again from the medical team's perspective: how likely is it that *not* implanting the child will prevent him or her from learning aural speech? Even with concerted effort on the part of the family it is far less likely that the child will obtain intelligible speech in the absence of a cochlear implant, and rare that he/she would obtain what would be considered successful speech in the hearing community.

There is also a technological aspect in this case that informs the consideration of both beneficence and nonmaleficence. How likely is the device to do the purported good? Exactly how effective are cochlear implants? The answers to these questions are, to some degree, moving targets given the evolving technology. Data on the subject inevitably lag behind as the age of implantation continues to decrease and the latest data are based on children implanted at older ages (Christiansen & Leigh, 2002). Thus, a data set reported for one group may not accurately apply to the children currently being implanted. As mentioned previously, there are many factors that contribute to a successful implant, some of which are known and others that have yet to be understood.

Legal cases

Two legal cases are also relevant to our discussion. The first took place in Michigan in 2002. The deaf sons of Lee Larson, a Deaf mother, were placed into foster care when she was charged with neglect. While custody was being resolved, the state sought to give the boys cochlear implants. Larson refused this intervention and was taken to court. The state used a beneficence argument, claiming that implants would give these children a more open future, increasing their educational and financial opportunities and choices. The court ultimately granted Larson the right to decide whether her two children would receive implants (D'Silva et al., 2004).

Recently, another case received a great deal of attention. Shaun McLaughlin, a Deaf father of a deaf child, shares custody of his daughter with the child's mother. McLaughlin's daughter has bilateral cochlear implants. The details still remain unclear but it seems that a court order required McLaughlin to ensure that his daughter keep her cochlear implants on at all times, except during sleep or when activities such as swimming or wearing a helmet would preclude their use (Boggs, 2010). In 2010 he faced contempt of court charges for failing to follow the court's order. The Deaf community expressed strong opposition to this ruling and the *News Tribune* quoted McLaughlin as saying, "I think it impacts them because deaf people feel like they don't have sufficient authority over their own lives. I guess I feel like, on the list of civil rights issues – we're kind of toward the bottom of the list."

Best interests and the harm principle

The discussion above makes it clear that differing perspectives on harms and benefits leave no easy solution to the question of whether cochlear implants offer the best option for a deaf child. So why not simply wait and let the child decide when he or she is older, ultimately honoring the principle of respect for persons? One problem with this approach is that the potential benefit of a cochlear implant decreases with age. Many scientists and educational specialists describe a language window – a sensitive period of time occurring between approximately 1 and 4 years of age during which the human central auditory system remains maximally plastic. Sharma et al. (2002) found that after age 7, this plasticity is greatly reduced. According to the analysis of Christiansen and Leigh (2002), evidence across studies demonstrates that the earlier a child is implanted the greater chance he or she has of learning to use and benefit from a cochlear implant. Kim and colleagues (2010, p. 6) state that children who receive implantation prior to 2 years of age can be expected to reach their age-equivalent developmental milestones. While deferring cochlear implantation until a child is capable of deciding for him/herself may honor the principle of respect for persons, the potential harm of lost opportunity through decreased effectiveness that results from waiting must be factored into any consideration of this option. In the end "ethical discussions on medical implantation must take into account the social and cultural notions of disease and the conditions under which patients both with and without implants will live" (Hansson, 2005, p. 524).

How much freedom should parents have to make decisions about cochlear implants? Lainie Friedman Ross (1998, p. 49) emphasizes the importance of respecting family decision-making "as long as there

is no agreed-upon definition of the good," noting that "parents will place different emphases on different primary goods ... Given that there is no consensus on what the good life entails, parents in a liberal society must be free to choose whether to expose their child to a wide or narrow array of coherent life plans."

Likewise, Diekema (2004) suggests that parents should be allowed to make decisions for their children unless there is strong consensus that the decision places the child at substantial risk of serious harm that can be prevented by overriding the parental decision. In the case presented in this chapter it is difficult to define what will be best for this deaf child since Deaf culture, the parents, and the medical team hold very different opinions on the matter. The child's best interest is "inherently a question of values" and these interests are multifaceted and include not only medical considerations but emotional and psychological factors. The child's best interest is not readily discernible in this case, and the decision of the parents should be honored.

Resolution of case and discussion

The issues raised by cochlear implants highlight the complexities of technology and medicine in the modern age, disagreements over the definition of disability, and the desires of people to choose different ways of life based on diverse values and beliefs. It is essential to fully understand the potential harms and benefits of this kind of decision from a variety of perspectives, to keep communication between parties open, to ultimately determine who the rightful decision-maker(s) should be, and then to either respect their decision or determine whether that decision should be challenged legally. In this case the parents are the rightful decision-makers and have made a decision based on their culture and values. Would a medical team be justified in forcing the parents to have the child implanted based on their differing perception of the harms and benefits? Diekema lists eight conditions for justified state interference with parental decision-making (see Chapter 3). The condition most pertinent to our case – Would any other option prevent serious harm to the child in a way that is less intrusive to parental autonomy and more acceptable to the parent? – suggests that the family's desire to wait until their child is old enough to make his own decision about whether or not to implant does not seem unreasonable. Therefore intervening against the wishes of the parents would not be appropriate. Although not ideal as far as maximizing the potential benefit of an implant, waiting for the child to decide would most honor other ethical principles related to respect for the family, their culture, and their language, while also minimizing the harm of disrupting the family's integrity.

References

Baynton, D.C. (1996). *Forbidden Signs: American Culture and the Campaign Against Sign Language.* Chicago, IL: University of Chicago Press, 150.

Berg, A.L., Herb, A., & Hurst, M. (2005). Cochlear implants in children: ethics, informed consent, and parental decision-making. *Journal of Clinical Ethics*, **6**(3), 237–248.

Berg, A.L., Ip, S.C., Hurst, M., & Herb, A. (2007). Cochlear implants in young children: informed consent as a process and current practices. *American Journal of Audiology*, **16**, 13–28.

Boggs, A. (2010). Spokane father won't force deaf daughter to wear required cochlear implants. *The News Tribune*, April 30. www.thenewstribune.com/2010/04/29/1168049/spokane-father-wont-force-deaf.html. Last accessed October 20, 2010.

Christiansen, J.B. & Leigh I.W. (2002). *Cochlear Implants in Children: Ethics and Choices.* Washington, DC: Gallaudet University.

Deaf President Now Protest (2010). Gallaudet University Website. http://president.gallaudet.edu/x42164.xml. Last accessed October 20, 2010.

Diekema, D.S. (2004). Parental refusals of medical treatment: the harm principle as threshold for state intervention. *Theoretical Medicine*, **25**, 243–264.

Drolsbaugh, M. (2008). *Deaf Again.* Springhouse, PA: Handwave Publications.

D'Silva, M.U., Daugherty, M., & MacDonald, M. (2004). Deaf is dandy: contrasting the deaf and hard of hearing. *Intercultural Communication Studies*, **13**(2), 111–117.

Hansson, S.O. (2005). Implant ethics. *Journal of Medical Ethics*, **31**, 519–525.

Hyde, M., Punch, R., & Komesaroff, L. (2010). Coming to a decision about cochlear implantation: parents making choices for their deaf children. *Journal of Deaf Studies and Deaf Education*, **15**(2), 162–178.

Kim, L.S., Jeong, S.W., Lee, Y.M., & Kim, J.S. (2010). Cochlear implantation in children. *Auris Nasus Larynx*, **37**, 6–17.

Lane, H. & Bahan, B. (1998). Ethics of cochlear implantation in young children: a review and reply from a Deaf-world perspective. *Otolaryngology – Head and Neck Surgery*, **119**(4), 297–313.

NAD (National Association of the Deaf). (2000). Position Statement on Cochlear Implants. www.nad.org/issues/technology/assistive-listening/cochlear-implants. Last accessed October 20, 2010.

NIDCD (National Institute on Deafness and Other Communication Disorders) (2009). Cochlear implants. www.nidcd.nih.gov/health/hearing/coch.asp. Last accessed October 18, 2010.

Okubo, S., Takahashi, M., & Kai, I. (2008). How Japanese parents of deaf children arrive at decisions regarding pediatric cochlear implantation surgery: a qualitative study. *Social Science*, **66**(12), 2436–2447.

Padden, C.A. & Humphries, T. (1988). *Deaf in America: Voices from a Culture.* Cambridge, MA: Harvard University Press.

Ross, L.F. (1998). *Children, Families, and Health Care Decision-Making.* New York: Oxford University Press.

Sharma, A., Dorman, M.F., & Spahr, A.J. (2002). A sensitive period for the development of the central auditory system in children with cochlear implants: implications for age of implantation. *Ear & Hearing*, **23**(6), 532–539.

Tuchler, D. (2009). A response to *Refusing cochlear implants: Is it child neglect?* Post by Julian Savelescu. Practical Ethics: Ethical perspectives on the news. University of Oxford. www.practicalethicsnews.com/practicalethics/2009/07/refusing-cochlear-implants-is-it-child-neglect.html. Last accessed October 20, 2010.

Weinberg, A. (2005). Pediatric cochlear implants: the great debate. *Penn Bioethics Journal*, **I**(1), 1–4.

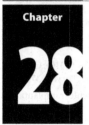

Ethical issues in the treatment of pediatric patients with disorders of sex development

Rebecca M. Harris and Joel Frader

Case narrative 1

Julie G, a 26-year-old banker, has a normal first pregnancy and goes into labor at 41 weeks. All proceeds normally. Her husband stays with her in the delivery room and she has the baby at approximately 4 a.m. When the obstetrician delivers the baby, she indicates that the infant is a boy. Later that morning, a pediatrician from the practice Julie and her husband have chosen arrives to speak with them and examine the newborn. She notices the urethral opening is at the base of the phallic shaft and the phallus seems somewhat short. She wonders if the child might have a disorder of sex development (DSD). Specifically, she wonders if the child might have normal female chromosomes and some form of virilizing congenital adrenal hyperplasia (CAH) – a relatively common form of DSD.

Dr. P sits down with the parents. She explains what she has observed and what it might mean. She emphasizes that the baby appears otherwise entirely normal and should be healthy, unless the child has a form of CAH with disturbed regulation of the body's important minerals. Both parents want to know whether their baby is "really" a boy or a girl. They have questions about picking a name for the child, what to tell those close to them, and what treatment the child will need.

Dr. P provides a general outline of contemporary thinking about virilized chromosomal girls. She acknowledges controversy about the gender of rearing and early surgery, but recommends that the parents have time to rest, and the physicians have time to gather more information about the baby. She says she will order some blood tests and imaging to begin the evaluation and will meet with the parents at the end of the day.

The baby's father telephones his parents, who live nearby, to discuss the news. The paternal grandfather

(PGF), a successful businessman, becomes agitated, says he will call a friend with whom he plays tennis, a semi-retired pediatric urologist. That afternoon, the PGF arrives with his physician friend who undresses the infant and, after a brief examination, declares that the child must be a virilized female who should be raised as a boy. He explains the "necessary" surgery.

A few hours later, the baby's pediatrician returns, having seen the ultrasound report indicating a normal appearing uterus and gonads consistent with ovaries. Cord blood has been sent for urgent karyotyping, the results of which should be available at the end of the next day. The parents relate what the grandfather's friend said and want to know when they should schedule the hypospadias repair ... the pediatrician hesitates before responding.

This case raises questions about the ethics of (1) gender assignment for newborns with DSDs and (2) surgical intervention in DSDs to "normalize" the genitals, especially when the surgery may affect future sexual experience (pleasure) or reproductive capacity before the patient can participate in decision-making.

Case narrative 2

A 17-year-old girl arrives at a reproductive endocrinologist's office for her first appointment. She has been referred because she has not yet had her first menstrual period. An attempt at a vaginal examination by the pediatrician produced considerable discomfort for the patient and confusion on the part of the pediatrician, who then ordered a pelvic ultrasound examination. The study failed to demonstrate typical female internal anatomy. The family felt a particular urgency to understand the situation, as the patient was a few months away from a marriage that was arranged

---

Clinical Ethics in Pediatrics: A Case-Based Textbook, ed. Douglas S. Diekema, Mark R. Mercurio and Mary B. Adam. Published by Cambridge University Press. © Cambridge University Press 2011.

years earlier. Both families of the betrothed expected the marriage to produce many children, beginning as soon as possible.

The obstetrician-gynecologist reviewed the history and family information, looked at the ultrasound images, examined the patient, and concluded that the patient most likely was a chromosomal male with complete androgen insensitivity syndrome (CAIS). The physician explained her thinking to the patient and her mother and indicated the tests needed to confirm the diagnosis. She told them that the patient was entirely healthy, that the vast majority of cases of CAIS became known with failure to develop menses, and that the patient would not be able to conceive or carry children. The patient began sobbing and after a few minutes asked if this meant she was "actually" male. The physician responded that it made little sense to think about her condition that way; biologically she had developed as a female and psychologically and socially she was entirely female, as well. The physician suggested it made more sense to think about herself as an infertile female. She acknowledged that the patient had intra-abdominal gonads and many physicians would recommend their removal because of the relatively small chance of malignant deterioration.

The patient's mother said she could not stop thinking about the coming marriage and what this would mean for their family economically and socially. After some discussion, the patient and her mother agreed to additional tests to confirm the diagnosis and made a follow-up appointment. At the next visit, during which the suspected diagnosis was confirmed, the patient's mother said she had decided against disclosing the information to anyone else, including her husband and her daughter's future husband. She asked the physician to promise not to provide diagnostic information if the patient's father inquired or if the patient's new husband called after the marriage.

This case points to ethical issues surrounding gender identity in adolescents and young adults and to physicians' duties to protect confidential information regarding the potential for reproduction when one member of a couple wishes to withhold medical information that may affect the other person in the relationship.

Ethical principles in context

Most in society assume that sex equals gender and we have only two "definitive" options: male and female.

However, many types of sex exist – gonadal, reproductive, chromosomal, genomic, genital, hormonal/endocrine, brain, genetic, etc. – and these sexes do not necessarily match up. Individuals with a DSD, previously called "intersex," fall along a spectrum of conditions of atypical development of the internal and/or external reproductive structures that affect approximately 1 in 4000 infants.

Historically, individuals with a DSD were called "hermaphrodites," after the Greek god Hermaphroditus, depicted as having a combination of male and female reproductive anatomy (Jospe & Florence, 2004). In modern medicine, influential study of DSDs began in the 1960s with John Money, PhD, a psychologist and founder of the Johns Hopkins Gender Identity Clinic. Money taught the separation of sex and gender, with sex following from one's gonads and gender being a matter of social and psychological roles (Money, 1985). Money believed that sociocultural constructs could overcome biology and anatomy (Money & Erhardt, 1996) and thus one could reassign gender to young patients with a DSD, regardless of their genetic makeup, until approximately 18 months of age. This notion guided medical practice regarding infants with "ambiguous genitalia" for decades. During this time, pediatric endocrinologists, geneticists, urologists, and others regarded newborns with a DSD as having a medical emergency. Physicians often withheld the declaration of the infant's sex and described the baby as "unfinished." The job of the subspecialist was to discover the "hidden" or "true" sex. Parents were advised to limit communication with friends and family. Professionals determined the gender of rearing based on anatomic and surgical considerations. Patients often endured multiple procedures without learning their diagnosis or its meaning until well into adulthood, if ever.

In the early 1990s psychologists, social scientists, and individuals with DSDs (Chase, 1998) challenged this culture of paternalism and secrecy. The response to medical practices in DSD cases stemmed from arbitrary sex assignment criteria, deception, and incomplete communication provided by physicians and poor outcomes for many reassigned individuals who had surgical interventions (lack of sexual pleasure, difficulty or inability to achieve orgasm, and painful intercourse). Patients and allied activists pointed to the lack of systematic, long-term studies supporting the medical and surgical practices. The extant studies often lacked rigor; they had few participants; failed to use comparative designs; did not differentiate between functional and cosmetic outcomes; and had confusing and conflicting conclusions.

In 1993, Anne Fausto-Sterling, a critic of Money, described sex and gender as cultural constructs (Fausto-Sterling, 1993). She denied that there were inherently male and female behaviors and identities. Instead, she postulated a genital "continuum" from penis to clitoris with everything in between representing a valid variant. Following a personally important conversation with Fausto-Sterling, Cheryl Chase, an individual with a DSD, founded the Intersex Society of North America (ISNA), an organization to support individuals with a DSD and their families and to advocate for changes in medical practice (ISNA, 2006; Weil, 2006).

Basic science

Over the past several decades scientific advances have identified over a dozen genes involved in sexual development (MacLaughlin & Donahoe, 2004). The products of these genes range from transcription factors to receptors to hormones; the gene mutations may result in forms of DSDs including gonadal dysgenesis, pseudohermaphroditism, and congenital adrenal hyperplasia. In addition, studies have provided new insight into neurological sex-dimorphism. Initially, scientists thought that postnatal environmental influences affected gender identity while prenatal sex hormones directed sex-dimorphic behavior (Ehrhardt & Meyer-Bahlburg, 1981). Through experiments with other species, new evidence showed that sex hormones affect the developing brain, though other factors such as the products of the sex-determining region Y gene (*Sry*) also influence sexual dimorphism in brain development (Dennis, 2004). Recently, Yang et al. (2010) completed a literature review to better appreciate how to advise families about gender identity in infants/children with DSDs. The authors found some solid evidence for the neurobiological role of the endocrine system in the development of sexual behaviors, but concluded that many published studies relied on anecdotes and presented somewhat contradictory findings. They recommended additional research with an emphasis on long-term studies.

Ethical issues

Nomenclature

While taxonomy and nomenclature may not themselves raise ethical issues, the history of social responses to those with DSDs demonstrates that terminology communicates value-laden fears and attitudes that may harm affected children and adults. Dreger et al. (2005) reviewed this issue and recommended discarding all terms based on the outdated, illogical word "hermaphrodite." The original nomenclature was developed in 1876 by Theodor Albrecht Edwin Klebs before the identification of sex chromosomes, and characterized individuals with a DSD based on their gonads. Although some alterations in the taxonomy occurred over the last century, the framework remained in use through the end of the twentieth century. Dreger et al. (2005) noted that a classification scheme relying on the anatomy of the gonads rarely provides practical clinical help, as gonadal biopsies incur risks, especially in newborns, and may provide inaccurate information in conditions such as mixed gonadal dysgenesis. In addition, a gonadal system may simply miss the point, engendering distress in a patient who considers himself a male despite the presence of ovaries or a young woman with androgen insensitivity syndrome. Second, the term "hermaphrodite" signifies a person with both female and male genitals – a concept that only exists in mythology and which may elicit confusion and/or fear in parents or patients. Third, terms such as "female pseudohermaphrodite" imply the patient is somehow fully described by her condition rather than being a person with a condition. Dreger and colleagues (2005) recommended a new taxonomy for DSDs based on valid scientific data about the origin of the conditions and clinical utility. The new system seeks to avoid associations with stereotypic male and female behaviors so as to separate the medical diagnosis from the complex issues of sociocultural and emotional factors which affect gender assignment.

Informed consent

Informed consent for interventions in children with a DSD involves legal and ethical concerns, especially regarding interventions made prior to the patient's ability to participate in decision-making and with regard to non-disclosure of the nature of the patient's condition and the reasons for treatment. Cosmetic genital surgery or surgery without clear medical indication should generally be deferred until the patient can express a clear preference for or against it. (A urovaginal fistula is an example of a DSD anomaly with a medical indication for early surgical repair.) All proposed interventions require a discussion of the risks, benefits, and alternatives, including the reasonable option of deferring surgery; the failure to provide such a full disclosure may violate informed consent laws and constitute a legal battery. If the child is capable of understanding even part of the situation, s/he should have an opportunity to hear the information in developmentally appropriate language and either assent to or refuse elective procedures (Lee et al., 2006).

Nonmaleficence

The Hippocratic dictum "primum non nocere," or "first do no harm," implies that physicians' actions may not benefit the patient and cautions physicians to take into account as much as possible about the patient's circumstances before acting. Surgery to normalize a patient's genitals in early childhood, without the full understanding of the child's eventual feelings and beliefs about surgery or the patient's sexual orientation, may well constitute the kind of harm Hippocrates contemplated. Psychological benefits of cosmetic genital surgery on young children have not been clearly demonstrated and many surgeries have negative consequences for future sexual fulfillment.

Culture and patient autonomy

In 2003, Diamond and others (2003) discussed a hypothetical case in which parents of a 13-year-old boy brought him to the hospital for hypospadias and breast development. The child had a chromosome complement of 46XX and was virilized. The family's culture favored males. The parents indicated discomfort about accepting their child if physicians undertook gender reassignment. Further, they suggested that if their child were homosexual he might be murdered. The father decided to preserve the child's gender identity and instructed the physician to perform surgeries necessary to make the boy appear fully male. Several experts provided commentary on this scenario. David Diamond emphasized the importance of family-centered (FC) decision-making and highlighted the role of culture. The FC model generally supports decisions by families with specific cultural perspectives even when the family's preferences deviate from those of "mainstream" medicine. However, the model may conflict with stricter notions of patient autonomy. A future-oriented approach, while recognizing that most DSD patients will present for care while still minors, looks to parents and clinicians to

consider deferring decisions about elective surgery out of respect for the autonomous individual the child will become. Many health care professionals now support shared decision-making among the patient with a DSD, when sufficiently mature, his parents, and the relevant clinicians to accept or reject optional surgery (Daaboul & Frader, 2001).

Summary

While some have suggested that individuals with DSDs constitute a third gender, achieving widespread acceptance of that view seems somewhat unrealistic. Many societies do not grant those falling outside typical dimorphic gender behavior, e.g., males who display exaggerated feminine characteristics, equal status. For this reason, most do not argue for a delay in gender assignment for newborns recognized to have a DSD. ISNA activists and many medical professionals stress the need for accurate medical diagnoses and appropriate condition-specific medical treatment, when indicated, as well as multidisciplinary counseling and support for parents and children with DSDs when they have the capacity to participate (Ahmed et al., 2004).

In 2006 the American Academy of Pediatrics *Consensus Statement on the Management of Intersex Disorders* recommended discontinuation of confusing and potentially pejorative terms such as "intersex" and "pseudohermaphrodite" and adoption of the neutral term "disorder of sexual development." The statement also outlined research and management recommendations (Lee et al., 2006). A separate statement emerged from a multidisciplinary group convened by the Hastings Center. Their paper provided guidelines for managing patients with DSDs, including comprehensive multidisciplinary assessment by relevant clinicians, such as a pediatric endocrinologist, a pediatric urologist and/or surgeon, a mental health professional, and a geneticist and/or medical ethicist, when appropriate. The paper recognized that families with children with DSDs require continuing support beginning immediately after diagnosis. Acknowledging that some still consider surgery an urgent matter, the group concluded that while current surgical techniques may produce less physical damage than older techniques, such progress does not justify early surgery to modify genital appearance. Such procedures generally require discussion with and approval of the patient. Moreover, the authors argue for disclosure of the diagnosis and its implications to the child with DSD in an age-appropriate manner. Finally, the group called for rigorous follow-up studies to achieve a more comprehensive understanding of the physical, sexual, and psychosocial experiences of those with DSD as well as improved education of health care professionals about DSD care (Frader et al., 2004).

Case resolution

In case 1, the ethical dilemma revolves around the recommendation of the family friend, a pediatric urologist, to raise as a boy a chromosomal girl who, while virilized from CAH, could have a normal female reproductive future should she so choose. The family's anxiety and the voice of a family friend providing a concrete recommendation may bring a temporary sense of relief. However, the parents do not fully understand the diagnosis, prognosis, available treatments, risks, and likely outcomes. The pediatrician must help the family appreciate the importance of taking time to learn about the complexities of DSDs before making a surgical decision. The pediatrician should coordinate the appropriate specialists, including a mental health professional with experience in the management of children with DSDs, to assist and support the family.

An aspect of case 2 that complicates treatment of the patient's DSD is the cultural context in which she and her family live. The patient's mother asked the physician not to disclose the diagnosis to the patient's father or fiancé, even after the marriage. For this patient, revelation of the diagnosis of CAIS could undermine her future, preventing the wedding and producing social and economic hardship for the family. The family's cultural commitments affect their medical compassion and flexibility. The patient's age, 17 years, requires the physician to involve her fully in discussions and make her preferences paramount, absent a compelling reason to do otherwise.

The physician might well tell the patient that her condition may make sexual intercourse painful (she has a short vagina) and her infertility will likely cause her future husband to press for an explanation; keeping secrets, such as her diagnosis, often proves difficult. If the husband then learns that the patient knew about her condition prior to the marriage and withheld the information, his anger and mistrust could prove very difficult indeed. In addition, there are multiple paths

to parenthood, including adoption, surrogacy with artificial insemination of a gestational mother with the husband's sperm, and so on. While the physician is legally and ethically bound to respect a request for confidentiality, she also has a moral obligation to help the patient and her mother think through the consequences of a decision to keep the diagnosis from her family and fiancé.

References

Ahmed, S.F., Morrison, S., & Hughes, I.A. (2004). Intersex and gender assignment; the third way? *Archives of Disease in Childhood*, **89**, 847–850.

Chase, C. (1998). Surgical progress is not the answer to intersexuality. *Journal of Clinical Ethics*, **9**, 385–392.

Daaboul, J. & Frader, J. (2001). Ethics and the management of the patient with intersex: a middle way. *Journal of Pediatric Endocrinology and Metabolism*, **14**, 1575–1583.

Dennis, C. (2004). Brain development: the most important sexual organ. *Nature*, **427**, 390–392.

Diamond, D.A., Sytsma, S., Dreger, A., & Wilson, B. (2003). Culture clash involving intersex. *Hastings Center Report*, **33**, 12–14.

Dreger, A.D., Chase, C., Sousa, A., Gruppuso, P.A., & Frader, J. (2005). Changing the nomenclature/taxonomy for intersex: a scientific and clinical rationale. *Journal of Pediatric Endocrinology and Metabolism*, **18**, 729–733.

Ehrhardt, A.A. & Meyer-Bahlburg, H.F. (1981). Effects of prenatal sex hormones on gender-related behavior. *Science*, **211**, 1312–1318.

Fausto-Sterling, A. (1993). The five sexes: why male and female are not enough. *The Sciences*, **33**(2), 20–25.

Frader, J., Alderson, P., Asch, A., et al. (2004). Health care professionals and intersex conditions. *Archives of Pediatrics and Adolescent Medicine*, **158**, 426–428.

Intersex Society of North America (2006). DSD Guidelines: Handbook for Parents. www.dsdguidelines.org/htdocs/parents/index.html. Last accessed October 28, 2010.

Jospe, N. & Florence, M. (2004). Hermaphroditus in Greco-Roman myth: lessons and hypotheses for intersex today. *Journal of Pediatric Endocrinology and Metabolism*, **17**, 1471–1479.

Lee, P.A., Houk, C.P., Ahmed, S.F., & Hughes, I.A. (2006). Consensus statement on management of intersex disorders. International Consensus Conference on Intersex. *Pediatrics*, **118**, e488–e500.

MacLaughlin, D.T. & Donahoe, P.K. (2004). Sex determination and differentiation. *New England Journal of Medicine*, **350**, 367–378.

Money, J. (1985). Gender: history, theory and usage of the term in sexology and its relationship to nature/nurture. *Journal of Sex and Marital Therapy*, **11**, 71–79.

Money, J. & Erhardt, A.A. (1996). *Man and Woman, Boy and Girl*. Northvale, NJ: Jason Aronson, Inc.

Weil, E. (2006). What if it's (sort of) a boy and (sort of) a girl? *New York Times Magazine*, September 24, 48–53.

Yang, J.H., Baskin, L.S., & DiSandro, M. (2010). Gender identity in disorders of sex development: review article. *Urology*, **75**, 153–159.

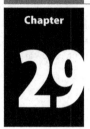

Chapter

29

Sterilizing procedures in minors with cognitive disabilities

Donald Brunnquell

Case narrative

Sherry is a 14-year-old who was born with a chromosomal interstitial deletion and diagnosed with autism and moderate mental retardation (IQ measured at 45, adaptive functioning range averaging about a 4-year-old level, but with a wide range of abilities). She lives at home with her parents and attends a full-time special education classroom at her local public school. Her adaptive abilities include feeding herself but not preparing meals, and dressing herself but not choosing appropriate clothing. Her vocabulary includes about 20 rarely used words, and she generally communicates with sounds and emotive vocalization. She wears adult diapers and remains incompletely toilet trained in spite of extensive training efforts at home and school. Despite extensive behavioral training, she will sometimes smear feces if not changed promptly. Menarche began about a year ago, and she has had inconsistent menstrual periods over the past year, with bleeding lasting 3–10 days. Training to use pads has been unsuccessful, and she will sometimes take them off and smear blood. Her school now refuses to allow her to attend during her menstrual periods because of the management difficulty and blood exposure to other students and staff. During her menstrual periods she seems to have significant pain, and shows behavior changes including increased aggression, social withdrawal, and refusal to cooperate. She has also shown an increase in sexual behavior in the past several months, including two episodes of removing her clothes on the school bus, masturbating in public, and spending increased time with one particular boy that includes holding hands and stroking arms.

Sherry's parents consulted with her pediatrician who suggested that they consider a hysterectomy to help with both menstrual management and prevention of pregnancy. The pediatrician referred her to an obstetrician/gynecologist and the ethics committee. The parents have articulated their concerns as:

1. Sherry shows an increase in sexual behavior, and they are concerned that she could become pregnant (a consulting geneticist says this is possible), and this would be awful for both Sherry and the unborn child.

2. Her periods have had a strong negative impact on her behavior and ability to take part in activities, especially school.

3. The increased aggression during her periods has raised questions about their continued ability to care for her at home.

4. While they intend to care for her at home as long as they are physically able to do so, they worry about the long-term risks for sexual abuse and pregnancy, if she ends up living in a group home or institution after they can no longer care for her at home.

Definitions: sterilization and cognitive disability

For the purposes of this chapter, sterilization will be considered to be a medical procedure with the primary goal of permanently and (likely) irreversibly removing the person's capacity to have a child by natural means. Tubal ligation is the most common form of surgical sterilization. Sterilization should also be distinguished from menstrual control, another goal which parents of children with cognitive disabilities sometimes feel are in the child's interest. Hysterectomy achieves the goal of sterilization and the goal of ending menstrual periods.

Clinical Ethics in Pediatrics: A Case-Based Textbook, ed. Douglas S. Diekema, Mark R. Mercurio and Mary B. Adam. Published by Cambridge University Press. © Cambridge University Press 2011.

Calibey's (1981) distinction between compulsory sterilization (legislatively required permanent sterilization for societal purposes), voluntary sterilization (free choice of the individual to permanently limit reproductive capacity), and involuntary sterilization (choice by a legitimate third party for an individual who cannot provide consent to permanently limit reproductive capacity) should be noted.

For the purposes of this chapter, cognitive disability is taken to mean a condition of impairment of the ability to reason that is severe and permanent, such that there is agreement among professionals that the person is not now and will never be able to:

1. have the capacity to judge any major decision about their own medical care (will not ever be competent to consent the medical procedures)
2. make rational decisions about their own sexual activity, and the harms and benefits of that activity
3. make rational decisions about the risks and benefits of pregnancy, and the harms and benefits of bearing or fathering a child
4. have the capacity to parent a child, and would not be allowed by society (e.g., child protective services) to take responsibility for parenting a child without continuous supervision.

While no single level of testing or adaptive behavior can be established to encompass these concerns, one can presume that diagnoses of moderate to profound mental retardation will generally meet these criteria, and mild mental retardation may in some instances meet these criteria. Individual assessment is needed in every case.

This chapter concerns involuntary, permanent reproductive sterilization of minors with cognitive disability based on individual decisions by legitimately empowered third parties, generally parents or the courts. Compulsory sterilization decisions by state rules, agency rules, hospital or other organizational rules should not be countenanced by medical professionals. Only when individual caregivers pursue this option because of their good faith belief that it is in the interest of the child should medical personnel consider their involvement in this procedure.

The history of compulsory sterilization and individual case decisions

Almost all women who have had sexual intercourse have at some time used contraception (Mosher & Jones,

2010). In 2003, Baill et al. noted that "female sterilization is the most commonly used 'modern' contraceptive in the United States … 27 percent of women who have chosen to use contraception have opted for tubal sterilization" (p. 1287).

The history of abuses of sterilization in the United States and internationally requires attention, as it represents a sad and tragic episode in medical practice (*Buck v. Bell*, 1927). Reilly (1987) estimates that between 1907 and 1963 more than 60 000 persons were sterilized in the United States pursuant to state laws. Many sterilizations were performed for eugenic reasons. The 23 sterilizations performed under state law in South Carolina were all "Negro females." The American eugenic movement was an encouragement to the even more horrific abuses in Nazi Germany from 1933 to 1945. (See Reilly, 1991 and Lombardo, 2008 for an in-depth discussion of this history.)

These grave abuses of sterilizing procedures constitute "compulsory sterilization," and individual requests for "involuntary sterilization" by legitimate guardians should be viewed differently. As with any request by a patient or a parent regarding a medical or surgical treatment, the interests of the patient should be the primary consideration for the provider. While including the interests of others directly involved in the patient's life and the potential societal implications for the group of people recognized as having cognitive disabilities may be secondary interests, assessing the aggregate balance of harms and benefits for the patient remains the primary concern. The history of compulsory sterilization has created an emphasis on the societal implications, often overriding any consideration of the actual interests of the patient and their direct caregivers. It is the interests of the patient, not the history of the procedure, that should dominate the discussion.

Principle-based analysis of requests for sterilization

Given the historical abuses of sterilization, it is appropriate to begin consideration of the issue by addressing the principle of respect for persons as a core duty. Respect for persons incorporates at least two ethical convictions: first, that individuals should be treated as autonomous agents, and second, that persons with diminished autonomy are entitled to protection (The Belmont Report [NCPHS BBR, 1979]). In the case of those with cognitive disability, the principle of respect for persons demands that their autonomy be evaluated, and those with insufficient capacity to act autonomously be protected. That protection requires that their substantive interests be addressed as individuals. They should have the same rights to access or refuse treatments as other individuals. That includes the range of choices regarding medical and surgical intervention in reproduction. Given that 27% of women choose surgical sterilization at some point in their reproductive life, clearly this option should be available to all women, including those with cognitive disability. Protecting each person includes assuring access to the treatments that are in their aggregate best interest.

While by definition we are discussing persons with diminished capacity, it is still important to address their autonomy interests. An essential element of any consideration of sterilization includes a careful determination that the person does not and will not have capacity to make decisions about sexual and reproductive functioning on their own or even with significant assistance. This requires careful assessment of the individual by professionals trained in the area of assessment of cognitive abilities, and assessment of the implications of this information by the legal decision-makers for the person. The fact of incapacity in sexual and reproductive decisions does not alone justify sterilization, but is a necessary condition. One formulation of the sterilization question for those with cognitive disability is whether preservation of the interest in reproductive autonomy is outweighed by other interests. Reproductive autonomy is a real interest, but not an absolute interest that must be maintained at all costs. Clearly many women at some point reach the conclusion that other interests outweigh this preservation of reproductive autonomy.

For persons with cognitive disability, considerations of justice are especially important for all health care decisions, including sterilization. One inadequate formulation of such protection is that any risky procedure or any procedure that alters life in a way that could be disadvantageous for that person at some point in the future should never be done. For some in society, sterilization falls into the category of a presumptively unjust procedure when the decision is not made by the person undergoing the procedure. This point of view fails to address the fact that each person, including those with cognitive disability, has many interests, and that all interests should be considered together if the legal decision-maker is to truly act in the person's aggregate best interest. To consider any procedure per se impermissible in fact denies

the person the basic respect they deserve as a human being. In each case an aggregate assessment of harms and benefits is needed.

In a principle-based system, the primary work of determining aggregate best interest is achieved through analysis of nonmaleficence and beneficence for the affected individual. Each potential treatment option should be considered in view of the burdens and risks it entails, and the possible benefits it brings. Treatments in and of themselves should never be required or impermissible, for it is their effect on the person that ultimately matters. Bringing the best available empirical knowledge to this analysis is essential. In the end, careful analysis must include what has value for the particular individual in view of the best available knowledge of reproductive interests in the context of all of the other interests of the person. Those other interests may include the risk of pregnancy; the interest in sexual activity without the fear of pregnancy; avoiding pregnancy that would be frightening, painful and not understood; avoiding the experience of bearing a child who would then be removed from the person's care; the realistic likelihood that future medical advances will permit the person to have capacity to make their own decisions; avoiding difficulties such as pain, confusion, and social isolation associated with menstruation that cannot be adequately controlled; the known and unknown effects of long-term hormonal control with nonpermanent methods of achieving contraception or menstrual control; and many other concerns specific to an individual. A principle-based approach calls for a careful weighing of all of these concerns for the individual.

The goals of requests for sterilization

In responding to any request from a parent regarding a sterilization procedure, an essential first step is to understand the goals for the child. Prevention of pregnancy is the clear result of sterilization, but parents often conflate this with the goal of menstrual control for hygiene reasons, and are also often concerned about preventing sexual abuse of their child. Abnormal uterine bleeding, mood and behavior issues associated with menstruation, and other medical conditions also provide reasons for intervention. Clearly sexual abuse and transmission of sexually transmitted diseases (STDs) cannot be prevented by sterilization, and are important issues that must be addressed through other means.

Patterson-Keels and colleagues (1994) provide the clearest evaluation of parental views on sterilization. In their survey of 88 parents, the most frequent reasons for sterilization were fear of pregnancy (65%), fear of sexual abuse (41%), and uncertainty about other methods of birth control (33%). When asked to choose among statements that best represented their attitude about sterilization, 54% said fear of pregnancy outweighed reservations about sterilization, 15% said difficulties with menstrual periods outweighed reservations about sterilization, 23% said they would consider sterilization only as a last resort, and 15% reported they would never agree to sterilization.

Given the frequent parental concerns about pregnancy as a result of sexual abuse for persons with cognitive disability, understanding the actual risks of this occurrence is important. This author could find no studies reporting pregnancy rates resulting from abuse in this population. Sexual abuse of the cognitively disabled, however, appears to be high. Sullivan and Knutson (2000) reviewed maltreatment in all children in schools in Omaha, NE in 1994–1995. They reported a 31% maltreatment rate among disabled children (compared with 11% of nondisabled). Of the group of maltreated disabled children, 248 were categorized with "mental retardation," and of those, 36.6% experienced some form of sexual abuse. Davis (2009) reports studies of sexual victimization of women with intellectual disabilities that find rates of 25% in one study and 49% in another study. The Disabled Persons Protection Commission of Massachusetts (2010) reports that 68–83% of women with developmental disabilities will be sexually assaulted in their lifetime. Clearly sterilization does not remove the risk of sexual assault, but the concerns of parents of a resulting pregnancy are at least a realistic concern to be considered.

The American College of Obstetricians and Gynecologists (ACOG) committee opinions on Sterilization of Women (2007) and on Menstrual Manipulation for Adolescents with Disabilities (2009), and the American Academy of Pediatrics (1999) recognize the complex set of goals that enter into the discussion of preventing pregnancy and achieving relief from the individual and social effects of menstruation on the adolescent with cognitive disabilities. In the 2007 Opinion, ACOG notes that "the presence of a mental disability does not, in itself, justify either sterilization or its denial" (p. 218). They propose careful procedural safeguards for people who cannot make their own decision, but recognize that sterilization may best achieve the goals of the patient in some instances. The ARC of the United States and the American Association on Intellectual and Developmental Disabilities (AAIDD) Position Statement on Sexuality (2008) notes that the presence of an intellectual disability, regardless of severity, does not, in itself, justify loss of rights related to sexuality. They hold that education and decisions should be individualized, and that those with intellectual or developmental disability should "be protected from sterilization solely because of their disability." The ACOG (2009) position contends that for menstrual control, "first-line treatment options should be safe, minimally invasive, and nonpermanent." They conclude that endometrial ablation is not indicated. They state that hysterectomy should "very rarely" be considered. The medical basis for this opinion remains unclear, since no good comparative studies of hysterectomy and the long-term risks of hormonal treatments for persons with cognitive disabilities have been conducted. All of these organizations argue for individualized decisions based on the overall interests of the person involved.

Sterilization of male minors with cognitive disabilities

Consideration of vasectomy for males is a more complex topic because the issue of direct harm to the patient from reproduction bears significantly different weight. For females the direct risks, discomforts, and psychological burden of pregnancy and delivery are significant, but for the male patient whose parents request sterilization, these direct health risks are not relevant. The considerations relevant to the male with cognitive disability include any psychological burden to the patient, any burden on a potential child, the burden to the woman bearing the child, the burden to family members who may be required to care for the resulting child personally or financially, and burden to society.

These are largely burdens to others, and so these must weigh against the risks of the vasectomy procedure itself. These procedural risks are generally seen as quite low, essentially the risks of infection and general anesthesia that may be required to perform the procedure on a person with cognitive disability. While some question regarding an association of vasectomy with later prostate cancer has been discussed, this risk, if it exists at all, is small and may not be causal (Schwingl & Guess, 2000; Dennis et al., 2002). As with females, the right to procreate is a basic presumptive right for all persons, but it is a relative good especially in situations in which it will never be meaningful to the person. Parents of young men in this situation reasonably argue that for someone who cannot have a concept of fatherhood and understand its joys and responsibilities, it does not represent a significant loss. It could be argued that for some young men with cognitive disability, vasectomy could represent an increase in opportunity for the person. The potential increase in freedom of association, possible sexual activity, and increased likelihood of living in less restrictive environments are real benefits to a young man.

In summary, with procedural protections in place that are similar to those for females undergoing sterilization, vasectomy for males with cognitive disabilities should be permissible when the decision is made by individual caregivers in the best interest of the child, there is agreement of professionals regarding the aggregate balance of harms and benefits in the case, a fair procedure is followed, and it includes the young person if he can participate and gives heavy weight to any preference he can articulate.

The interests of the person with cognitive delays in sterilization

All people, including those with cognitive disabilities, have a presumptive positive interest in reproduction. Similarly, there is a presumptive interest in sexuality as a basic form of human functioning. These interests are described as presumptive because, all other things being equal, the interests should be maintained. Clearly not all people experience or exercise these interests in the same way. The courts recognize these basic interests in cases such as *Skinner* v. *Oklahoma*, yet these are not absolute interests, as noted in other court cases (Reilly, 1987).

There are also negative interests for all people, such as avoidance of unwanted pregnancy, avoiding parental responsibilities, and avoiding the burdens of pain and distress associated with menstrual periods and hygiene. The frequency of use of birth control and sterilization methods clearly demonstrates that many women perceive the interest in avoiding pregnancy as realistic for persons whether or not they have a cognitive disability.

For a person with cognitive disability, both sets of the interests exist, and all these options should continue to be available. As noted by Pham and Lerner (2001), "Laws forbidding sterilization of the mentally

incompetent may be nearly as dehumanizing as the forced sterilization laws they replaced" (p. 283). ACOG (2007) notes that "sterilization should not be denied to individuals simply because they also may be vulnerable to coercion" (p. 2).

It is important to note that the interests of the child interact with those of family members and caregivers. Parents are expected to make significant sacrifices for their child, and they gain much in the way of satisfaction in helping their child. If parents conclude that the burdens of continuing child care are so great they can no longer have the child in their home, the interests of the child are affected. One can and should take into account the overall balance of harms and burdens. That may mean weighing the burdens of sterilization against the burdens of the child being placed outside the home.

The interests of others

It is important to note that while the direct interests of the child should remain primary, interests of others often interact with the interests of the child and may be considerable. The American Academy of Pediatrics (AAP) (1999) notes that issues of reproduction and menstrual control can affect the abilities of those who provide care for children with cognitive disabilities to effectively continue their care. The effort to prevent pregnancy, for example, could detract from caregivers' efforts to promote interests in social interaction or appropriate sexual activity. Furthermore, they note that caregivers "have substantive and reasonable concerns" about their own interests being affected by caring for a person with cognitive disability who becomes pregnant and in caring for children who may result from such a pregnancy. In addition, the ACOG Committee on Ethics (2007) states that "The well-being of a child potentially conceived also should receive consideration."

Relative risk and assessment of medical burdens and benefits

Risk associated with the proposed treatments and the resulting risk–benefit assessment for the patient is an essential concern. As in other discussions of risk, the existence of even significant risk does not rule out a procedure. In each instance the best estimate of relative risks should be the basis of decisions. Assuming the risks of pregnancy are assessed as real and significant, one must then ask about the relative risks of varying forms of preventing pregnancy.

This question revolves especially around the relative risks of long-term hormonal treatment versus surgical treatment. Unfortunately there are at best incomplete data on the risks of either option for girls with major developmental delays, and little by way of direct assessment of relative risk for the general population. The effort of individual assessment of risk in each case is necessary.

The history of abuses of sterilization in the past has brought significant social pressure to choose the least invasive and most reversible options. This is generally construed to mean hormonal contraception. A review of the literature reveals that it is not clear that the long-term risk to the patient is less with long-term hormonal treatment than with surgical treatment. (See Baill et al., 2000; Paransky & Zurwain, 2003; Arvio et al., 2009; Savasi et al., 2009 for further discussion of these risks.)

Risks of general anesthesia or other aspects of the procedure should be taken into account. It should be noted that it is common for persons with cognitive disabilities to have dental and routine medical procedures under anesthesia, and this may provide some information regarding the individual's risk.

While a complete description of all studies that bear on the question of relative risk of achieving the goals of prevention of pregnancy and suppressing menstruation is beyond the scope of this chapter, one can clearly conclude that significantly more study is needed in the population of adolescents with cognitive disability. Given that significant risks and differences in efficacy exist for all options, it is reasonable to conclude at this time that individual assessment of each patient is needed, and that allowing a range of options to the legal guardians who must make the choice is the approach that corresponds to similar situations where no clinically clearly superior option exists.

Oversight and procedural justice

Since involuntary sterilization involves a person who is by definition not competent, procedural safeguards must be in place to assure that the interests of the individual are the driving force behind each decision. For minors with cognitive disabilities, parents are the presumptive decision-makers and presumed legitimate moral agent for the child, since they generally live with the child, know her or him the best, and have natural bonds of affection with the child. Parents are not without conflicts of interest, however, and oversight is appropriate. While some states require judicial

oversight and practitioners should clearly follow this requirement if it exists, it is more appropriate that a group of professionals with expertise exercise the primary oversight role, recognizing their obligations to advance the interests of the child and to prevent abuse and neglect.

The AAP (1999) and ACOG (2007), as well as numerous authors (Pham & Lerner, 2001; Diekema, 2003; Paransky & Zurwain 2003) have written about the ethical issues and compiled substantive criteria for decisions about sterilizing procedures. While these organizations and authors list varying procedural concerns, these procedural protections can be condensed to include the following:

1. Compulsory sterilization, that is, sterilization authorized by state, agency, or organizations (rather than individual decisions by caregivers who are legitimate individual moral agents for the child) should not be allowed. Sterilization should be considered only if individually requested by the parents or other legal guardians of the child.

2. The affected person's opinion should always be solicited and they should be included in the discussions to the extent they are capable; if they can state a clear preference their preference should presumptively carry the greatest weight.

3. Professionals with expertise in the child's general medical condition (generally a pediatrician), the gynecologist (or urologist for a male), other medical specialists with relevant expertise to the child's situation, a psychologist or mental health professional who can evaluate current and future capacity, and a social worker to evaluate the capacity to act as a parent should all independently evaluate and reach a conclusion that the proposed procedure is in the aggregate overall interest of the patient.

4. There must be agreement that the person is not now and would never have the capacity to decide for themselves about reproduction.

5. Alternative approaches should be considered by parents (or legal guardians) and medical professionals, and the relative balance of risks and benefits of those approaches should be compared. This comparison should take into account indirect interests such as future caregiving, and the interests of family and others affected by the decision. Uncertainty about harms and benefits of specific procedures should be weighed, but the

simple existence of uncertainty should not prevent decision-making.

6. State and local laws should be assessed and followed, including court involvement when required.

7. There should be unanimous agreement among the parents/guardians and medical professionals that the proposed procedure is in the child's overall interests.

Case resolution

After the initial request from Sherry's parents, information and formal written opinions were gathered from her pediatrician, other medical consultants, a psychologist, a social worker, and a behavioral specialist. Medical specialists believed that in spite of her genetic condition there was a real possibility of fertility. All agreed that her increase in sexual behavior suggested real risk to her. At a meeting to assess the case, the parents and convened professionals agreed that a hysterectomy under general anesthesia was acceptable and in her aggregate best interest. The procedure could be authorized by parents under state law. The procedure was scheduled and carried out a few months later without complications. Intermediate-term follow-up indicated that there were no medical complications, and that aggression had decreased and school attendance increased.

References

American Academy of Pediatrics (AAP) Committee on Bioethics (1999). Sterilization of minors with developmental disabilities. *Pediatrics*, **104**(2), 337–340. Reaffirmed August 1, 2009.

American College of Obstetricians and Gynecologists (ACOG) (2007). Committee Opinion 371: Sterilization of Women, Including Those With Mental Disabilities. *Obstetrics and Gynecology*, **110**, 217–220.

American College of Obstetricians and Gynecologists (ACOG), Committee on Adolescent Health Care (2009). Committee Opinion 448: Menstrual Manipulation for Adolescents with Disabilities. *Obstetrics and Gynecology*, **114**, 1428–1431.

Arc of the United States and American Association on Intellectual and Developmental Disabilities (2008). Position Statement: Sexuality. Available at www.thearc.org/page.aspx?pid=2376. Last accessed November 5, 2010.

Arvio, M., Kilpinen-Loisa, P, Tiitenen, A., Huovinen, K., & Makite, O. (2009). Bone mineral density and sex hormone status in intellectually disabled women on progestin-induced amenorrhea. *Acta Obstetrica et Gynecologica*, **88**, 428–433.

Baill, C., Cullins, V., & Pati, S. (2003). Counseling issues in tubal sterilization. *American Family Physician*, **67**(6), 1287–1294.

Buck v. Bell (1927). 274 US 200.

Calibey, K. (1981). Nonconsensual sterilization of the mentally retarded – analysis of standards for judicial determinations. *Western New England Law Review*, **33**(4), 689–714.

Davis, L. (2009). People with intellectual disabilities and sexual violence. *The Arc Q & A*. Available at www.thearc.org/document.doc?id=2995. Last accessed December 12, 2010.

Dennis, L.K., Dawson, D.V., & Resnick, M.I. (2002). Vasectomy and the risk of prostate cancer: a meta-analysis examining vasectomy status, age at vasectomy, and time since vasectomy. *Prostate Cancer and Prostatic Disease*, **5**(3), 193–203.

Diekema, D. (2003). Involuntary sterilization of persons with mental retardation: an ethical analysis. *Mental retardation and Developmental Disabilities Research Reviews*, **9**, 21–26.

Disabled Persons Protection Commission, Commonwealth of Massachusetts (2010). Prevalence of violence. Available at www.mass.gov/?pageID=dppcterminal&L=2&L0=Home&L1=Recognizing+Abuse+%26+Neglect&sid=Idppc&b=terminalcontent&f=recognizing_prevalence_of_violence&csid=Idppc. Last accessed December 20, 2010.

Lombardo, P. (2008). *Three Generations, No Imbeciles: Eugenics, the Supreme Court, and Buck v. Bell*. Baltimore, MD: Johns Hopkins University Press.

Mosher, W.D. & Jones, J. (2010). Use of contraception in the United States: 1982–2008. *Vital and Health Statistics*, Series 23, No. 29.

National Commission for the Protection of Human Subjects of Biomedical and Behavioral Research (1979). The Belmont Report. Available at www.hhs.gov/ohrp/humansubjects/guidance/belmont.htm. Last accessed November 3, 2010.

Paransky, O.I. & Zurwain, R.K. (2003). Management of menstrual problems and contraception in adolescents with mental retardation: a medical, legal, and ethical review with new suggested guidelines. *Journal of Pediatric and Adolescent Gynecology*, **16**, 223–235.

Patterson-Keels, L., Quint, E., Brown, D., Larson, D., & Elkins, T. (1994). family views on sterilization for their mentally retarded children. *Journal of Reproductive Medicine*, **39**(9), 701–706.

Pham, H. & Lerner, B. (2001). In the patient's best interest? Revisiting sexual autonomy and sterilization of the developmentally disabled. *Western Journal of Medicine*, **175**, 280–283.

Reilly, P.R. (1987). Involuntary sterilization in the United States: a surgical solution. *Quarterly Review of Biology*, **62**(2), 153–170.

Reilly, P.R. (1991). *The Surgical Solution: A History of Involuntary Sterilization in the United States*. Baltimore: Johns Hopkins University Press.

Savasi, I., Spitzer, R.F., Allen, L.M., & Ornstein, M.A. (2009). Menstrual suppression for adolescents with developmental disabilities. *Journal of Pediatric and Adolescent Gynecology*, **22**, 143–149.

Schwingl, P. & Guess, H. (2000). Safety and effectiveness of vasectomy. *Fertility and Sterility*, **73**(5), 923–936.

Sullivan, P. & Knutson, J. (2000). Maltreatment and disabilities: a population-based epidemiological study. *Child Abuse and Neglect*, **24**(10), 1257–1273.

Chapter

30

Parental requests for intervention in children with lethal conditions

Benjamin S. Wilfond and John C. Carey

Case narrative

Annie is born at full term with good Apgar scores, but weighs only 2350 grams. On physical exam, she is alert but has somewhat low tone. She has abnormal facial features, a short sternum, and over-riding digits. After failure to pass a nasogastric tube, a tracheal–esophageal fistula (TEF) is diagnosed. Chromosome studies confirm trisomy 18, and an echocardiogram shows a moderate ventricular septal defect (VSD) and moderate pulmonary valvular dysplasia.

Ellen, the neonatologist, and Mary, the surgeon, meet Annie's parents, Bill and Liz, to discuss treatment options. They explain that trisomy 18 is a lethal condition and that most children die within the first few weeks to months. The team does not recommend surgery, explaining that surgery is not in the child's best interest and will result in unnecessary suffering for Annie. They offer the services of the neonatal palliative care team and reassure Bill and Liz that the palliative care team can assist the family in the grieving process. They can provide comfort care for Annie by keeping an IV in place for hydration and pain relief.

Bill and Liz are devastated by the news. They are both 36 years of age and have been together for 18 years. They met in college, and now Bill is a carpenter and Liz is a special education teacher. This is their first child. They had prenatal care, but did not have any prenatal screening for fetal anomalies, including ultrasounds, serum screening, or amniocentesis. Their midwife was concerned when they declined the first ultrasound and referred them to a genetic counselor who she hoped could better explain the pregnancy risks. When the genetic counselor met with Bill and Liz, they gave several reasons for not wanting an ultrasound. First, they were very committed to the health of their child and were concerned that the ultrasound might expose the child to unnecessary risks. They had read that prenatal ultrasounds may cause autism. Second, they generally wished to limit technology in their life. They do not own a TV, computer or cell phones, and only use a "flex car" when necessary. Third, they were very committed to making this baby part of their family. Liz had undergone an abortion when she and Bill were in college. They do not regret that decision, but before this pregnancy, she was anxious that they might not be able to conceive. Finally, they are comfortable with disability and understand its impact. Bill has a younger brother with Down syndrome.

Bill and Liz tell Ellen and Mary that they would like to take Annie home and request surgery to repair the TEF so they can feed their baby. Mary agrees to repair the TEF. Ellen is left speechless when she hears the parents' request and after they walk out of the room she says to Mary, "Look, this child is going to die soon, and I don't think that this is medically appropriate. My job is to help patients, and all this will do is cause unnecessary pain and suffering. Further, she has a VSD that will increase her surgical and anesthetic risk for repairing the TEF, and we know the cardiothoracic surgeons won't take her to the operating room. I took an oath to do what is best for my patient, and this feels so wrong!" Ellen contacts the ethics consultant for advice.

Ethical issues and analysis

This case raises many issues that are addressed in other chapters. These include palliative care, prenatal testing, futility, parent–provider disagreement, cultural attitudes, conscientious objections, allocation of scarce resources, and social justice. This chapter will touch on these issues as they relate to this case, but will focus specifically on how to approach parental requests for interventions that providers think are not justified

Clinical Ethics in Pediatrics: A Case-Based Textbook, ed. Douglas S. Diekema, Mark R. Mercurio and Mary B. Adam. Published by Cambridge University Press. © Cambridge University Press 2011.

because they arise in the context of a lethal condition. Focusing on the question of when medical and surgical interventions are appropriate in children with lethal conditions draws attention to an uncomfortable discourse about the value of children who will never function independently, an issue that needs to be addressed at personal, professional, and societal levels.

Lethality

In pediatrics, "lethal anomalies" is a term usually reserved for a variety of conditions that have two key features (Koogler et al., 2003). First, children with these conditions exhibit profound intellectual impairments, and their behavior is not likely to develop beyond that of a one- or two-year-old. Second, these conditions result in structural anomalies (heart, airway, gastrointestinal) or physiological complications from neurological impairments (aspiration, apnea, seizures) that, if left untreated, will likely result in death.

Many health care providers are uncomfortable using interventions such as neonatal resuscitation, TEF repair, VSD repair, gastrostomy, or tracheostomy in children with lethal anomalies: interventions that are routinely performed on other children. Not performing these surgeries or forgoing other so-called aggressive interventions to manage pneumonia, seizures, apnea, cardiac failure, or respiratory failure may contribute to the lethal prognosis becoming a self-fulfilling prophesy.

In this chapter, trisomy 18 illustrates this broader category of lethal conditions and represents an instructive example because there are more data and more diverse views expressed about this condition than for other, similarly lethal conditions such as mitochondrial disorders (e.g., Leigh disease), lysosomal storage disorders (e.g., Tay–Sachs disease), and skeletal dysplasias (e.g., campomelic dysplasia). The 2010 American Heart Association guidelines state that for conditions "associated with almost certain early death and when unacceptably high morbidity is likely among the rare survivors, resuscitation is not indicated" (Kattwinkel et al., 2010). Trisomy 13, anencephaly, and birth weight <400 g are cited as conditions for which resuscitation is not indicated. The determination of "unacceptably high morbidity," however, is a value judgment. The problem with describing a condition as lethal is that it translates the value judgment into a clinical determination. But parents, such as Bill and Liz, might have different values than members of the medical team.

Physician attitudes about lethal trisomies

Historically, the conventional approach for trisomy 13 and 18 has been to not provide interventions (Paris et al., 1992). An article in *The Lancet* about avoiding surgery in these children states, "We believe that, because of their limited life expectancy or profound mental retardation, such patients ought to be transferred from the intensive-care unit and be allowed to die … But letting such children die may be insufficient; perhaps we ought to help them to die, and change the aim of treatment from cure into comforting care in their terminal state …"(Bos et al., 1992). More recently, McGraw and Perlman (2008) found in a survey of New York neonatologists that only 44% would be willing to initiate resuscitation in babies born with trisomy 18. The primary reasons offered were maternal preference (70%), appearance of the neonate in the delivery room (46%), and legal concerns (25%). They write, "The vast majority of respondents (~90%) who would consider resuscitation indicated that they would do so despite knowing that the life span of infants with trisomy 18 is invariably short. These observations raise the concern that some neonatologists are abandoning the best-interest standard, which would require that providers agree only to treatment strategies that are consistent with furthering the good of the infant, and instead are adopting an 'ethic of abdication' in their approach to difficult treatment/non-treatment decisions"(McGraw & Perlman, 2008). They conclude by saying, "We contend that having intensive care measures such as intubation and corrective surgery available as potential options for infants with a confirmed lethal trisomy gives the impression to parents that these are reasonable interventions to consider and downplays the invasive painful nature of these therapies."

Futility

The attitudes expressed above certainly track Ellen's concerns. As discussed in other chapters, physicians are not obligated to provide, let alone offer, every intervention to every patient. Often this issue is discussed as a concern about futility (Truog et al., 1992). *Physiologic futility* applies to situations in which an intervention will not work. Providing penicillin for diabetic ketoacidosis, for example, is futile. *Quantitative futility* is often described as a treatment that offers less than a 1% chance of success. Yet historically, physicians – particularly neonatologists – have been willing to provide quantitatively futile interventions, using innovations to improve outcomes over time. As a result, the gestational age of viability has declined substantially since 1963, when John F. Kennedy's son died at 34 weeks' gestation in a hyperbaric oxygen chamber at 2 days of age (a futile intervention).

Ellen's concerns are most appropriately labeled as a concern about *qualitative futility*; in other words, what is and what is not "worth" doing. While her concerns about pain and suffering are legitimate, they are based on a subjective assessment of the benefits and burdens of the proposed interventions. Underlying these concerns is an inherently normative claim about the value of a life based on an anticipated short life and low potential for future interaction. Many parents and pediatricians would concur with Ellen and make decisions to forgo otherwise standard pediatric interventions, such as TEF or VSD repair, or choose no neonatal resuscitation in a child with trisomy 18.

The historical context of treatment decisions for children with disabilities

Identifying the boundaries surrounding when parents should be permitted to make decisions *to withdraw support* is a classic issue in pediatric bioethics. In the 1970s and 1980s, this debate played out for Down syndrome (trisomy 21) and spina bifida. Duff, a neonatologist, argued that parents should be able to make medical decisions precisely because these are quality of life decisions, and a family-centered response is ethically appropriate for children whose lives will be forever tied to their parents. He described the parents' situation as a "Medical Vietnam," suggesting that parents need a way to get out of this intractable situation (Duff, 1981). His argument was countered by Bartholome and Fost, two pediatric bioethicists, who noted that Duff was mischaracterizing the life of children with Down syndrome (Bartholome, 1981; Fost, 1981). In their view, the experience of children with Down syndrome was not so bleak that parents should be able to make decisions to deny otherwise routine medical and surgical care. The procedural resolution to this debate in the 1980s led to the development of hospital ethics committees, which were considered a better place to bring disagreements than the courts.

The asymmetry between the classic debate about trisomy 21 and the contemporary debate about trisomy 18 is that today's debate is about whether parents should be permitted to make decisions to *provide treatment* when the medical team advises against it. Should parents be permitted to make requests for interventions that may prolong their child's life, even if only by a few weeks, months, or years, particularly if the profound intellectual and developmental issues will persist? Duff's argument in support of parental discretion ironically could be applied to support treatment of children with trisomy 18, even though his writings suggest an implicit view that children with disabilities may be better off without otherwise life-sustaining interventions. Further, Wilkinson (2010) recently observed that many do not think that non-human animals with equivalent cognitive capacities are harmed by their existence and thus, parental preferences for interventions for children with profound disabilities should be supported since parental love can transcend species, let alone disabilities.

Negotiating parent and provider disagreements

In this case, the physicians did not recommend surgery because Annie will likely not have a long life, and even if she does live a year or longer, she will have profound intellectual impairments. Provider recommendations in this setting are helpful and even desirable for guiding parental decision-making (Ross, 2003). Before making such recommendations, however, providers may want to inquire about the family's cultural values and beliefs. Bill and Liz might say, "We love our Annie, just as you love your children, and we value the time that we have together. We don't want to put Annie through interventions that might not help her, or that would only cause pain. But we know that some children with trisomy 18 can live for months and occasionally years. We would like to give Annie that chance. As her parents, we owe her that much. We respect that you do not share our values about children with disability. We see her life as important and fulfilling to our family. We hope you will honor our request for the TEF repair, and if she thrives but starts showing signs of heart failure, we will consider repairing her VSD."

The decision about whether to pursue surgical interventions essentially hinges on whether parents believe the quality of this life is meaningful or worthwhile. Why should parents be privileged in such decisions? After all, doctors and nurses are moral agents and should not be expected to provide interventions that they sincerely believe to be ethically inappropriate. There is a rich literature on the issue of conscientious objection and a consensus that providers should not be expected to participate in socially contested interventions such as abortion, euthanasia, and the treatment of the profoundly disabled (Curlin et al., 2007; Ross & Clayton, 2007; Mercurio et al., 2008; Ross & Frader, 2009). Yet these and other authors are clear that when providers claim a conscientious objection, they are obligated to explain the reason(s) that they are not willing to provide such interventions and to inform parents of other options or alternative providers. In this case, Ellen could say to Liz and Bill, "Look, I appreciate that you love and care for your daughter, but if I was in your position, I would make a different decision. I disagree so strongly with your decision that I can not in good conscience, take care of your daughter. I will ask one of my colleagues to assume her care."

That would be an uncomfortable yet honest conversation. Yet, there are several asymmetries that might push Ellen back towards respecting the family's wishes. First, providers have ultimate control over whether the interventions will take place. Ellen intimated this point when she suggested that the cardiothoracic surgeon would not repair the VSD. The point is not whether or not she was correct, but simply that the physician possesses the "power" to say no. Arguably, it is precisely because of this imbalance of power that the provider should be willing to take a few extra steps toward the parents. Second, the parents will live with this experience and the consequences of whatever decisions are made, one way or another, for the rest of their lives. Parents of children with trisomies have described feeling abandoned by their providers and losing trust in them following their experiences with end-of-life decisions (Farlow, 2009; Thiele, 2010). Third, determining whether it is in the child's interest to live longer because of medical interventions proves difficult to determine. For this reason, parents should necessarily be involved in these decisions (Koogler et al., 2003; Carey, 2009). Arras (1984) has argued even further that a "best interests" standard is not even appropriate because such children do not have interests in the traditional sense. He proposed that a "relational potential" standard should be used. This family-centered solution suggests that, for children with "lethal" conditions, their primary meaning of life is related to their ability to form relationships with their parents and thus the parents' views about those relationships should guide the decision.

One approach to persistent disagreement is to involve ethics consultants and committees to provide a process for resolving disagreements collectively. Mercurio (2011) recently described two discussions and analyses from hospital ethics committees, one that resulted in a decision to provide VSD surgery to a child with trisomy 18, as well as another decision to withdraw support over parents' objections, illustrating how ethics committees can guide decisions in different directions.

Resource scarcity

Resource scarcity is an external constraint on parental decision-making. Scarcities exist on many different levels. Organ availability for transplant remains the most pressing example of an *explicit scarcity*. Explicit scarcity forces us to acknowledge that tragic choices must be made and that processes must be developed to facilitate transparency and fairness. Hospital *resource scarcity* is generally less acute, but pandemic infection planning underscores that such decisions must be made occasionally. For children with profound disabilities, the issue is primarily *fiscal scarcity*. Given ever increasing health care expenditures, should we provide care for children who will not live a long time, rather than spending that money in other ways?

Concerns about financial costs are often raised in discussions about trisomy 18 (Courtwright et al., 2010). Ellen did not make this claim and instead focused on her concerns about Annie's interests. However, cost may provide a more socially acceptable justification. This is a claim that these children will never contribute anything "meaningful" to society or become independent, and therefore we cannot afford to provide them with expensive medical interventions. Some may argue that this is most compelling when such children might actually live for a long time because the financial cost associated with their highly dependent care is even greater. Others may ague that this is most compelling when life is expected to be very short because a short life is even less valuable and any expense paid to extend it is more wasteful. That cost concerns can be raised regardless of whether the length of life is short or long suggests that the underlying concern is not the costs per se, but the value of the life with profound disabilities.

The policy debate about providing standard pediatric care for children with lethal conditions should occur publicly, as part of open political discourse, rather than at the bedside, where disabled children and their parents will have a muted voice. Of course, even within public debate, others must represent the interests of children with intellectual impairments since they cannot speak for themselves. If this political debate were to occur, it is not clear how it would play out.

The proportion of health care costs from such children is modest compared with the costs of adult end-of-life care (Levinsky et al., 2001; Feudtner et al., 2005). More importantly, when scarce resources and uncertain futures require difficult decision-making, we should offer special protections to the people in our society who are most vulnerable. Throughout human history, people have rarely been willing to collectively forgo their interests when they are in a position to take advantage of those less fortunate and less powerful. It has only been during the latter half of the last century, and only with political pressure from advocacy groups, that some societies have begun to approach people with disabilities with respect and equal treatment. However, far less discussion has occurred about people with profound intellectual disabilities as opposed to physical disabilities. Many people have limited exposure to persons with intellectual disabilities, and even health care providers have limited experiences with them outside of health care settings. This limits the ability of most people to see the full range of interactions that occur between persons with intellectual disabilities and their family members.

Natural history of trisomy 13 and 18

More than 90% of children with trisomy 13 and 18 do not live more than a year, and about 50% do not live past the first week of life (Carey, 2010; Vendola et al., 2010). The most common clinical causes of death are central apnea, aspiration, pulmonary hypertension, or heart failure, and often a combination of all of these. Ellen refers to the cardiothoracic surgeons who she believes would not perform surgery. Many surgeons are unwilling or at least reluctant to repair a VSD (the most common cardiac anomaly) in children with trisomy 13 and 18. A series of papers describing intensive management, including surgery, of approximately 100 children have clarified that cardiac surgery can facilitate discharge, reduce clinical symptoms, and extend life. In the United States, Graham and colleagues reported a 91% discharge rate (2004). Reports from Japan describing aggressive management in the NICU and cardiac surgery repair resulted in a 1-year survival rate of approximately 25% (Kosho et al., 2006; Kaneko et al., 2008, 2009; Kosho, 2008). Among children with trisomy 13 and 18 who live more than a year, many required limited interventions in the first few months of life, while others survived following surgical or otherwise

aggressive interventions (Bruns, 2010). These children make modest but progressive developmental improvements. Over time, children with trisomy 13 and 18 acquire skills of late infancy such as self-feeding, understanding cause and effect, and vocalizing, but older children rarely attain expressive language skills or walk independently. Overall the average school-age child with trisomy 18 has an age-equivalent skill level of less than one year, even though many individual abilities will exceed the 12-month level (Baty et al., 1994).

Suggestions and recommendations

Below are several recommendations for engaging with parents who have children with lethal conditions and who request interventions that providers think are not appropriate. *Most importantly, providers should avoid using the term "lethal" and acknowledge directly that the discussion is about differing views about quality of life.*

1. *Clarify the facts about clinical and developmental prognosis.* It is simply not true that death is imminent for *all* children with these conditions. Most conditions are heterogeneous. Discussions about prognosis should be supported by what data are available for the particular condition in question.

2. *Listen to parents' concerns and reasons.* Put yourself in their shoes and consider any requests from their perspective. What is their goal in asking for a given intervention? Is that goal important to the family and can it be reasonably attained? Think about how you would want to be treated by a clinician whose values were different than yours and on whom you had to rely for help.

3. *Share your views with the parents and acknowledge that your values conflict with their views.* Doing this respectfully may allow for a more engaged conversation, which may enhance the possibility of reaching a mutually agreeable solution.

4. *Involve the full clinical team in such conversations.* This may include nurses, social workers, respiratory therapists, genetic counselors, intensivists, surgeons, developmental pediatricians, neurologists, cardiologists, pulmonologists, and geneticists. The differing experiences and perspectives of these many professionals may allow all members of the health

care team to broaden their understanding of the situation at hand. These conversations may also create a forum for regular engagement about complex and controversial issues.

5. *Involve ethics consultants and ethics committees when disagreement persists.* The role of ethics consultants and committees is discussed in the final chapter of this book. Ethics committees can provide an opportunity for diverse views to be aired and offer a process for resolving disagreements. In many institutions, this formal process is a necessary step in the event that the institution wishes to withhold the interventions requested by the parents.

6. *Learn more about the experience of families with children who have profound disabilities.* If your experience with children with profound disabilities is limited to the clinical setting, talk with families about what their life is like outside the hospital and if feasible, make arrangements to visit a family in their home.

Resolution of case and conclusion

Ellen discusses her concerns with her team and finds that most members of the team share her views. One team member suggests asking the developmental pediatrician to talk to Annie's family. He arranges for Liz and Bill to meet with two families: one who made the decision to not resuscitate their child on the third day of life and another whose child had a VSD repaired and then lived at home for 4 years before dying. Both children had a lasting impact on their families, and both sets of parents cherished their time with their child.

Ellen talks further with the ethics consultant. She does not change her view about what *she* would do if she were similarly situated, but she appreciates that "lethality" is not a clinical diagnosis but a normative concept. She understands that lethality is not a trump card that she can invoke when she does not agree with a family's request.

Ellen cares for Annie after her TEF repair and talks with Bill and Liz often. Several months later, when Annie begins to show signs of heart failure, Ellen has a long discussion with Bill and Liz, and they decide together not to proceed with the VSD repair.

What Ellen learned from Annie is that the value of life cannot be measured in years or big achievements, but from the strength of personal relationships, no matter how fleeting in duration.

References

Arras, J.D. (1984). Toward an ethic of ambiguity. *Hastings Center Report*, **14**(2), 25–33.

Bartholome, W.G. (1981). Decisions on death and dying. *Pediatrics*, **68**(6), 910–911.

Baty, B.J., Jorde, L.B., Blackburn, B.L., & Carey, J.C. (1994). Natural history of trisomy 18 and trisomy 13: II. Psychomotor development. *American Journal of Medical Genetics*, **49**(2), 189–194.

Bos, A.P., Broers, C.J., Hazebroek, F.W., et al. (1992). Avoidance of emergency surgery in newborn infants with trisomy 18. *Lancet*, **339**(8798), 913–915.

Bruns, D.A. (2010). Neonatal experiences of newborns with full trisomy 18. *Advances in Neonatal Care*, **10**(1), 25–31.

Carey, J.C. (2009). Attitudes of neonatologists toward delivery room management of confirmed trisomy 18: potential factors influencing a changing dynamic. *Pediatrics*, **123**(3), e547–548.

Carey, J.C. (2010). Trisomy 18 and trisomy 13 syndromes. In *Management of Genetic Syndromes*, ed. B. Cassidy & J.E. Allanson. New York: John Wiley & Sons.

Courtwright, A.M., Laughon, M.M., & Doron, M.W. (2010). Length of life and treatment intensity in infants diagnosed prenatally or postnatally with congenital anomalies considered to be lethal. *Journal of Perinatology* (16 December). Online prepublication at www.nature.com/jp/journal/vaop/ncurrent/suppinfo/jp2010124s1.html.

Curlin, F.A., Lawrence, R.E., Chin, M.H., & Lantos, J.D. (2007). Religion, conscience, and controversial clinical practices. *New England Journal of Medicine*, **356**(6), 593–600.

Duff, R.S. (1981). Counseling families and deciding care of severely defective children – a way of coping with Medical Vietnam. *Pediatrics*, **67**(3), 315–320.

Farlow, B. (2009). Misgivings. *Hastings Center Report*, **39**(5), 19–21.

Feudtner, C., Villareale, N.L., Morray, B., et al. (2005). Technology-dependency among patients discharged from a children's hospital: a retrospective cohort study. *BMC Pediatrics*, **5**(1), 8.

Fost, N. (1981). Counseling families who have a child with a severe congenital anomaly. *Pediatrics*, **67**(3), 321–324.

Graham, E.M., Bradley, S.M., Shirali, G.S., Hills, C.B., & Atz, A.M. (2004). Effectiveness of cardiac surgery in trisomies 13 and 18 (from the Pediatric Cardiac Care Consortium). *American Journal of Cardiology*, **93**(6), 801–803.

Kaneko, Y., Kobayashi, J., Yamamoto, Y., et al. (2008). Intensive cardiac management in patients with trisomy 13 or trisomy 18. *American Journal of Medical Genetics A*, **146A**(11), 1372–1380.

Kaneko, Y., Kobayashi, J., Achiwa, I., et al. (2009). Cardiac surgery in patients with trisomy 18. *Pediatric Cardiology*, **30**(6), 729–734.

Kattwinkel, J., Perlman, J.M., Aziz, K., et al. (2010). Part 15: Neonatal Resuscitation 2010 American Heart Association Guidelines for Cardiopulmonary Resuscitation and Emergency Cardiovascular Care. *Circulation*, **122**(18), S909–S919.

Koogler, T.K., Wilfond, B.S., & Ross, L.F. (2003). Lethal language, lethal decisions. *Hastings Center Report*, **33**(2), 37–41.

Kosho, T. (2008). Care of children with trisomy 18 in Japan. *American Journal of Medical Genetics A*, **146A**(11), 1369–1371.

Kosho, T., Nakamura, T., Kawame, H., et al. (2006). Neonatal management of trisomy 18: clinical details of 24 patients receiving intensive treatment. *American Journal of Medical Genetics A*, **140**(9), 937–944.

Levinsky, N.G., Yu, W., Ash, A., et al. (2001). Influence of age on Medicare expenditures and medical care in the last year of life. *JAMA*, **286**(11), 1349–1355.

McGraw, M.P. & Perlman, J.M. (2008). Attitudes of neonatologists toward delivery room management of confirmed trisomy 18: potential factors influencing a changing dynamic. *Pediatrics*, **121**(6), 1106–1110.

Mercurio, M.R. (2011). The role of a pediatric ethics committee in the newborn intensive care unit. *Journal of Perinatology*, **31**(1), 1–9.

Mercurio, M.R., Peterec, S.M., & Weeks, B. (2008). Hypoplastic left heart syndrome, extreme prematurity, comfort care only, and the principle of justice. *Pediatrics*, **122**(1), 186–189.

Paris, J.J., Weiss, A.H., & Soifer, S. (1992). Ethical issues in the use of life-prolonging interventions for an infant with trisomy 18. *Journal of Perinatology*, **12**(4), 366–368.

Ross, L.F. (2003). Why "doctor, if this were your child, what would you do?" deserves an answer. *Journal of Clinical Ethics*, **14**(1–2), 59–62.

Ross, L.F. & Clayton, E.W. (2007). Religion, conscience, and controversial clinical practices. *New England Journal of Medicine*, **356**(18), 1889–1892.

Ross, L.F. & Frader, J. (2009). Hypoplastic left heart syndrome: a paradigm case for examining conscientious objection in pediatric practice. *Journal of Pediatrics*, **155**(1), 12–15.

Thiele, P. (2010). He was my son, not a dying baby. *Journal of Medical Ethics*, **36**(11), 646–647.

Truog, R.D., Brett, A.S., & Frader, J. (1992). The problem with futility. *New England Journal of Medicine*, **326**(23), 1560–1564.

Vendola, C., Canfield, M., Daiger, S.P., et al. (2010). Survival of Texas infants born with trisomies 21, 18, and 13. *American Journal of Medical Genetics A*, **152A**(2), 360–366.

Wilkinson, D.J.C. (2010). Antenatal diagnosis of trisomy 18, harm and parental choice. *Journal of Medical Ethics*, **36**(11), 644–645.

Chapter 31

Genetic testing and screening of minors

Lainie Friedman Ross

Case narrative

Mr. and Mrs. Smith come to your office with your patient Susan, who is 14 years old, and her little brother Sam, 7 months of age. The last 2 years have been a roller coaster for the Smiths. After 10 years of trying to conceive a second child, they finally succeeded. Although Sam is growing well and appears healthy, he was diagnosed with cystic fibrosis (CF) as part of the state's newborn screening (NBS) program. More recently, Mrs. Smith was diagnosed with breast cancer and is undergoing chemotherapy. She is the third of three sisters to develop breast cancer by age 40, and genetic testing found that all three sisters have a BRCA mutation.

The Smiths come for Susan's routine exam. After discussing adolescent immunizations (Tdap, Menactra, and Gardasil), you ask if they have anything they would like to discuss. They ask whether Susan can be tested for CF. On further inquiry, it is clear that they are not worried that she has CF as she is quite tall and has never had any respiratory problems, but they are concerned about whether she is a CF carrier. Mrs. Smith asks whether you can test Susan for the family's BRCA mutation on the same blood sample.

The case raises several important ethical issues about the appropriate timing of genetic testing and screening of minors. The case involves three different genetic testing and screening scenarios: NBS for CF for Sam, carrier genetic testing, and predictive genetic testing for an adult-onset condition for Susan. There are some overlapping and different ethical issues raised by each scenario. NBS raises a concern of justice because historically there was wide variability in conditions included in each state's NBS panel. There is also concern about the moral justification for mandatory NBS. These concerns depend in part on how one defines best interest and the definition of benefit. Predictive genetic testing and carrier genetic testing raise ethical questions about whether there is a duty to know or a right not to know one's genetic risk factors, whether minors have a right to privacy against their parents, whose consent is necessary and who gets to decide if and when genetic testing is in a minor's best interest.

Newborn screening

Newborn screening began in the 1960s after Dr. Robert Guthrie developed the bacterial inhibition assay to screen for phenylketonuria (PKU) and the filter paper card on which to collect the samples. Until the mid-1990s, most states included between three and ten conditions in their state panels. However, with the development and application of tandem mass spectrometry (MS/MS) to NBS, some states expanded to include over 40 conditions, creating wide disparities between states. Parent advocacy groups argued that a child's well-being should not depend on where a child is born. The Health Resources and Services Administration (HRSA) funded the American College of Medical Genetics (ACMG) to develop a list of conditions that should be included in all NBS programs (ACMG/HRSA, 2005). The Secretary's Advisory Committee endorsed the HRSA/ACMG proposed uniform panel that included 29 primary conditions and 25 secondary conditions.

The parental argument that a child's well-being should not depend on the state in which a child is born is a justice argument. This argument is compelling if the conditions included in the NBS panel meet the criteria of offering direct benefit to the child. Traditionally that was understood to mean that there was an early diagnosis and treatment for each condition that would reduce morbidity and mortality (Wilson & Jungner, 1968). However, the uniform panel includes some conditions

Clinical Ethics in Pediatrics: A Case-Based Textbook, ed. Douglas S. Diekema, Mark R. Mercurio and Mary B. Adam. Published by Cambridge University Press. © Cambridge University Press 2011.

that may not be disorders but merely variants and other conditions for which the natural history and need for medical treatment are unknown (Natowicz, 2005). Advocates argue in favor of expanded screening using an expanded concept of benefit to include benefit to parents (for reproductive planning) and benefit to society (improved knowledge about rare conditions) (Bailey et al., 2006).

The controversy over expanded NBS is further fueled by the fact that NBS is mandatory in 48 of the 50 states, although most states permit refusals based on religious or philosophical objections. The reason for mandatory screening is historical: Guthrie was a parent of a child with mental retardation and became a political advocate for universal screening to prevent disability. Guthrie and the National Association for Retarded Children (now known as the ARC) were frustrated by what they perceived to be the slow uptake of screening by physicians. They successfully lobbied for mandatory universal screening.

The main moral argument against mandatory screening is that voluntary consent is more consistent with cultural values that give great deference to individual decision-making about health care matters, and in the realm of pediatrics, the deference given to parents about how they raise their children (Goldstein et al., 1979; Buchanan & Brock, 1989; Ross, 1998). Those who support parental autonomy and the right to refuse NBS concede that screening for conditions like PKU has significant benefits, but current NBS panels also include conditions of questionable significance and for which treatment may cause iatrogenic harm (Natowicz, 2005). Those who support parental autonomy may concede that it is not in a child's best interest for a parent to refuse PKU screening, but they argue that overriding parental authority is very difficult to justify when the likelihood of a bad outcome is quite remote (the risk of PKU is one in 10 000 infants) (Newson, 2006). The threshold for state intervention is not whether a parent's action is less than ideal, but whether a parent's decision is so bad as to be described as abusive or neglectful (Goldstein et al., 1979; Buchanan & Brock, 1989; Ross, 1998). Given that the likelihood of a true positive screen is quite low, parental refusal does not fall below this threshold. Thus, mandatory screening implies that the state knows what is best for a particular child better than the child's parents.

The second objection to mandatory screening is that it is not necessary. Data from Maryland show that virtually all parents consent (Faden et al., 1982). And

there may be legitimate reasons that a parent refuses screening, based on religious reasons or based on their own assessment of risks and benefits. For example, parents are more likely to receive a false positive result than a true positive, and repeat testing can be stressful for parents. As screening expands to include more conditions, this concern grows in significance (Waisbren et al., 2003; Tarini et al., 2006).

The Smiths do not express any negative concerns about NBS for CF, although they do feel that they should have received information about NBS prenatally, an omission that has been well documented in the literature. While Susan was born before CF was included in many NBS panels (fewer than a dozen states screened for CF prior to 2000), her growth and health are not consistent with CF. Her parents want testing because they understand that she has a high risk of being a carrier (since both parents are carriers and she is not affected, she has a 2/3 chance of being a carrier).

You explain that there are no known associated health risks of being a carrier for CF. You suggest that she is still quite young and can choose to get tested as an adult. You explain that testing Susan when she is an adult gives her the choice about whether or not to get tested and allows her to have some privacy and control about her reproductive health risks. You explain that many individuals and couples choose not to be tested – sometimes based on religious grounds that any intervention would be interfering with God's plans; and others choose not to be tested because they reject the quest for the perfect child. The Smiths respond that Susan has a moral obligation to know her own reproductive risks in order to make informed reproductive choices.

You all look at Susan. She tells you that her cousins were tested for CF at their school (they live in Australia where high school carrier screening programs exist), and they have shared their test results widely both within the family and at their school. She is not sure why you are so concerned about privacy. "It is what it is. It won't make me any less of a person," she responds. She realizes that knowing this information now will increase her reproductive choices. Since most carrier testing occurs in pregnant women and couples and not antenatally, couples have to decide whether or not to continue a pregnancy with an affected child. In contrast, if the information is known antenatally, Susan can ask her partner to be tested and make informed reproductive decisions accordingly.

Susan's brother was diagnosed with CF because of NBS. In the United States, several different CF NBS methodologies exist. All begin with screening for immunoreactive trypsinogen (IRT). In some states, an elevated IRT leads to a request for a second IRT test several days to weeks later. If the IRT remains elevated, then a sweat test is recommended. In other states, an elevated IRT leads to DNA testing. If one or more mutations are identified, the child is referred for a sweat test. In most states fewer than 60 mutations are included in the newborn screening despite there being >1600 mutations. Thus a negative DNA test does not ensure the lack of CF and in some states, those with very elevated IRT and no DNA mutation still undergo a sweat test.

The Smiths live in a state that uses the double IRT methodology and so they do not know Sam's mutations. Neither parent has elected to undergo carrier testing because they do not plan to have more children. You are concerned that testing Susan may not be definitive. If a mutation is found, then she will be a known carrier. But if she tests negative, it is unknown whether she is a true negative or whether the mutations that run in the family are rare and not included in routine panels. You suggest that it is most appropriate to wait until adulthood, but if they insist upon testing before Susan reaches majority, you would only test Susan after the family mutations are identified.

Several professional organizations wrote policy statements regarding genetic testing and screening of minors between 1994 and 2001. The Working Party of the Clinical Genetics Society (UK), the American College of Medical Genetics and the American Society of Human Genetics (ACMG/ASHG), and the American Academy of Pediatrics (AAP) all state that carrier testing for reproductive purposes should generally wait until adulthood (Working Party CGS, 1994; ASHG/ACMG, 1995; AAP, 2001). There are two pragmatic concerns with this position. First, this position fails to notice that carriers are routinely identified in NBS for hemoglobinopathies and now, for some carriers, as part of NBS for CF. In 1994, the Institute of Medicine published a report arguing in favor of disclosing carriers identified in NBS to parents (Andrews et al., 1994), and today this practice is almost universal. Second this position assumes that there are no health risks in being a carrier, an assumption that is being challenged for at least some genetic conditions (Ross, 2010).

The main moral argument in favor of delaying carrier testing until adulthood is the right to privacy and the right not to know. Many women and couples do refuse to undergo prenatal testing. The main moral

arguments in favor of carrier testing in childhood are that it may be easier to incorporate this knowledge into one's self-concept at a younger age and that it may allow individuals to have wider options (having knowledge antenatally).

Susan does raise the point that there are several countries around the world where carrier testing is done in high schools. In Australia and Canada, the focus has been on ethnic communities (Tay–Sachs disease and CF carrier testing in Ashkenazi Jews who attend Jewish day schools), but in other countries, the focus has been broader (thalassemia screening in certain parts of the Mediterranean and the Middle East). Such screening programs would meet great resistance here in the United States (Ross, 2010). First, we are a more heterogeneous country. The Canadian program was active at a time where most of the Ashkenazi Jewish adolescents in Montreal attended one of several high schools. Interestingly, the French Canadian children were not offered this service although Tay–Sachs disease is also common in that community. In Australia, the focus has been on Jewish teenagers who attend a Jewish day school. There would be serious concerns about stigmatization if Jewish children were targeted in more diverse high schools. Second, there are serious flaws in targeted screening because it assumes a knowledge and purity of ethnic ancestry that does not exist. For example, studies by Dyson in the UK show that both self-identification and health care provider-identification of those at risk for hemoglobinopathies resulted in a number of false positives and false negatives (Dyson, 2005).

The Smiths agree to consider testing of themselves and will report back to you regarding carrier testing of Susan. They then ask about testing Susan for BRCA. They point out that Mrs. Smith and her sisters all have the same known mutation. Since the family mutation is known, testing is simplified. Like CF, there are many mutations in the BRCA gene that are associated with increased risk. When there is no known mutation in a family, a negative test may mean that the individual has a mutation that has not yet been associated with disease.

You suggest that there is nothing that health care providers would do differently in childhood if Susan's BRCA status were known, and so testing can wait until she is an adult and can decide for herself. You point out that if she tests herself as an adult, she has the right to privacy regarding her health risks and has the choice about whom to inform and when. The Smiths are adamant that they want to know Susan's BRCA status because it will help them counsel their daughter at the "right moments." Susan is ambivalent. She has just gone through puberty and is not sure whether she wants to perceive her breasts as future cancer buds. You explain to the Smiths that testing is clearly not urgent and that maybe they should get some formal genetic counseling and even psychological counseling regarding this issue. You state that you will not order such testing without Susan's active permission.

Mrs. Smith is a bit bewildered. She thought that parents made health care decisions for their children and does not understand why Susan needs to be actively engaged. You explain that all professional organizations have argued to generally defer predictive genetic testing until adulthood (Working Party CGS, 1994; ASHG/ACMG, 1995; AAP, 2001). The reason for this policy position is that predictive genetic testing for an adult-onset condition is not like deciding whether or not her daughter needs antibiotics for pneumonia, but that it is an elective medical procedure. You explain that the AAP believes that the maturing adolescent should have a greater role in her health care, particularly for elective decisions when it is not clear whether the benefits outweigh the risks (AAP, 1995). This shows respect for the child's developing autonomy and competency, and respects the fact that some people just don't want to know whether they are at risk for a genetic condition.

Mrs. Smith dismisses the right not to know. She argues that since there are preventions and treatments available for individuals with BRCA mutations, it would be irresponsible not to know. She points out that if Susan tests positive, she would be counseled to have earlier and more frequent mammograms. You explain that the recommendation is to begin mammography 5 years before the earliest detection of breast cancer in the family. Since Mrs. Smith and her sisters all developed cancer in their mid to late 30s, Susan would not need to undergo mammography until her late 20s.

Mrs. Smith then states that if Susan were known to be BRCA positive, she would encourage her to get married and have children quickly. You respond that since neither of you would encourage Susan to have a child now, these issues can be deferred for at least another 4 years at which point Susan should have some say about the timing of such testing. She may not want to undergo testing until she is done with schooling or has a serious boyfriend, although other young women choose to undergo testing at age 18 to avoid living with ambiguity.

Mrs. Smith is annoyed and wonders whether she should just seek out direct-to-consumer testing. You express a very negative reaction, because the testing does not allow Susan and her parents to obtain appropriate pre- and post-test counseling about the benefits and risks of testing, the clinical and psychosocial meaning of the test, and the limitations of the testing (Tabor & Kelley, 2009). You encourage the Smiths to discuss their concerns with a genetic counselor and a psychologist as they are raising many concerns, and it is important that these issues be explored with someone who has the proper skills. You also offer to discuss testing again in 2 months at her next appointment to continue her adolescent immunization series.

Key points

Newborn screening: Although NBS is mandatory in most jurisdictions, we have an obligation to inform parents about why we screen and what they should do if they receive notification about an abnormal screen. When carrier status is identified, the parents should be informed.

Carrier testing: In general, carrier testing of children is not medically indicated. It should not be done on a routine population basis, particularly in the schools where there may be great peer pressure to conform and to share results. Still, in high-risk families, parents and their children may want to know. In some cases, carriers may have some mild symptoms and carrier identification may be useful. In other cases, parents may want to know carrier status in order to counsel their children for reproductive planning. In general, while it is morally permissible to perform carrier testing on healthy minors, pediatricians should recommend delaying carrier testing until the child can be a part of the decision-making process.

When carrier identification occurs in NBS, parents should be informed, and they should be encouraged to share their child's carrier information with health care providers and with the children themselves as they mature.

The pregnant adolescent and the teenager trying to get pregnant should be offered carrier screening like any other obstetrical patient.

Predictive genetic testing for adult-onset conditions: In general, predictive genetic testing for adult-onset conditions is not medically indicated and should be deferred until adulthood. Still, in high-risk families, parents and their children may want to know, and there may be scenarios where the stress of waiting may cause more harm than testing. At minimum, predictive genetic testing should be deferred until the adolescent can participate and actively assent to testing.

Case resolution and discussion

Mr. and Mrs. Smith meet with a genetic counselor. They explore the pros and cons of undergoing carrier testing. Using a common prenatal CF panel, Mr. Smith is found to have the most common mutation, delta-F508, but Mrs. Smith's test is inconclusive. She is offered full-gene sequencing, but defers due to the costs. On these grounds, they agree that it makes sense to defer testing of Susan.

The counselor also discusses the pros and cons of predictive genetic testing of teenagers for BRCA. Given Susan's ambivalence and the stress of chemotherapy, the Smiths agree to defer testing although they do think it is important that Susan has testing as a young adult in order to make both reproductive and life planning decisions.

References

American Academy of Pediatrics (AAP) Committee on Bioethics (1995). Informed consent, parental permission and assent in pediatric practice. *Pediatrics*, **95**, 314–317.

American Academy of Pediatrics (AAP) Committee on Bioethics (2001). Ethical issues with genetic testing in pediatrics. *Pediatrics*, **107**, 1451–1455.

American College of Medical Genetics/Health Resources and Services Administration (ACMG/HRSA). (2005). Toward a Uniform Screening Panel and System. ftp://ftp.hrsa.gov/mchb/genetics/screeningdraftforcomment.pdf (last accessed November 19, 2010).

American Society of Human Genetics (ASHG)/American College of Medical Genetics (ACMG) (1995). Points to consider: ethical, legal, and psychosocial implications of genetic testing in children and adolescents. *American Journal of Human Genetics*, **57**, 1233–1241.

Andrews, L.L., Fullarton, J.E., Holtzman, N.A., & Motulsky, A.G. (eds.) and the Committee on Assessing Genetic Risks, Institute of Medicine (IOM) (1994). *Assessing Genetic Risks: Implications for Health and Social Policy*. Washington, DC: National Academy Press.

Bailey, D.B. Jr., Beskow, L.M., Davis, A.M, & Skinner, D. (2006). Changing perspectives on the benefits of newborn screening. *Mental Retardation & Developmental Disabilities Research Reviews*, **12**, 270–279.

Buchanan, A. & Brock, D. (1989). *Deciding for Others: The Ethics of Surrogate Decision Making*. New York: Cambridge University Press.

Dyson, S. (2005). *Ethnicity and Screening for Sickle Cell/Thalassaemia. Lessons for Practice from the Voices of Experience*. Edinburgh, UK: Elsevier Churchill Livingstone.

Faden, R., Chwalow, A.J., Holtzman, N.A., & Horn, S.D. (1982). A survey to evaluate parental consent as public policy for neonatal screening. *American Journal of Public Health*, **72**, 1347–1352.

Goldstein, J., Freud, A., & Solnit, A. (1979). *Before the Best Interests of the Child*, Vol. II. New York: The Free Press.

Natowicz, M. (2005). Newborn screening – setting evidence-based policy for protection. *New England Journal of Medicine*, **353**, 867–870.

Newson, A. (2006). Should parental refusals of newborn screening be respected? *Cambridge Quarterly of Healthcare Ethics*, **15**, 135–146.

Ross, L.F. (1998). *Children, Families, and Health Care Decision-making*. Oxford, UK: Oxford University Press.

Ross, L.F. (2010). Carrier detection in childhood: a need for policy reform. *Genome Medicine*, **2**, 25. Available at: http://genomemedicine.com/content/2/4/25.

Tabor, H.K. & Kelley, M. (2009). Challenges in the use of direct-to-consumer personal genome testing in children. *American Journal of Bioethics*, **9**, 32–34.

Tarini, B.A., Christakis, D.A., & Welch, H.G. (2006). State newborn screening in the tandem mass spectrometry era: more tests, more false-positive results. *Pediatrics*, **118**, 448–456.

Waisbren, S.E., Albers, S., Amato, S., et al. (2003). Effect of expanded newborn screening for biochemical genetic disorders on child outcomes and parental stress. *JAMA*, **290**, 2564–2572.

Wilson, J.M. & Jungner, G. (1968). Principles and practice of screening for disease. *Public Health Papers* 34. Geneva: World Health Organization.

Working Party of the Clinical Genetics Society (UK) (1994). The genetic testing of children. *Journal of Medical Genetics*, **31**, 785–797.

Chapter 32

The introduction of innovative technology into practice

John D. Lantos

Introduction

Stories of clinical innovation in medicine are generally stories of fits and starts, of irrational exuberance and of avoidable tragedy, of skill, luck, science, and serendipity. Such stories are often transformed, in retrospect, into orderly, semi-fictional narratives that show science as a rational process. These narratives portray medical progress as the result of carefully designed experiments that test specific hypotheses. The results of such experiments, so the story goes, are then incorporated into clinical practice. The real history of innovation is both more fun and more frightening than such myths might suggest.

In the real world, progress is non-linear and messy because every innovation is a frightening gamble. When innovations are first tried, we know little about them. We don't know whether they will work, for whom, or with what associated harms. We don't know whether the benefits will ultimately outweigh the risks. We don't know the comparative effectiveness of innovative and standard therapies. We aren't even sure exactly when it is ethically permissible to study a new therapy, or which research methodology is best, or when it has been studied enough. Even when good studies are done, it is often hard to interpret the results.

Furthermore, practitioners are famously erratic in their willingness or reticence to adopt new therapies. They sometimes adopt therapies when there is little or no evidence of their efficacy, and fail to adopt therapies that have proven to be beneficial. In this chapter, I will present some case studies of particular innovative therapies and examine the unique issues raised by each. Finally, I will generalize about some of the lessons learned by these cases.

Supplemental oxygen for respiratory distress in newborns

The history of the use of supplemental oxygen in neonatology illustrates the complex dynamic of medical innovation in pediatrics. Supplemental oxygen therapy for respiratory distress syndrome (RDS) is a mainstay of modern neonatology. Over the last 70 years, it was tried, widely adopted, criticized, studied, modified, and studied again and again. Its use has always been surrounded by controversies, and continues so to this day.

In 1942, Wilson and colleagues showed that the irregular breathing patterns of premature babies could be converted to regular respirations by giving supplemental oxygen to the babies (Wilson et al., 1942). This was heralded as a potential major breakthrough but its widespread adoption was hindered by the fact that the therapy was unwieldy. Incubators at the time were not airtight, so a steady concentration of oxygen could not be maintained.

By the 1940s, newly designed incubators made it possible for doctors to provide and maintain high concentrations of oxygen for prolonged periods of time (Dunham et al., 1940). Many nurseries immediately adopted the combination of supplemental oxygen and incubators.

Shortly afterwards, some doctors noticed that the babies who survived had developed a new type of blindness. In 1951, Crosse labeled this blindness "retrolental fibroplasia." She suspected that excess oxygen might be the cause, and suggested that this hypothesis be tested in a randomized trial (Crosse, 1951).

In 1952, an alternate-assignment, parallel treatment trial of high versus low oxygen regimens was con-

Clinical Ethics in Pediatrics: A Case-Based Textbook, ed. Douglas S. Diekema, Mark R. Mercurio and Mary B. Adam. Published by Cambridge University Press. © Cambridge University Press 2011.

ducted. Babies in the high-oxygen arm had higher rates of retrolental fibroplasia (Patz et al., 1952).

The next year, an NIH consensus conference recommended a prospective trial of high-dose oxygen to more rigorously test whether oxygen was the cause of retinopathy. The study was carried out. It showed that oxygen curtailment led to a two-thirds reduction in eye disease with no appreciable increase in mortality for babies in the low oxygen arm (Kinsey, 1955). Many nurseries started using lower oxygen levels. Some noticed higher mortality rates. This led to a reanalysis of the data from the earlier trial. The reanalysis showed strikingly different results. Mortality was much higher for the infants in the low-oxygen arm. There were 16 excess deaths for every case of retinopathy prevented (Bolton & Cross, 1974).

This led to controversy about the optimum dose of oxygen to balance its beneficial effects on survival with its detrimental effects on the eye. The controversy was difficult to resolve, in part, because, in those days, it was difficult to measure the level of oxygen in the blood. All that could be measured accurately was how much oxygen was delivered, not how much was absorbed.

In the decades that followed, better technology allowed doctors to follow not just the delivery of oxygen but the partial pressure of oxygen in the baby's blood. These were also the years when positive-pressure ventilation was first introduced (more on that below). Still, no prospective studies of different oxygen regimens were carried out. Instead, the results of retrospective studies were used to develop consensus recommendations for treatment. Different doctors and different NICUs used different oxygen regimens and had different results.

In 2002, Tin (2002) reviewed the available data and concluded, "Oxygen must have been given to more infants than any other medicinal product in the last 60 years. Despite that, we still know very little about how much infants actually need, or how much it is wise to give. The depth of our ignorance is really quite embarrassing." A few years later, Silverman (2004) echoed these sentiments, "There has never been a shred of convincing evidence to guide limits for the rational use of supplemental oxygen in the care of extremely premature infants. For decades, the optimum range of oxygenation (to balance four competing risks: mortality, ROP blindness, chronic lung disease, and brain damage) was, and remains to this day, unknown."

Since Silverman's editorial, two randomized trials have been published. A study of low versus high oxygen saturations for babies with chronic lung disease showed no difference in mortality or developmental outcomes between the two arms (Askie et al., 2003). But a prospective, multicenter randomized trial of low (85–89%) versus high (91–95%) oxygen saturation in premature babies showed that those in the low-saturation group had higher mortality rates but that survivors had lower rates of retinopathy (SUPPORT Study Group, 2010).

The story of supplemental oxygen in neonatology illustrates all the key dilemmas of innovation. A new therapy is introduced in an uncontrolled way. Some clinicians immediately adopt it. Others call for more studies. Studies may or may not be done, or done well. The results are not straightforward and lead to more debate. Different doctors in different centers develop different clinical protocols. Outcomes vary. New technologies change the risk–benefit ratio of old therapies. Practice patterns develop that are hard to change.

This story plays out again and again. The story of the development of mechanical ventilation for premature babies is similar.

The development of mechanical ventilation

Positive-pressure ventilation was first used as a desperate innovative measure for dying infants. In 1965, Delivoria-Papadopoulos et al. (1965) "demonstrated the possibility of reversing at least temporarily the biochemical changes of terminal asphyxia in patients dying with RDS." In other words, she and her colleagues intubated dying babies and showed that they could be temporarily kept alive. But the babies all went on to die. There were no NICUs to provide the intensive care necessary to monitor babies on mechanical ventilation.

These initial studies of the physiologic feasibility of mechanical ventilation led to the belief that the therapy might be clinically useful if it was initiated sooner, before the patients were "terminal." This change from treating babies who were "dying" to treating babies who were judged "unlikely to benefit from standard therapy" can be thought of as a change in the "eligibility criteria" for their clinical trial. (The investigators did not describe it that way.) The new, relaxed eligibility criteria would allow patients into the clinical trial of mechanical ventilation who might, in fact, have survived without it, but it might also allow doctors to save babies who would have been too sick to save if they waited until death was imminent. This illustrates a crucial question that arises in the study of any innovation. Who, exactly, should be eligible for an initial trial? The eligibility criteria may determine the results of a trial. If they are too restrictive, then a potentially beneficial therapy might appear useless because patients are too sick to benefit. If they are not restrictive enough, then patients who did not need the innovative therapy might be unnecessarily exposed to risk (Lantos & Frader, 1990).

The paper describing the initial trial by Delivoria-Papadopoulos is cautiously optimistic. Eight babies who were ventilated in the first 24 hours of life all died. Babies who did not require ventilation until they were over 24 hours of age did better – 7/13 survived. No baby who weighed less than 1800 grams at birth survived. From these findings, the authors conclude, "Our results suggest that if infants over 1800g with failing respirations after 24 hours of age are placed on (ventilation), and before a damaging degree of metabolic acidosis has developed, approximately one-half will survive with our present methods."

This analysis reveals another key feature of innovation. The innovators did not develop hypotheses, design experiments to test them, or limit their analyses to a particular study question. That sort of clinical research generally occurs at a later stage – when two well-accepted therapies are tested against one another. Instead, they did what innovators usually do at earlier stages – innovate, retrospectively analyze the results of those innovations, use those analyses to refine the innovations, and eventually end up with something that seems to work. This process is both messier and more fertile than the classic hypothesis-testing approach.

There were few randomized trials of mechanical ventilation, though there was some argument about the relative risks and benefits of using continuous positive airway pressure, as opposed to intermittent ventilation. Chernick (1973) discussed the difficulties in assessing the different techniques that were being used to treat respiratory disease in the newborn, the different studies that were being reported, and the rapid changes that were overtaking the field of newborn medicine. "It is noteworthy that all of the published reports … to date have been noncontrolled studies. Proponents of these approaches to therapy were too much impressed with their results to attempt a controlled trial." He thought that was okay. "One or two controlled studies of the use of distending pressure in severe hyaline membrane disease, although daring, are welcome; many more would be foolish. Since this method of therapy has been clearly proved to increase arterial pO_2, the potential risk of *not*

treating infants is too great to be denied." These concerns represent the flip side of concerns about which patients are eligible for enrollment in a trial. They suggest how difficult it is to continue to study a therapy that has shown promising results in initial trials. Instead, these early trial results often shape practice and make further, definitive studies impossible to carry out.

The development of total parenteral nutrition (TPN)

The development of TPN differed from that of mechanical ventilation in a number of ways. First, mechanical ventilation had been used successfully in other clinical circumstances before it was applied to premature babies. TPN, by contrast, had never been successfully used in older patients. Many doctors thought that it would be impossible to provide complete nutrition for any patient intravenously. Dudrick (2003), one of the pioneers of TPN, wrote, "The prevailing dogma among clinicians in the 1960s was that feeding a patient entirely by vein was impossible. Even if it were possible, it would be impractical; even if it were practical, it would be unaffordable. Indeed, TPN was considered a 'Gordian Knot' or a 'Holy Grail' pursuit by most physicians and surgeons."

Second, TPN was developed primarily by surgeons rather than by pediatricians. Many of the earliest reports were in surgical journals. The goal of the treatment was initially to treat babies with complications of surgery, particularly the surgery that led to the "short-gut" syndrome. While this should not have influenced the rigor of the evaluation, it did lead to more skepticism from neonatologists than it might have had the pioneering work been done by one of their own.

Third, although initially created for the rare situation of short-gut syndrome, TPN would eventually be used as a preventative and supportive treatment for all premature babies. Ventilation, by contrast, was used only for a specific indication – respiratory failure. For such patients, death is imminent and treatment is lifesaving. Nutritional support, by contrast, is something that can lead to improvements in survival rates but not in so dramatic a way. Each of these differences would be important in the way that TPN developed.

Most of the research that led to the successful clinical use of TPN took place at the University of Pennsylvania. Researchers there developed the infusates and the techniques of TPN in laboratory experiments using dogs. Once these animal studies showed that the technology was feasible, they considered trying it in humans. One of the first human patients to be given TPN was a newborn baby who had a near-total bowel atresia. Dudrick (2003) describes the case as follows:

> After massive intestinal resection, her duodenum had been anastomosed to the terminal 3 cm of ileum; her weight had declined from 2.5 kg at birth to 1.8 kg at 19 days of age; she appeared catabolic, hypometabolic, and moribund, and it was obvious that she was dying of starvation. After extensive consideration of the medical, moral, and ethical aspects of her problems, an *ad hoc* diverse committee of lay and professional people discussed, pondered, and debated every conceivable aspect of the proposed monumental and unprecedented experimental undertaking and were in accord that the risks of attempting to provide TPN by means of a central venous catheter in this infant were justifiable as the only reasonable option to save her life.

This description of the process contains many of the same fundamental features as the descriptions of the early trials of mechanical ventilation – that is, the clinical assessment that the patient was dying, a risk–benefit assessment that TPN was as likely to help as to harm, cognizance of the ethical as well as the clinical issues, and, ultimately, a decision to venture into unknown clinical territory.

The infant almost immediately began to gain weight and to emerge from her moribund state, leading the investigators to conclude that the TPN treatment was successful. Although the baby was never able to eat by mouth, she was fed by vein for 22 months before she died.

The success with this infant encouraged further clinical, uncontrolled trials. A 1969 paper reported the results of TPN for 18 babies with congenital anomalies of the gastrointestinal tract (Wilmore et al., 1969). TPN was given for "7–400 days." The paper describes three of the infants in detail. All have good outcomes – two infants were described as having been discharged from the hospital, the third was reported to be gaining weight. They conclude that "few complications occurred in the use of total parenteral nutrition."

These results in full-term neonates suffering from surgical complications were of enormous interest to neonatologists whose techniques of mechanical ventilation were now making it possible to keep tiny premature babies alive. Often, the babies were too small to take enteral nutrition. TPN saved the lives of these babies. By 1975, Winters, one of the pioneers of TPN, would report that,

> At present, there are clear definitions of indications and expectations of results for this method of therapy in two well-defined

groups of patients – i.e., selected surgical neonates and infants with chronic intractable diarrhea. In addition, we have suggestive evidence of another potentially valuable application in the nutritional management of very low birth weight infants. However, in this group, a controlled study will be necessary before the role of total parenteral nutrition (TPN) in neonatal care of such infants can be determined precisely. (Winters, 1975)

In spite of Winters' exhortation, TPN, like mechanical ventilation, diffused into clinical practice largely without any formal randomized trials. Instead, innovation continued and papers described interesting cases or the practices of particular NICUs and the good and bad outcomes they observed. There was widespread practice variation. At some centers, innovations were carefully studied. At other centers, no such studies were carried out. Clearly, innovation without careful study has been the norm in much of pediatrics.

Surprisingly, there are also situations in which careful studies are done that ought to change practice, but they do not lead to the innovations that should follow. Two examples of this are the introduction of antenatal steroids to reduce the severity of lung disease in premature babies, and the use of maternal screening and treatment for group B streptococcal infections.

Antenatal steroids and screening for group B streptococcus

In 1972, Liggins and Howie (1972) conducted a prospective, randomized clinical trial of glucocorticoid treatment for pregnant women. Early neonatal mortality was 3.2% in the mothers who were treated and 15% in the controls ($p = 0.01$). Respiratory distress syndrome occurred in 9% of the babies whose mothers were treated, compared with 26% of controls. They advocated further study of "antenatal corticosteroids" to prevent the complications of respiratory distress syndrome. After this classic study, over a dozen similar studies showed dramatic improvements in outcomes (NIH Consensus Development Panel, 1995). Surprisingly, these studies did not lead to rapid or widespread changes in obstetric practice. In 1985, over a decade later, only 8% of women in preterm labor received such treatment (Meadow et al., 2003). It wasn't until nearly 20 years after Liggins and Howie's study, and after a 1994 National Institutes of Health consensus conference recommended antenatal steroids, that practice began to change. Following that conference, change came rapidly. By 1995, 55% of women in preterm labor were given steroids. By 2000, nearly 30 years after the first scientific studies, that number had finally risen to 75% (Meadow et al., 2003).

The story of the development of protocols to prevent neonatal infections with group B streptococcus (GBS) has some similarities to the story of antenatal steroids. In pregnant women, GBS often causes asymptomatic bacteriuria. It can also cause urinary tract infection or infections of the uterus or amniotic fluid. After labor and delivery, it can cause endometritis and wound infections (Baker & Edwards, 1995). Mothers who carry the bacteria may be completely asymptomatic but can transmit the infection to their newborn babies. In the newborn, GBS can cause severe pneumonia, sepsis, and meningitis. The Centers for Disease Control and Prevention (2007) estimated that GBS caused 7600 cases of sepsis and 310 infant deaths in 1990.

Yow and colleagues (1979) showed that perinatal transmission of GBS could be dramatically reduced by giving ampicillin to mothers who were colonized with GBS. A number of studies over the next decade showed similar results (Allardice et al., 1982; Boyer & Gotoff, 1986). Some doctors and hospitals implemented protocols for screening and treatment of pregnant women. They saw and reported dramatic decreases in the incidence of invasive GBS disease in neonates (Velaphi et al., 2003). Nevertheless, most physicians were quite slow to adopt universal screening protocols (Jafari et al., 1995). It wasn't until 2002 that the American College of Obstetrics and Gynecology endorsed universal screening for GBS. This partial adoption of GBS screening led to a dramatic decline in neonatal deaths from sepsis. In a national study, death rates were cut nearly in half, from 24.9/100 000 live births from 1985 through 1991 to 15.6 from 1995 through 1998 (Lukacs et al., 2004). The CDC reported that the overall incidence of GBS fell another 33% between 2000 and 2005 (Centers for Disease Control and Prevention, 2007).

The slow adoption of antenatal steroids or GBS screening into routine clinical practice contrasts with the far more rapid adoption of supplemental oxygen, mechanical ventilation, or TPN. One can hypothesize about the reasons for these differences. One reason might be that treatment with ventilation or oxygen led to immediate, easily perceivable improvements whereas the effects of steroids or screening were more subtle. Another might be that both steroids and screening required cooperation of obstetricians for a treatment that ultimately was for the benefit of the baby, not the pregnant woman. Whatever the explanation, it

was clearly not because of the lack of high-quality, prospective, randomized clinical trials.

Debates continue: hypothermia for hypoxic brain injury

The dynamic illustrated by these examples continues in more current controversies, such as the debate about the efficacy of hypothermia for hypoxic brain injury.

In 2005, three studies of hypothermia for the treatment of hypoxic brain injury in neonates were published in high-impact, peer-reviewed journals (Eicher et al., 2005; Gluckman et al., 2005; Shankaran et al., 2005). All showed that babies who received hypothermia had better outcomes (lower rates of a combined variable of "death or disability") than control babies. This led to controversy about whether or not this evidence was sufficient for this therapy to be considered standard care, or whether further study was needed. The American Academy of Pediatrics Committee on the Fetus and Newborn noted, "Therapeutic hypothermia is a promising therapy that should be considered investigational until the short-term safety and efficacy have been confirmed in the additional human trials underway. Long-term safety and efficacy remain to be defined" (Blackmon et al., 2006). Around that time, Papile (2005) wrote of hypothermia, "This treatment is best considered an experimental technique for which informed parental consent should be obtained. Widespread application of brain cooling in the care of neonates with hypoxic–ischemic encephalopathy would be premature." An NICHD workshop concluded that although, "… hypothermia appears to be a potentially promising therapy for HIE, long-term efficacy and safety are yet to be established" (Higgins et al., 2006).

By 2007, expert opinion had begun to shift. A meta-analysis showed that hypothermia improved outcomes for many asphyxiated babies (Shah et al., 2007). As a result, some neonatologists argued that the benefits of hypothermia were great enough, the risks small enough, and the rigor of the studies high enough so that hypothermia should now be considered the standard of care for babies who have suffered asphyxia. The corollary claim would be that further randomized trials, in which some babies were randomized to normothermia, would be unethical. For example, Wilkinson and colleagues (2007) noted, "We believe that the strength of the existing evidence warrants careful consideration of whether the risks to participants involved in continuing trials are justified." Gunn and colleagues (2008) observed that, "robust evidence for benefit from current meta-analyses, the remarkable safety profile, the strong foundation in basic science, and supporting evidence from related disease states such as encephalopathy after cardiac arrest" all dictate that practicing physicians, in consultation with patients and families, should use hypothermia as a treatment for neonatal encephalopathy.

Still, the debate continued. Schulzke and colleagues (2007) cautiously noted that, "Therapeutic hypothermia seems to have a beneficial effect on the outcome of term neonates with moderate to severe hypoxic ischemic encephalopathy. Despite the methodological differences between trials, wide confidence intervals, and the lack of follow-up data beyond the second year of life, the consistency of the results is encouraging. Further research is necessary to minimize the uncertainty regarding efficacy and safety of any specific technique of cooling for any specific population." Kirpalani and colleagues (2007) echoed these sentiments, noting that while "exciting potential exists in hypothermia for cooling," serious questions remain. They wrote, "We should demand strong evidence of robust, consistent effects in highly valid studies that have enrolled adequate numbers of patients before mandating a new therapy for management of all relevant patients. The evidence for cooling fails to meet this standard."

Conclusions

Evaluation of innovative therapies is a messy business, particularly in pediatrics, for a few reasons. First, regulations governing clinical research appropriately treat infants and children as a vulnerable population. These regulations require that studies not be done in children or babies if they can be done, instead, in consenting adults. That makes sense for certain clinical studies. It does not, however, make much sense for diseases of the newborn for which clinical trials in adults are inapplicable.

A second reason why the evaluation of innovation is particularly difficult in pediatrics is that clinical trials in children require a long follow-up in order to look for rare and – by definition – unknown long-term side effects. The story of diethylstilbestrol (DES) is an example of this problem. The risks of DES did not show up for 20 years, and then they occurred in the offspring of the women who were treated. Most clinical trials look for short-term risks and benefits.

Finally, clinical research is difficult in pediatrics because of the unique complexities of parental consent. Many innovative therapies must be tested in children who are critically ill. Parents whose children may die face severe emotional stress and are not in the best position to give informed consent (Hulst et al., 2005). In such cases, it is often possible to get parents to sign a consent form, but it is likely that they don't really understand what their consent means (Eder et al., 2007).

These complex considerations often lead to a tense stalemate in pediatrics between those who quite rationally and persuasively argue against the widespread adoption of particular treatments on the basis of promising preliminary data and those who argue against continued clinical research on therapies whose promise seems to create an ethical imperative for their use based upon reasonable inference from existing data.

The recurrence of such dilemmas suggests that our categories for thinking about the evolution of new pediatric therapies may be wrong. Treatments are seldom either straightforwardly "experimental" or unambiguously "standard." All therapies are in constant evolution. Thus, ongoing evaluation of all therapies is essential, and the use of these same therapies in routine day-to-day care is also essential.

An ideal system of understanding innovation in pediatrics (or the many other areas of medicine where new approaches are being tried) would acknowledge that everything is somewhat "experimental." There is no "standard" therapy anymore. Every promising innovation changes the relative risks and benefits of every existing innovation. Decisions about treatment should always be based upon the best available evidence, but the only way to generate evidence is through a commitment to gather high-quality data. That is to say that we need to do ongoing evaluation of every clinical intervention. Health care is most effective when data about the efficacy of therapy are being constantly gathered and constantly evaluated. That is the only way to improve our clinical care and make the best possible decision for each patient.

References

Allardice, J.G., Baskett, T.F., Seshia, M.M., Bowman, N., & Malazdrewicz, R. (1982). Perinatal group B streptococcal colonization and infection. *American Journal of Obstetrics and Gynecology*, **142**(6 Pt 1), 617–620.

Askie, L.M., Henderson-Smart, D.J., Irwig, L., & Simpson, J.M. (2003). Oxygen-saturation targets and outcomes in extremely preterm infants. *New England Journal of Medicine*, **349**, 959–967.

Baker, C.J. & Edwards, M.S. (1995). Group B streptococcal infections. In *Infectious Diseases of the Fetus and Newborn Infant*, 4th edn, ed. J. Remington & J.O. Klein. Philadelphia, PA: WB Saunders Co., 980–1054.

Blackmon, L.R., Stark, A.R., & the Committee on Fetus and Newborn, American Academy of Pediatrics (2006). Hypothermia: a neuroprotective therapy for neonatal hypoxic-ischemic encephalopathy. *Pediatrics*, **117**, 942–948.

Bolton, D.P.G. & Cross, K.W. (1974). Further observations on the cost of preventing retrolental fibroplasia. *Lancet*, **1**, 445–448.

Boyer, K.M. & Gotoff, S.P. (1986). Prevention of early-onset neonatal group B streptococcal disease with selective intrapartum chemoprophylaxis. *New England Journal of Medicine*, **314**, 1665–1669.

Centers for Disease Control and Prevention (CDC) (2007). Perinatal group B streptococcal disease after universal screening recommendations – United States, 2003–2005. *MMWR*, **56**, 701–705.

Chernick, V. (1973). Continuous distending pressure in hyaline membrane disease: of devices, disadvantages, and a daring study. *Pediatrics*, **52**, 114–115.

Crosse, V.M. (1951). The problem of retrolental fibroplasia in the City of Birmingham. *Transactions of the Ophthalmological Societies of the United Kingdom*, **71**, 609–612.

Delivoria-Papadopoulos, M., Levison, H., & Swyer, P.R. (1965). Intermittent positive pressure respiration as a treatment in severe respiratory distress syndrome. *Archives of Disease in Childhood*, **40**, 474–479.

Dudrick, S.J. (2003). Early developments and clinical applications of total parenteral nutrition. *Journal of Parenteral and Enteral Nutrition*, **27**, 291–299.

Dunham, E.C., Dickinson, H.C., Gowens, G.J., & Witters, J. (1940). Incubators for premature infants. *American Journal of Public Health*, **30**, 1415–1421.

Eder, M.L., Yamokoski, A.D., Wittmann, P.W., & Kodish, E.D. (2007). Improving informed consent: suggestions from parents of children with leukemia. *Pediatrics*, **119**, e849–e859.

Eicher, D.J., Wagner, C.L., Katikaneni, L.P., et al. (2005). Moderate hypothermia in neonatal encephalopathy: efficacy outcomes. *Pediatric Neurology*, **32**, 11–17.

Gluckman, P.D., Wyatt, J.S., Azzopardi, D., et al. (2005). Selective head cooling with mild systemic hypothermia after neonatal encephalopathy: multicentre randomised trial. *Lancet*, **365**, 663–670.

Gunn, A.J., Hoehn, T., Hansmann, G., et al. (2008). Hypothermia: an evolving treatment for neonatal hypoxic ischemic encephalopathy. *Pediatrics*, **121**, 648–649.

Higgins, R.D., Raju, T.N., Perlman, J., et al. (2006). Hypothermia and perinatal asphyxia: executive summary of the National Institute of Child Health and Human Development workshop. *Journal of Pediatrics*, **148**, 170–175.

Hulst, J.M., Peters, J.W., van den Bos, A., et al. (2005). Illness severity and parental permission for clinical research in a pediatric ICU population. *Intensive Care Medicine*, **3**, 880–884.

Jafari, H.S., Schuchat, A., Hilsdon, R., et al. (1995). Barriers to prevention of perinatal group B streptococcal disease. *Pediatric Infectious Disease Journal*, **14**, 662–667.

Kinsey, V.E. (1955). Etiology of retrolental fibroplasia and preliminary report of the Cooperative Study of Retrolental Fibroplasia. *Transactions of the American Academy of Ophthalmology and Otolaryngology*, **59**, 15–24.

Kirpalani, H., Barks, J., Thorlund, K., & Guyatt, G. (2007). Cooling for neonatal hypoxic ischemic encephalopathy: do we have the answer? *Pediatrics*, **120**(5), 1126–1130.

Lantos, J.D. & Frader, J. (1990). Extracorporeal membrane oxygenation and the ethics of clinical research in pediatrics. *New England Journal of Medicine*, **323**, 409–413.

Liggins, G.C. & Howie, R.N. (1972). A controlled trial of antepartum glucocorticoid treatment for prevention of the respiratory distress syndrome in premature infants. *Pediatrics*, **50**, 515–525.

Lukacs, S.L., Schoendorf, K.C., & Schuchat, A. (2004). Trends in sepsis-related neonatal mortality in the United States, 1985–1998. *Pediatric Infectious Disease Journal*, **23**, 599–603.

Meadow, W.L., Bell, A., & Sunstein, C.R. (2003). Statistics, not memories: what was the standard of care for administering antenatal steroids to women in preterm labor between 1985 and 2000? *Obstetrics and Gynecology*, **102**, 356–362.

NIH Consensus Development Panel on the Effect of Corticosteroids for Fetal Maturation on Perinatal Outcomes (1995). Effect of corticosteroids for fetal maturation on perinatal outcomes. *JAMA*, **273**(5), 413–418.

Papile, L.A. (2005). Systemic hypothermia – a "cool" therapy for neonatal hypoxic-ischemic encephalopathy. *New England Journal of Medicine*, **353**, 1619–1620.

Patz, A., Hoeck, L.E., & De La Cruz, E. (1952). Studies on the effect of high oxygen administration in retrolental fibroplasia: nursery observations. *American Journal of Ophthalmology*, **35**, 1248–1253.

Schulzke, S.M., Rao, S., & Patole, S.K. (2007). A systematic review of cooling for neuroprotection in neonates with hypoxic ischemic encephalopathy: are we there yet? *BMC Pediatrics*, **7**, 30.

Shah, P.S., Ohlsson, A., & Perlman, M. (2007). Hypothermia to treat neonatal hypoxic ischemic encephalopathy:

systematic review. *Archives of Pediatrics and Adolescent Medicine*, **161**, 951–958.

Shankaran, S., Laptook, A.R., Ehrenkranz, R.A., et al. (2005). Whole-body hypothermia for neonates with hypoxic-ischemic encephalopathy. *New England Journal of Medicine*, **353**, 1574–1584.

Silverman, W.A. (2004). A cautionary tale about supplemental oxygen: the albatross of neonatal medicine. *Pediatrics*, **113**, 394–396.

SUPPORT Study Group of the Eunice Kennedy Shriver NICHD Neonatal Research Network (2010). Target ranges of oxygen saturation in extremely preterm infants. *New England Journal of Medicine*, **362**, 1959–1969.

Tin, W. (2002). Oxygen therapy: 50 years of uncertainty. *Pediatrics*, **110**, 615–616.

Velaphi, S., Siegel, J.D., Wendel, G.D. Jr., et al. (2003). Early-onset group B streptococcal infection after a combined maternal and neonatal group B streptococcal chemoprophylaxis strategy. *Pediatrics*, **111**, 541–547.

Wilkinson, D.J., Casalaz, D., Watkins, A., Andersen, C.C., & Duke, T. (2007). Hypothermia: a neuroprotective therapy for neonatal hypoxic-ischemic encephalopathy. *Pediatrics*, **119**, 422–423.

Wilmore, D.W., Groff D.B., Bishop H.C., & Dudrick, S.J. (1969). Total parenteral nutrition in infants with catastrophic gastrointestinal anomalies. *Journal of Pediatric Surgery*, **4**, 181–189.

Wilson, J.L., Long, S.B., & Howard, P.J. (1942). Respiration of premature infants; response to variations of oxygen and to increased carbon dioxide in inspired air. *American Journal of Diseases of Children*, **63**, 1080–1085.

Winters, R.W. (1975). Total parenteral nutrition in pediatrics: the Borden award address. *Pediatrics*, **56**(1), 17–23.

Yow, M.D., Mason, E.O., Leeds, L.J., et al. (1979). Ampicillin prevents intrapartum transmission of group B streptococcus. *JAMA*, **241**, 1245–1247.

33

Human subjects research involving children

Valarie Blake and Eric Kodish

If we knew what it was we were doing, it would not be called research, would it? (Albert Einstein)

Introduction

Pediatric research presents a number of different ethical challenges when compared with the clinical practice of pediatrics. Clinical practice is focused on caring for the individual patient using proven methods of diagnosis and treatment, while research embarks on the journey to find new treatments for future patients. This core difference in purpose is the ethical foundation for distinguishing between research and clinical practice (Litton & Miller, 2010). Most of the literature in research ethics uses a particular clinical trial or research dilemma as a starting point. We have opted to present a case study that arises in the clinical context to help highlight the distinctions between what is clinical practice and what is research. We contend that clinical practice and research should be treated differently from an ethics perspective, particularly when the questions involve children.

Case narrative

Colin, a 16-year-old boy, presents at the local emergency room with vomiting, high fever, and possible internal bleeding. Colin has a complex medical history and is well known to the hospital service. He was born in a difficult quintuplet birth and suffered a perinatal anoxic event, which has left him severely developmentally delayed. Colin smiles and makes eye contact and he communicates through simple language and gestures. Physicians estimate his level of understanding and cognitive abilities to be at the level of a 10-year-old. Physicians project that Colin could continue to benefit from participation in a vigorous program of therapy and rehabilitation, though progress would be slow.

At the emergency room, Colin's mother tells the nurse that Colin just got back from Mexico. Further questioning reveals that Colin has received unregulated stem cell infusions while in Mexico over the weekend, and that he has received these infusions two other times in the past year as well. Colin's mother is a health teacher at an area high school and has a fairly sophisticated understanding of medicine. She explains that the stem cells are derived from a donor and are injected via a femoral catheter that is threaded up to the circle of Willis in Colin's brain. They are intended to promote neural growth and repair damage done by the anoxic event, thus improving Colin's symptoms of developmental delay. While Colin's mother agrees that there is no scientific evidence yet to support these procedures in patients like her son, she believes that she has seen progress in Colin since the first infusion and she feels that modern medicine provides no other options to advance the health and interests of her child. She is thinking about discontinuing Colin's regularly scheduled rehabilitation sessions, so as to better focus on the stem cell infusions.

Overview of ethical issues

Stem cells are a promising new tool in the battle to fight disease. Their arrival has resulted in "high hope for cures ... on the part of individuals and families ... advocacy groups, stem cell research supporters, and scientists" (McCormick & Huso, 2010). However, while stem cells may have significant treatment potential in the future, they are in their infancy with respect to what we know and understand about them. Like any other treatment, significant research will be necessary to safely discover and harness the potential healing powers of stem cell therapies. However, given the hype around stem cells, "the public may not quite appreciate

Clinical Ethics in Pediatrics: A Case-Based Textbook, ed. Douglas S. Diekema, Mark R. Mercurio and Mary B. Adam. Published by Cambridge University Press. © Cambridge University Press 2011.

the many years of preclinical and clinical research that are required to establish … [these] therapies"(Hyun, 2010). Some patients and families have already begun pursuing unregulated stem cell treatments, often in foreign countries. The instance of unregulated stem cell therapy raised in this case demonstrates how robust research ethics can guide us in the search for finding new cures.

In Colin's case, there is no scientifically founded reason to believe that the stem cell infusions will benefit Colin and, moreover, these infusions could in fact harm Colin. First, because the effects of these stem cells have not yet been studied in humans, we do not know whether they will cause some physiological harm to Colin. Also because the treatment is unregulated, we do not know whether these stem cells are being produced and retrieved in a safe way, free of blood-borne illness. Additionally, Colin may be indirectly harmed by these therapies if his mother stops taking him to a proven treatment (like rehabilitation) in favor of an unproven and possibly unsuccessful treatment like the stem cell infusions. Because these infusions are unfounded and may even be harmful, providing them as part of clinical care is ethically problematic.

However, these treatments may be given in research if a number of ethical criteria are met. As Einstein's quote suggests, the very definition of research is that we are dealing with the unknown. Research ethics is designed to balance the interests of developing innovative new therapies against protecting research participants from potentially harmful and unproven treatments. Though stem cell infusions are not currently shown to benefit patients like Colin, providing these treatments in a way that satisfies benchmarks of ethical research may ensure that future children like Colin have better treatments available to them. To satisfy ethical standards of research and resolve some of the safety and ethics issues discussed above, a number of requirements must be met. Among these are ensuring that the data sought from the study are generalizable and useful, ensuring proper balance of risks and harms against benefits raised by research, and ensuring that participants are knowingly and voluntarily participating in the research given the possible lack of benefit to them.

Generalizable and useful data

Research is intended to "develop generalizable knowledge to improve health and/or increase understanding of human biology" (Emanuel et al., 2000). Ethical research should be both scientifically valid (thus generating reliable data) and of value (thus being some use in society) in order to serve its purpose (Freedman, 1987a). Only then can it "yield fruitful results for the good of society, unprocurable by other methods or means of study, and not random and unnecessary in nature" (Nuremberg Code, 1947). To be scientifically valid, the study must be designed statistically and scientifically in a manner that ensures that the data produced will actually tell us something about the efficacy or lack thereof of the given treatment that can be generalized across a wider population and used to tailor clinical practice. Proper scientific design also ensures that as few people as necessary are exposed to the harms of unproven treatments, while also ensuring that enough people are enrolled to safely project answers about the nature of that treatment in overcoming illness. Additionally, a properly designed study will only subject research participants to treatments that have strong scientific or theoretical preliminary support for why the treatment may be potentially efficacious in treating disease.

To be ethical, the study must also provide scientific value by combating relevant problems. To justify exposing participants to harm, the study should be practically oriented to target a real issue in society. Peer review is also an important aspect of ethical research. The International Society for Stem Cell Research (ISSCR) (2008) has highlighted this point: "Given the novelty and unpredictability of early stem cell-based clinical research, it is of utmost importance that the peer review process be conducted with the highest possible rigor and integrity." Lastly, it is important to note that ethical research must be recorded. Because research purports to gather new knowledge about a particular issue, it must be possible to catalogue the experiences of the researcher in a way which can be examined for future use; thus recording must be both accurate and truthful.

In Colin's case, these research ethics standards could help to justify exposing Colin to the potential risks of unproven treatments. Ultimately, if the stem cell infusions had been initiated in a properly designed study, the findings would be subject to peer review prior to publication. If the data showed the treatment to be effective and safe as judged by the expert scientific community, Colin's risks would have been justified by ensuring that possibly both Colin as well as others like him would receive a better treatment for their condition. If by contrast the treatment was shown to be overly toxic, dangerous, or ineffective, at least no other persons would need to be exposed to the direct or indirect harms of the infusions. In this way, children as a class benefit from the fruits of evidence-based pediatrics.

Balancing risk and benefit

Ethical research also requires a favorable risk/benefit ratio. While not all research is likely to garner benefit for the individual, it must be designed to at least provide knowledge that will benefit society. Ethical research requires the following: that the potential risk to the individual research participant is minimized, that potential benefit to the individual is enhanced, and that potential benefits to both the individual and society outweigh or be proportionate to the risks (Emanuel et al., 2000). Clinical equipoise is present where there is genuine uncertainty in the field of medicine, and not just in the mind of the individual investigator, about a preferred treatment. Once clinical equipoise is disturbed and a treatment is preferred, then the preferred treatment must be provided (Freedman, 1987b).

Balancing risk against benefit is particularly important in the pediatric context. In the past, children have been the "unwitting and unwilling subjects of medical experiments" and have suffered much harm at the hands of research. The root cause of past abuse and exploitation of children in medical research may have been a result of their status in society, their limited ability to give consent, and/or other factors (Lederer, 2003). However, excluding children from research is not a reasonable option because it would "cripple society's ability to ensure medical interventions are safe and effective for children" (Wendler & Varma, 2006). Thus the dangers of children participating in research must be weighed against the interests of developing proper clinical treatments for children. This involves ensuring that children's risk in research is minimized, that societal interests not outweigh the interest of the individual child, and permitting only those trials which use treatments that are at least as good risk/benefit-wise as other established treatments. Subpart D of the Code of Federal Regulations at 45 CFR 46 is intended to provide children with "additional protections" beyond those provided in the regulations as they apply to competent adults (Department of Health and Human Services, 1991). This approach executes its function by limiting the types of research which Institutional Review Boards (IRBs), the committees that review research protocols to protect research participants, may approve. Most

importantly, the risks of research are limited and linked to potential benefit to the child-subject in a manner that is intentionally and appropriately restrictive compared with competent adults (Kodish, 2005).

In Colin's case, the stem cell infusions exposed him to a number of potential harms without sufficient evidence for prospect of direct benefit to him. Moreover, because the infusions were administered outside a properly designed and IRB-approved research protocol, potential benefit to other children is highly unlikely. If conducted as research, exposing Colin to some level of risk may be justified to ensure that society reaps the benefit of new treatments for a previously incurable disorder. These benefits, however, must be balanced against any risks to Colin himself and, also, must be balanced against the risks and benefits he could achieve through already established treatments (like rehabilitation).

Properly informing research participants

Lastly, because research is designed to discover new treatments and benefit future patients, properly informing participants about the goals of research and possible risks and benefits is imperative (Kodish, 2003). Informed consent and voluntariness are important requirements for ethical research because they respect the individual's values in regard to the research, while ensuring they only participate where they wish to (Vanderpool, 1996). This is particularly crucial in the instance of children because of their limited decision-making capacity (Ungar et al., 2008). Because research is targeted not at improving the health of that given child but of future children, parental permission is required for a child to participate in research and in most instances the researcher must also seek the assent of the child to solicit his or her "affirmative agreement" to participate in the research (Department of Health and Human Services, 1991; Unguru et al., 2006). Assent demonstrates an appreciation for the dignity and respect of the child and also helps them to develop the ability to make autonomous decisions in the future (Diekema, 2003).

The therapeutic misconception is also a concern that must be addressed in ethical research. In therapeutic misconception, the research participant, or his or her parent/guardian does not understand the difference between the goals of research and the goals of clinical care. Thus it is important for researchers to explain to subjects the different obligations, goals, and responsibilities of the investigator as compared with the clinician to better ensure that parents and participants can appropriately weigh the risks and benefits of participating in research (Henderson et al., 2006).

In Colin's case, his mother consented to the treatment believing that it would ameliorate Colin's symptoms and thus serve his best interests. If the infusions had been proposed under a research protocol, Colin's mother would have more likely been informed that the treatment was yet unproven and that Colin might not see any clinical benefit. In this scenario, an IRB would have reviewed the risks, benefits, and alternatives prior to approval and study initiation. Colin's mother could then choose whether she wished to accept a certain level of individual risk in exchange for potential benefit to Colin and the societal benefit of gathering new knowledge. Furthermore, Colin's mother would have fully understood that the purpose of the infusions would be to gain knowledge and not necessarily to benefit her son, thus helping to resolve concerns of therapeutic misconception. In this particular case, Colin could possibly participate in making these decisions through assent. At an approximately 4th grade level, Colin could have been informed about the study and its potential benefits and risks at a developmentally appropriate level, demonstrating respect for him. He might also, if appropriate, be invited to participate in decision-making at an age-appropriate level.

Conclusion

Research ethics requires a careful balance between promoting innovation in medicine and science while also protecting the persons who are subjected to these new and unproven innovations. Colin's case highlights both of these points. Colin's anoxic encephalopathy is a highly debilitating condition for which modern medicine currently has no magic bullet. However, this does not justify exposing Colin to risks which can be minimized and which could be conducted in a manner that might benefit him directly and/or generate data that might benefit persons with his condition in the future. Research ethics and regulation help to address this balance. While studies of innovative therapies are crucial in developing our understanding of disease and contributing to progress in treatment, the studies must be designed to collect data which are generalizable and

which will be of benefit to society. Additionally, ethical research requires that we minimize harms to the individual participant, while maximizing benefit to both individual and society. Colin and his parent(s) must also be willing to assume the risks of a study that might not benefit him in the way that a proven treatment would. An investigator with ethical integrity must make sure that Colin and his mother understand that the stem cell infusions he is receiving are not treatment; they are experimental and unproven. Research ethics clarifies these complex issues. The fiduciary obligation of the pediatrician to his/her patient in clinical practice is relatively simple when compared with the competing obligations that arise in the ethics of pediatric research. Robust pediatric research ethics and regulation can help safeguard individual children and optimize the health of future children, balancing the needs of progress and protection.

References

Department of Health and Human Services (1991). Subpart D: Additional protections for children involved as research subjects. 45 CFR 46.401–45CFR 46.409.

Diekema, D. (2003). Taking children seriously: what's so important about assent? *American Journal of Bioethics*, **3**, 25–26.

Emanuel, E., Wendler, D., & Grady, C. (2000). What makes clinical research ethical? *JAMA*, **283**, 2701–2711.

Freedman, B. (1987a). Scientific value and validity as ethical requirements for research: a proposed explication. *IRB*, **9**, 7–10.

Freedman, B. (1987b). Equipoise and the ethics of clinical research. *New England Journal of Medicine*, **317**, 141–145.

Henderson, G.E., Easter M.M., Zimmer, C., et al. (2006). Therapeutic misconception in early phase gene transfer trials. *Social Science and Medicine*, **62**, 239–253.

Hyun, I. (2010). The bioethics of stem cell research and therapy. *Journal of Clinical Investigation*, **120**, 71–75.

International Society for Stem Cell Research (ISSCR) Task Force for the Clinical Translation of Stem Cells (2008). Guidelines for the Clinical Translation of Stem Cells. www.isscr.org/clinical_trans/pdfs/ ISSCRGLClinicalTrans.pdf (last accessed September 30, 2010).

Kodish, E. (2003). Informed consent for pediatric research: is it really possible? *Journal of Pediatrics*, **142**, 89–90.

Kodish, E. (2005). *Ethics and Research with Children: A Case-Based Approach*. New York: Oxford University Press, chapter 1.

Lederer, S. (2003). Children as guinea pigs: historical perspectives. *Accountability in Research: Policies & Quality Assurance*, **10**, 1–16.

Litton, P. & Miller, F.G. (2010). What physician-investigators owe patients who participate in research. *Journal of the American Medical Association*, **304**, 1491–1492.

McCormick, J. & Huso, H. (2010). Stem cells and ethics: current issues. *Journal of Cardiovascular Translational Research*, **3**, 122–127.

Nuremberg Code (1947). http://ohsr.od.nih.gov/guidelines/nuremberg.html (last accessed October 1, 2010).

Ungar, D., Joffe, S., & Kodish, E. (2006). Children are not small adults: documentation of assent for research involving children. *Journal of Pediatrics*, **149**, S31–S33.

Unguru, Y., Coppes, M.J., & Kamani, N. (2008). Rethinking pediatric assent: from requirement to ideal. *Pediatric Clinics of North America*, **55**, 211–222.

Vanderpool, H.Y. (1996). *The Ethics of Research Involving Human Subjects*. Frederick, MD: University Publishing Group, 45–58.

Wendler, D. & Varma, S. (2006). Minimal risk in pediatric research. *Journal of Pediatrics*, **149**, 855–861.

Resource allocation and triage in disasters and pandemics

Jeffrey P. Burns and Christine Mitchell

Case narrative

A children's hospital has formed a disaster planning committee to develop and implement a formal disaster policy. The committee's work proceeds uneventfully until deliberations begin on a framework for triage. The committee struggles to reach consensus on a framework for determining who should receive limited resources and how those resources should be allocated following a mass casualty incident. Should those with the highest risk of mortality receive intervention? How should their prognosis be determined? Who should make the allocation decisions; should it be someone other than the actual caregivers? Under what conditions will caregivers who participate in reallocation of resources face civil and criminal penalties? In particular, the committee becomes highly polarized when it begins discussions around the following hypothetical scenario.

A pandemic from influenza has caused severe shortages of mechanical ventilators and other life-sustaining treatments across the country. All of the intensive care unit (ICU) beds in the hospital are occupied by infants and children requiring mechanical ventilation, many of whom are critically ill from influenza. All non-emergency surgical cases have been canceled, and all step-down units and post-anesthesia recovery areas are being utilized. In addition, all of the hospitals in the region are experiencing the same shortages and therefore cannot provide any assistance. All but one of the hospital's ventilators are being used by patients who would die without them. Given these circumstances, which of the following three patients in the hospital's emergency department should be prioritized to receive the one available ventilator?

- A 5-year-old girl, previously healthy, with severe pneumonia.

- An 18-year-old boy with Duchenne muscular dystrophy, dependent on tracheostomy and mechanical ventilation for neuromuscular respiratory failure, wheelchair bound, and now with severe acute respiratory distress syndrome.
- A 5-month-old infant with Down syndrome (trisomy 21), now with sepsis and multi-organ failure.

Introduction

The term influenza emerged from the Latin word *influentia* because medieval doctors believed that the cyclical epidemics of flu were influenced by stars and planets revolving toward and away from the earth. While the real cause of influenza escaped medieval physicians, what they did correctly understand was that pandemics are a recurring threat to humanity. According to the World Health Organization, the world has experienced an average of three pandemics per century since the sixteenth century, occurring at intervals of 10–50 years (World Health Organization, 2007). Thus, the need to anticipate and plan a response to this potential threat to the health of the entire population remains a reality.

Yet, as recent events across the world tragically reveal, a pandemic is just one kind of a disaster, and children are among the most vulnerable victims of many mass casualty incidents. Accordingly, comprehensive planning must account for unique vulnerabilities of children – their inability to care for themselves or get themselves to sites for care in addition to particular infections, diseases, or accidents that may disproportionately affect the young. Moreover, public trust, or at minimum "acceptance," of official procedures following a mass casualty disaster will be essential to allocating limited resources most effectively (Altevogt et al., 2009). When triage decisions mean that some will

Clinical Ethics in Pediatrics: A Case-Based Textbook, ed. Douglas S. Diekema, Mark R. Mercurio and Mary B. Adam. Published by Cambridge University Press. © Cambridge University Press 2011.

receive limited life-saving treatment and others will be denied, what allocation process will be perceived as fair?

Ethical criteria for allocation of scarce resources

Sickest first

Many believe, and clinicians generally agree, that medical attention and treatment should be based on need such that the sickest get priority. This is sometimes called the "rule of rescue" or, by philosophers, "prioritarianism" – that is, favoring the worst-off by first treating those with the worst prospects if left untreated. This is the primary criterion used in emergency rooms (although in emergency rooms when the neediest are treated first the expectation is that others will also receive treatment later) and by the US United Network for Organ Sharing in choosing recipients for transplantation of scarce organs – not all who are listed will be transplanted; some will die. One criticism of the "sickest first" criterion is that they may be so sick that they are not able to benefit from treatment that might help a somewhat less desperately ill person. Thus the refinement of this criterion on battlefields, for example, involves a modified triage system that combines "need" with "ability to benefit" from treatment, selecting those who are sickest *and* who will most reliably survive by being treated first.

Saving the most

Historically, allocation decisions in public health have been driven by an implicit or explicit utilitarian rationale of accomplishing the "greatest good for the greatest number," typically translated into a maximizing strategy for saving the most lives (Winslow, 1982). Indeed, many recent proposals for allocating resources following a mass casualty incident have formulated this utilitarian principle by stating that triage should "maximize the number of people who survive to hospital discharge."

While saving more lives makes moral sense, it is not so obvious that we should save two older adults who might each live only another 10 or 20 years rather than saving a 5-year-old who might live to be 70. Should we save the most lives or the most life-years? Maximizing life-years would generally lead to saving the youngest first if they had a good prognosis for long life. By this

criterion, assuming equal chances of short-term survival, priority for life-saving treatment would go to a 5-year-old who is otherwise healthy over a 5-year-old with a limited life expectancy from severe co morbid conditions. While intuitively appealing, critics of this approach contend that in actual practice during a mass casualty – when the demand to make rapid decisions will be enormous, and when the flow of accurate information will be limited – making accurate assessments about prognoses and co-morbidities may be difficult. Moreover, preferentially allocating resources to the youngest seems unfair to older others who also have as-yet-unfulfilled lives and projects, leading us to question whether maximizing life-years is, by itself, the best way to formulate an ethical response to the allocation of scarce life-saving resources, in part because many older persons have responsibilities for others (including children) and a proven ability to make social contributions that children may or may not make in the future.

Social value criteria

Proponents of social value criteria argue that priority for receiving scarce health care resources should be determined by evaluation of a person's contributions to society. Such criteria were infamously applied in the early 1960s by the Seattle Dialysis Committee who decided that priority for the first generation of scarce dialysis treatment should be given to heads of families and professional workers over others. Critics of this approach argue that it is inherently subjective and ethically indefensible to calculate that one individual is intrinsically more worthy of saving than another, especially in a pluralistic society with a multiplicity of important social values where "social worth" criteria would lead to favoring conventional mainstream values (Alexander, 1962). Indeed, the public outcry over the Seattle committee's use of such criteria was so strong that Congress passed the first legislation guaranteeing access to life-saving renal dialysis for all, publicly funded by Medicare. Nevertheless, many note that certain individuals – physicians and nurses, for example – are unusually essential during mass health crises such as an influenza pandemic – and argue that they be saved first so they can save others.

Instrumental value criteria

Instrumental value, also referred to as "narrow social utility" or the "multiplier effect," has also been proposed as a framework for allocation decisions. Instrumental value refers to a person's ability to carry out a specific function that is essential to society (typically health care providers, law and public safety personnel, or sailors on a lifeboat after a shipwreck). Prioritizing them is not based on their greater inherent social worth but on their specific "multiplier" ability to enable more people to survive a disaster. An example of this ethical reasoning can be seen in recommendations from the US National Vaccine Advisory Committee. Their current policy on the allocation of vaccines and antiviral medications during a pandemic gives first priority to workers in vaccine manufacturing and health care providers. While this is more defensible than prioritizations based on general social worth criteria, it should be noted, as a possible matter of fact, that the recovery of anyone during a mass casualty event may be so long or unpredictable that we may not be able to accurately anticipate which persons with essential functions could return to their duties in time to meaningfully contribute to the multiplier effect (White et al., 2009). That, however, is more relevant to scenarios involving adults and vaccines than children and ventilators.

Life-cycle criteria

Under the life-cycle principle, also known as the "fair innings" argument and the "intergenerational equity" principle, the goal is to allocate health resources so that each person has an equal opportunity to live through the various phases of a normal life span, thereby favoring younger persons because they will have had the least opportunity to live a full life.

A refinement of the life-cycle criteria is the "investment refinement criteria," allocating limited life-saving treatment based on the societal "investment" in a person and not merely their age (Emanuel & Wertheimer, 2006). This criterion rejects a pure version of the life-cycle principle that would grant priority to 6-month-olds over 1-year-olds, for example, and instead advocates for gradations within a life span. Thus, early adolescents and young adults are prioritized over infants and younger children, on the basis of the extent already invested in a person's life *balanced* by the amount left to live.

Recent surveys reveal that most people believe younger patients should be prioritized over older ones in a mass casualty incident. Indeed, this was the spontaneously chosen principle of triage in the *Titanic* disaster recalled in the maxim, "women and children

first." Critics contend that these approaches discriminate against older persons, do not take into account the person's state at the time of allocation, and are based solely on outcomes rather than also considering process and resources (White et al., 2009). While length of life is important, so also is its quality as well as the social investment in it. And what if it were to take greater and longer use of scarce resources to save someone with a whole life ahead of him/her?

Conservation criteria

This criterion focuses on the amount of resources required, advocating that the likelihood of benefit using minimal resources should take precedence in order to maximize the efficient utilization of scarce medical supplies. By the principle of conservation, priority for scarce life-saving treatments would go to those who will benefit most from the fewest resources. In this case, we might think about allocating the ventilator on the basis of who is most likely to need it the shortest number of days.

Treating persons equally

Egalitarians, in contrast to utilitarians, argue that there should always be equal regard for individual persons and their lives. From this perspective, the conceptual foundation of the allocation of scarce resources should not be guided by seeking to benefit the greatest number at the expense of some, but that each person should be given the same *chance* to survive (Childress, 2003; Peterson, 2008). Proponents of this approach argue that our collective moral intuition – even in a pluralistic society – is formed by a sense of prior social agreement deeply rooted in the notion of equal treatment for all. Hence egalitarians advocate a lottery or queuing processes ("first come, first served") that embody the value of equal treatment for all, or at least equal opportunity to line up for treatment. Supporters of this position note that individuals from diverse backgrounds when forced by circumstances into a small community invariably resort to a lottery in order to distribute scarce resources. Critics, on the other hand, note the overlooking of morally relevant considerations (such as whether a person might be too sick to be saved) in giving a scarce resource to persons less likely to benefit, the inequalities inherent in learning about the locations of care, getting to locations of care, and being able to queue. We think that the relevant expression should be "treating persons fairly" rather than the attractive but too simplistic "treating persons equally."

Issues unique to children

The unique vulnerabilities of children raise issues following a mass casualty incident not encountered in planning for the care of adult patients. In mass casualty incidents that result in a surge of pediatric casualties in addition to adults, a disaster plan would have to anticipate the needs of a mixture of pediatric and adult patients. Since care for children requires greater staff/patient ratios, a disaster that affects infants, children, and adults will likely place a disproportionate strain on existing pediatric resources that subsequently would require some use of adult resources and adult providers unfamiliar with pediatric patients. A mass casualty incident that only affects pediatric patients would require even further alteration in hospital disaster plans to include adult providers caring for pediatric patients in adult units with adult equipment, thus placing children at an even greater disadvantage as a result not only of the disaster but also of the unspecialized staff and equipment (Markenson, 2009).

Second, medical triage of children in a mass casualty incident will be even more difficult than for adult patients as there is currently no validated scoring system for predicting pediatric survival upon presentation that could be used to "objectively" guide triage decisions. Many adult triage protocols use the Sequential Organ Failure Assessment (SOFA) score to predict medical prognosis and determine the ethical allocation of resources in a disaster, yet this clinical evaluation system has not been validated for pediatrics (White et al., 2009). Moreover, reliance on severity of illness scoring systems and prognostic models to objectively and fairly allocate scarce resources, while appealing, is problematic as the primary basis for individual patient triage and decision-making. For example, the two most widely used severity-of-illness scores in pediatrics are the Pediatric Risk of Mortality (PRISM) and the Pediatric Index of Mortality (PIM). Both are dependent on information collected after admission to a pediatric ICU, making them impractical as emergency triage tools to determine who should gain access to the ICU and receive limited life-saving treatments. More fundamentally, the conceptual foundation of severity of illness scores is that they generate probabilities for a population of patients, but are not precisely predictive for each individual patient. For example, PRISM

III or PIM applied to an individual patient may predict a hospital mortality rate of 46% for that child. The actual meaning of this statistic, however, is that for a group of 100 patients with a similar severity of illness, 46 patients are predicted to die; but these models cannot predict whether a particular patient is included in the 46% who will eventually die or in the 54% who will eventually survive.

Last, disaster plans for pediatrics must address the role of families in accompanying and potentially caring for their child. On the one hand, having a parent present at a child's bedside in a disaster seems appropriate for many reasons, and will likely aid the staff at a time of limited resources. On the other hand, the presence of additional family members, such as siblings of the patient, may pose additional burdens on limited hospital resources, resulting in diminished capacity to care for other children.

Clearly, health care providers have multiple moral duties: (1) most importantly, the duty to care, but also (2) the stewardship duty of using resources efficiently and effectively, (3) allocating limited resources fairly, sometimes called the duty of distributive justice, (4) the duty to respect the responsibilities of parents for participation in their child's care and decisions, (5) the duty to plan and prepare for pediatric mass casualties, and (6) the duty to inform the public about how allocation decisions will be made and where care can be obtained (Kinlaw et al., 2009).

As evident in the allocation criteria described here, several might need to be combined to arrive at an ethically justifiable allocation schema under conditions of scarcity (Persad et al., 2009).

Summary and case resolution

Which child should receive the last available ventilator in our scenario? Inability to meet the basic needs of equally deserving persons inevitably creates a sense of ethical quandary and moral tragedy. Yet there is currently no ethical consensus about such allocations in our society. And without prior ethical deliberation and agreement, the risk is that individuals or small communities will devise their own triage schemes that may be judged unfair after the fact. In order to preserve the moral foundations of social collaboration, the criteria used in this situation and similar shortages should be developed with broad societal input, and be publicly articulated and defended in advance of a crisis. While we lack a broadly accepted framework for allocating scarce life-saving treatments, we believe there are some things that are *not* ethically justifiable.

- Triage decisions should not be made on the basis of socioeconomic status, gender, race, or ethnicity.
- Coexisting conditions that do not affect short-term prognosis should not bar consideration for allocation of life-sustaining resources.
- Disabilities and handicaps should not be automatic barriers to receiving life-saving resources. Rather, the rights of the most vulnerable warrant protection, especially children whose conditions do not preclude survival, relationships with others, and living an enjoyable life.
- Decisions should not be made covertly or in secret. The criteria for decisions and the process for making them should be transparent and publicly shared.

Allocating the "last" ventilator should take into consideration those conditions for which it will be most helpful in restoring health and preserving a longer rather than shorter life span. We would like to think that the teen with Duchenne muscular dystrophy, who is described as dependent on mechanical ventilation, would already have a ventilator, and we do not believe it is justifiable to remove and reallocate it since he needs it and presumably owns it. If he does not currently have a ventilator, it seems likely that he would require ventilation for the rest of his life and is less likely to survive than the previously healthy 5-year-old with pneumonia and, perhaps, than the septic 5-month-old with multi-organ failure.

It is not possible here to evaluate the severity of the 5-year-old's pneumonia or the treatability of the 5-month-old's multiple organ failure and sepsis. If it can be known whether either would require prolonged ventilation with a poor prognosis for survival, then the criteria of treating the sickest with the best ability to survive with a shorter period of mechanical ventilation should be applied. We have, thus, applied a combination of criteria in which intervention would be distributed according to greatest need, modified by ability to benefit (in terms of surviving and living longer) and conservation of resources. However, if both patients are equally treatable with mechanical ventilation and other available resources, we do not think the difference between 5 months and 5 years is sufficiently substantial to select between those two by

any method other than equal opportunity – that is, a lottery.

It must also be acknowledged that the triage that will be required in a mass casualty incident may not allow time for thoughtful moral reflection, or indeed any serious and consistent reflection, and that decisions will need to be made quickly in the context of much uncertainty. The chaos and unpredictability of the moment, and the unyielding rush of mental and physical demands upon health care providers in a public health crisis, may make it difficult to apply the criteria described here. In such a case a lottery would likely be the triage process perceived most fair and effective by both the public and caregivers.

References

Alexander, S. (1962). They decide who lives, who dies: medical miracle and a moral burden of a small committee. *LIFE magazine*, November 9, 102–125.

Altevogt, B.M., Stroud, C., Hanson, S.L., Hanfling, D., Gostin, L.O., & the Institute of Medicine Committee on Guidance for Establishing Standards of Care for Use in Disaster Situations (2009). Guidance for Establishing Crisis Standards of Care for Use in Disaster Situations: A Letter Report. Washington, DC: National Academies Press. Available at www.iom.edu/~/media/Files/Report%20Files/2009/DisasterCareStandards/Standards%20of%20Care%20report%20brief%20FINAL.pdf (last accessed January 31, 2011).

Childress, J.F. (2003). Triage in response to a bioterrorist attack. In *In the Wake of Terror: Medicine and Morality in a Time of Crisis*, ed. J.D. Moreno. Cambridge: MIT Press, 77–93.

Emanuel, E.J. & Wertheimer, A. (2006). Public health. Who should get influenza vaccine when not all can? *Science*, **312**(5775), 854–855.

Kinlaw, K., Barrett, D.H., & Levine, R.J. (2009). Ethical Guidelines in Pandemic Influenza: Recommendations of the Ethics Subcommittee of the Advisory Committee of the Director, Centers for Disease Control and Prevention. *Disaster Medicine and Public Health Preparedness*, **3**(Suppl. 2), S185–S192.

Markenson, D. (2009). Developing consensus on appropriate standards of hospital disaster care: ensuring that the needs of children are addressed. *Disaster Medicine and Public Health Preparedness*, **3**(1), 5–7.

Persad, G., Wertheimer, A., & Emanuel, E.J. (2009). Principles for allocation of scarce medical interventions. *Lancet*, **373**(9661), 423–431.

Peterson, M. (2008). The moral importance of selecting people randomly. *Bioethics*, **22**(6), 321–327.

White, D.B., Katz, M.H., Luce, J.M., & Lo, B. (2009). Who should receive life support during a public health emergency? Using ethical principles to improve allocation decisions. *Annals of Internal Medicine*, **150**(2), 132–138.

Winslow, G.R. (1982). *Triage and Justice: The Ethics of Rationing Life-Saving Medical Resources*. Berkeley, CA: University of California Press.

World Health Organization (2007). Ethical Considerations in Developing a Public Health Response to Pandemic Influenza. Geneva, Switzerland: World Health Organization. Available at www.who.int/csr/resources/publications/WHO_CDS_EPR_GIP_2007_2c.pdf (last accessed January 31, 2011)

Parental refusals of vaccination and school vaccine mandates: balancing parental freedom, child welfare, and public health

Douglas J. Opel and Douglas S. Diekema

Case narrative

A 4-month-old boy is brought in by his mother for his well-child check. The child's health care provider asks how he has been since his 2-month check-up, and his mother says he's been generally healthy. Since the mother had been a little hesitant in agreeing to have him receive his 2-month immunizations, the provider makes sure to also ask her how things went with the immunizations after the last visit. "Terrible," she says, "he cried for about 4 hours straight, and this is a baby who doesn't cry. Then he was fussy for 18 to 24 hours. I am thinking it is better for him to get one shot from now on instead of three." The provider discusses the common side effects of immunizations and reassures the mother that the self-limited symptoms her son experienced were nothing serious. She is not convinced and states that she doesn't want to take the chance that he will have a similar experience. The boy's physical exam is unremarkable and he appears to be happy, healthy, and thriving. The provider tries to have a further discussion with the mother about the benefits of timely immunization for her son, yet he is met with continued resistance. "I don't want to do any vaccinations," she says with decisiveness. "None?" the provider says somewhat surprised, since he thought she felt that one shot was acceptable. "I don't want to take any chances," the boy's mother replies. The provider decides to drop the issue, and asks her to return for the 6-month visit or earlier if it's convenient for her. She agrees, but the provider leaves the room feeling defeated.

Introduction

Provider discussions with parents who are hesitant about childhood immunizations are difficult conversations. Consequently, they do not always go well (Bryant et al., 2009). Parents report difficulty in openly discussing their concerns about vaccines with their child's provider and feeling alienated when vaccines are discussed. Providers often provide little information to parents about immunizations, rarely validate parental concerns, and discredit parental sources of immunization information. Too much information and a lack of time, resources, and knowledge constrain a provider's ability to effectively communicate with concerned parents during health supervision visits.

Maintaining a therapeutic alliance with a parent is a common ethical challenge for providers (Moon et al., 2009). In conversations where parents want to refuse or delay immunizations, the therapeutic alliance can be strained by the difficulty in reconciling disagreement. Providers are required to navigate conflicting intuitions to respect parental authority yet protect the health of the child, and ultimately must determine whether intervening against a parent's decision to refuse or delay immunizations is justified. Furthermore, it seems unfair for one parent to excuse their child from assuming the risks of vaccines yet still be able to take full advantage of the benefits of herd immunity because other parents are willing to assume those risks. Lastly, the standard by which providers generally judge parents' medical decisions for their children is the best interest standard (Beauchamp & Childress, 2001), but since this standard ultimately rests on value judgments, it can exacerbate the provider–parent relationship by pitting the providers' conception of the child's best interest against that of the parents' (Diekema, 2004).

Ethical principles and discussion

The US preschool immunization program has been remarkably successful (Orenstein et al., 2005). Vaccination coverage levels are at near-record highs,

---

Clinical Ethics in Pediatrics: A Case-Based Textbook, ed. Douglas S. Diekema, Mark R. Mercurio and Mary B. Adam. Published by Cambridge University Press. © Cambridge University Press 2011.

and mortality from most vaccine-preventable diseases (VPDs) has been reduced by ≥99% in the United States (Roush & Murphy, 2007). Despite this success, national coverage levels for the 15-dose series continue to fall short of the *Healthy People 2010* goal of 80%, and vaccination levels vary considerably at the state, county, and local levels (Omer et al., 2008). An effect of this patchy and persistent under-immunization is a remaining disease burden: there are still >4000 cases of VPD per year in children <5 years old resulting in an estimated 300 deaths in the United States annually (Institute of Medicine, 2000).

Parental attitudes and beliefs contribute to about 15% of the under-immunization of 19- to 35-month-old US children (Gust et al., 2004). Nearly 12% of parents have refused at least one recommended childhood vaccine (Freed et al., 2010) and 28% of parents are unsure about, delayed, or decided not to have their child receive a vaccination (Gust et al., 2008). Further erosion of parental acceptance of immunizations is evident in the increasing number of parents who are claiming philosophical exemptions from required childhood vaccines (Omer et al., 2006).

Although there are several factors that influence a parent's decision to accept or refuse childhood immunization (Sturm et al., 2005) – such as perceptions of vaccine benefits, risks, and efficacy, cultural beliefs about disease and immunization, and Internet and media coverage of vaccine-related issues – a parent's interface with health care and their child's provider is emerging as very important. Parents consistently report that their child's provider remains their most important influence when deciding about childhood immunizations (Smith et al., 2006). Not only do most parents state that they most commonly seek immunization information from providers (Gust et al., 2004), but they change their minds about delaying or refusing a vaccine after receiving information or assurances from their child's provider (Gust et al., 2008). Provider–parent communication about immunizations is vital to the translation of the scientific benefits of vaccines into practice.

There is no standard clinical approach to communicating with parents who have concerns about childhood immunizations. Some pediatricians consider immunization as so essential to the practice of pediatrics that it cannot be compromised (Flanagan-Klygis et al., 2005). Others believe a "strong stance" is effective, advocate for "open communication," or simply feel they "cannot convince parents about the value of certain vaccines" (Fierman, 2010). As a result of this lack of a communication standard, some pediatric practice groups accommodate parents who refuse some or all immunizations out of respect for parental decision-making, while others do not offer pediatric care to patients whose parents chose to delay or refuse most immunizations. Despite the AAP Committee on Bioethics' recommendation against discontinuing care with families who refuse or delay immunization (Diekema & AAP, 2005), nearly 30% of pediatricians surveyed would do so (Flanagan-Klygis et al., 2005).

The primary ethical issue illustrated by this varied response to parental immunization refusal by health care providers is the tension between respecting parental autonomy and protecting the child's and the public's health. Should parental autonomy always be respected? If yes, why? If not, at what point might it be ethically justifiable to intervene against a parent's wishes in order to protect the child's and the public's health?

To begin to answer these questions, let's first consider the concept of autonomy. Autonomy refers to the ability to make one's own decisions free from constraints by others and according to one's desires, plans, and values. The ethical principle of respect for autonomy, therefore, is an acknowledgment that an autonomous person has the "right to hold views, make choices, and to take actions based on personal values and beliefs" (Beauchamp & Childress, 2001). This principle establishes the obligation for health care providers to allow autonomous individuals to make their own health care decisions.

Our obligation to respect an autonomous individual's decision, however, is contingent upon that individual being autonomous. Infants are not autonomous individuals. Rather, their developmental immaturity renders them incapable of understanding, deciding, and deliberating, processes that are associated with attributes of autonomous individuals. As such, they and other non-autonomous individuals need surrogates to make decisions on their behalf.

Under US law, parents are the legal surrogates for their children and are thereby empowered to make decisions on behalf of their children. In general, we give wide discretion to parents with respect to these decisions, since they know their child best, are able to weigh competing family interests best, and can instill in their children the values they have deemed the best (Diekema, 2004). However, parental autonomy is not absolute. As surrogate decision-makers for their children, the standard that parents are expected to adhere to when making decisions for their children is the best interest standard. According to this standard, parents are obligated to maximize the well-being of their child by minimizing risks, pain, suffering, and loss of functioning (Beauchamp & Childress, 2001). Therefore, a parent's decision that puts their child's health, well-being, or life in jeopardy violates the best interest standard for surrogate decision-making.

In the context of the case presented above, it is reasonable to ask whether a mother's decision to refuse or delay one or more immunizations for her 4-month-old child is in violation of the best interest standard. If so, this would provide reason to override the mother's decision because it clearly threatens the child's best interests. If not, we would be inclined to not interfere with the mother's decision out of respect for parental autonomy given her status as the legal surrogate decision-maker for her child.

Attempts to answer this question, however, are met with the realization that the best interest standard provides us with little guidance primarily because of the inherently subjective nature of what is "best" for the child. A parent may in fact be adhering to the best interest standard by making a decision that maximizes what she believes is best for her child, yet what the parent thinks is best for the child may be quite different from what the health care provider thinks is best for the child. This is possible because parents may have different values than a health care provider and therefore assign different weights to risks, benefits, and outcomes. The risks of a vaccine, for instance, might be weighed more heavily by a parent than they are by a health care provider because of different perceptions of the severity and likelihood of side effects. Alternatively, parents might have a different belief system in which naturally obtained immunity (i.e., that obtained by contracting the actual disease) is better than immunity obtained from a vaccine. Therefore, since the best interest standard ultimately rests on value judgments, it provides little direction in determining whether or not to intervene against a parent's wishes and instead tends to pit a health care provider's conception of the child's best interest against that of the parents (Diekema, 2004).

We argue that the harm principle offers a better foundation from which to determine whether it is justifiable to override a parent's decision (Diekema, 2004). Specifically, in situations where a parent's refusal of an intervention proven to be efficacious (in this case, vaccination) places the child at significant and imminent risk of serious harm compared with the option chosen by the parents (in this case, to not vaccinate), it is

justifiable for the provider to seek state intervention to override the parent's refusal.

When applying the harm principle to our case, we must decide whether the parent's refusal of the intervention (vaccination) poses significant risk of serious harm to the child, thereby providing a justification for overriding the parent's decision. To try and quantify the risk and harm associated with refusing a vaccine, let's suppose the mother is refusing the diphtheria and tetanus toxoids and acellular pertussis (DTaP) vaccine. Each antigen within the DTaP vaccine is meant to prevent a disease that has its own incidence rate. The incidence in the United States of diphtheria and tetanus is about 0.01 cases per 100 000 population, while the incidence of pertussis is about 4 cases per 100 000 population (Plotkin et al., 2008). Therefore, even though diphtheria and tetanus are rare, because these antigens are given in combination with pertussis, the incidence rate most relevant to the consideration of the risks and harms associated with the refusal of the DTaP vaccine is that of pertussis. Of those children <1 year of age who contract pertussis, over 60% require hospitalization (Broder et al., 2006). In addition, almost a quarter of infants <6 months of age suffer major complications from pertussis (categorized as either pulmonic, encephalitic, or nutritional) (Heininger et al., 1997). Lastly, there are risks associated with the DTaP vaccine itself. These risks and their frequencies include fever (<1%), crying for 3 or more hours (1–2%), hypotonic–hyporesponsive episode (<1%), and seizure (<1%) (Ciofi degli Atti & Olin, 1997).

While this information suggests that the risks of pertussis are greater than the risks of the DTaP vaccine, we would argue that a parent's decision to refuse the DTaP vaccine does not reach a harm threshold at which we would be justified in overriding their refusal. Although a child is *more likely* to contract pertussis if un-immunized than if immunized (Feikin et al., 2000), the incidence of pertussis still makes this likelihood quite low. In addition, if a child does contract pertussis before 6 months of age, he or she is more likely than not to avoid any major sequelae from the disease. We don't mean to suggest that children who contract pertussis do not suffer any harm. Undoubtedly, they do. However, the level of harm they are likely to experience is not serious enough to justify intervening against a parent's wishes.

This calculation of risk and harm will differ for each antigen or vaccine and will vary with time and geography. As such, there are situations where it is conceivable that the harm threshold would be reached if a parent refused an immunization. For instance, if the community in which a parent is refusing the DTaP vaccine is experiencing a pertussis outbreak, the risk of contracting the disease is much higher for an un-immunized child. Similarly, parental refusal of DTaP in communities with low herd immunity for pertussis, such as those that have high exemption rates from immunizations required for school entry, requires a different calculation of risk of contracting the disease. Finally, if the child has an underlying cardiac or pulmonary disease, the risk of harm should he or she contract pertussis might be higher, altering the threshold for overriding a parent's refusal.

The harm principle can also be interpreted broadly to extend beyond harm to one's own child and include harm to the general public. It is this interpretation that serves as the basis for vaccine mandates. The government's authority in the health arena arises primarily from its constitutionally sanctioned "police power" to protect the public's health, welfare, and safety (Dover, 1979). Therefore, the state can justifiably require vaccination for children entering child care and/or school when having unvaccinated children in the school could (1) place the health of other school children in jeopardy, (2) threaten the state's economic interests (through the cost of managing vaccine-preventable disease outbreaks and the costs of care for those who contract vaccine preventable illness or suffer related disability or death), or (3) impair the state's duty to educate children.

Since 1980, all 50 states have had school-entry immunization laws. School-entry laws are effective at both decreasing disease incidence and increasing vaccination coverage (Briss et al., 2000). Each state, however, allows parents to opt out of required immunizations for school-entry for medical reasons, 48 states have opt-out provisions for religious reasons, and 20 states allow parents to opt out for philosophical reasons. These opt-out provisions are primarily meant to diffuse perceptions of state coercion and to enhance the sustainability and acceptability of school immunization requirements. A consequence of these opt-out provisions is that school-entry immunization requirements cease to be a "mandate" and begin to look more like a strong suggestion that parents are free to ignore. Because parents can lawfully refuse immunizations on behalf of their child for non-medical reasons in all but two states, many do so. In Washington State, for example, where both religious and philosophical

exemptions from school-entry immunization requirements are allowed, the number of children exempted from required immunizations for philosophical reasons has almost doubled since 2003 (3.6% in 2003–2004, 4.1% in 2006–2007, 5.7% in 2007–2008, and 6.8% in 2008–2009) (Centers for Disease Control and Prevention 2009). Parents who don't comply with state laws that require them to either file for an exemption from immunization or provide evidence that their child has received the required immunizations, however, can be susceptible to strict enforcement. In 2007, for example, the parents of 2300 students in Prince George County, Maryland were ordered to appear in a special court hearing because they had failed to file for a state-approved immunization exemption or arrange for home-schooling, the two legal alternatives for complying with Maryland school immunization laws (Diekema, 2008).

Opting out of immunizations required for school-entry for philosophical reasons, although legal in some states, raises questions of fairness. Parents who opt out – so-called free-riders – still receive a vaccine's protective benefits through herd immunity even though they refuse to contribute to herd immunity by vaccinating their own children. The parents of immunized children, therefore, are left to shoulder the risks, cost, and inconvenience of vaccination.

Practical summary

Parental refusal of immunization raises ethical issues related to the limits of parental autonomy, obligations to protect the health of individual children and the surrounding community, and fairness. In general, we give wide discretion to parents as they make decisions on behalf of their children, but expect them to adhere to the best interest standard of surrogate decision-making. More importantly, the harm principle helps identify those situations when a parent's decision should be challenged: does a parent's refusal of an intervention proven to be efficacious place the child at significant and imminent risk of serious harm compared with the option chosen by the parents? If so, intervening against a parent's wishes is ethically justifiable.

Parental refusal of childhood immunizations rarely meets a harm threshold, suggesting that the parental decision should be respected in most situations. In rare cases, a failure to vaccinate a child might constitute a serious threat to the child's health. One example of such a situation would be a 5-year-old unvaccinated child who presents with a deep, contaminated wound sustained while walking barefoot in an abandoned lot. In such a case, the risk of tetanus (which is nearly always fatal unless treated prior to the onset of symptoms) rises well above baseline and can be prevented with tetanus immunoglobulin and vaccination. In such a case, involving state child protective agencies to assure treatment of the child would be justified. Some states have opt-out provisions that make it legal for parents to refuse immunizations required for school-entry for philosophical reasons. This, however, raises concerns of fairness, as those parents who opt out still reap the benefits of herd immunity without assuming any of the risks inherent to vaccines themselves. While this latter issue raises important ethical issues, it represents an issue for which the solution rests not with the individual health care provider, but at the policy level.

Case resolution and discussion

Family-centered care (FCC), the endorsed approach in pediatrics, offers a model for difficult conversations such as the one in this case. Grounded in collaborative communication between providers, patients, and families, FCC is fundamentally about valuing and incorporating child and family perspectives into clinical decision-making. The collaborative communication inherent to FCC meets the expectations parents have of providers in an immunization discussion, such as a whole-person approach; concerned, nonjudgmental listening; and being treated as individuals with individual needs. In addition, the use of FCC in immunization discussions is supported by consensus recommendations that promote collaborative communication as a best practice with parents who have concerns about immunizations (Diekema, 2005). FCC has also been applied in other settings where difficult conversations are common, such as pediatric palliative care (Feudtner, 2007) and critical care (Meyer et al., 2009), and has been associated with improved patient outcomes (Stewart, 1995).

The mother returned to the same provider for her child's 6-month visit and was open to discussing immunizations during this visit. While she didn't agree to all the recommended shots, she accepted a select few. The child's provider felt that her refusal, while unfortunate and raising her child's risk of contracting and transmitting a vaccine-preventable disease, did not constitute a significant risk of serious harm. The provider therefore respected the parent's decision and maintained the

therapeutic relationship with the mother. The mother continued to seek care from her provider and express her immunization concerns at future visits. The provider was able to acknowledge and carefully address those concerns. By the time the child turned 3 years old, she was fully immunized.

References

Beauchamp, T. & Childress, J. (2001). *Principles of Biomedical Ethics*, 5th edn. New York: Oxford University Press.

Briss, P.A., Rodewald, L.E., Hinman, A.R., et al. (2000). Reviews of evidence regarding interventions to improve vaccination coverage in children, adolescents, and adults. The Task Force on Community Preventive Services. *American Journal of Preventive Medicine*, **18**(1 Suppl.), 97–140.

Broder, K.R., Cortese, M.M., Iskander, J.K., et al. (2006). Preventing tetanus, diphtheria, and pertussis among adolescents: use of tetanus toxoid, reduced diphtheria toxoid and acellular pertussis vaccines recommendations of the Advisory Committee on Immunization Practices (ACIP). *MMWR*, 55 (RR-3), 1–34.

Bryant, K.A., Wesley, G.C., Wood, J.A., Hines, C., & Marshall, G.S. (2009). Use of standardized patients to examine physicians' communication strategies when addressing vaccine refusal: a pilot study. *Vaccine*, **27**(27), 3616–3619.

Centers for Disease Control and Prevention (2009). The School Entry Immunization Assessment Report. www2.cdc.gov/nip/schoolsurv/rptgmenu.asp. Last accessed April 11, 2009.

Ciofi degli Atti, M.L. & Olin, P. (1997). Severe adverse events in the Italian and Stockholm I pertussis vaccine clinical trials. *Developments in Biological Standardization*, **89**, 77–81.

Diekema, D.S. (2004). Parental refusals of medical treatment: the harm principle as threshold for state intervention. *Theoretical Medicine and Bioethics*, **25**(4), 243–264.

Diekema, D.S. (2008). Public health, ethics, and state compulsion. *Journal of Public Health Management and Practice*, **14**(4), 332–334.

Diekema, D.S. & The Committee on Bioethics, American Academy of Pediatrics (2005). Responding to parental refusals of immunization of children. *Pediatrics*, **115**(5), 1428–1431.

Dover, T.E. (1979). An evaluation of immunization regulations in light of religious objections and the developing right of privacy. *University of Dayton Law Review*, **4**(2), 401–424.

Feikin, D.R., Lezotte, D.C., Hamman, R.F., et al. (2000). Individual and community risks of measles and pertussis associated with personal exemptions to immunization. *JAMA*, **284**(24), 3145–3150.

Feudtner, C. (2007). Collaborative communication in pediatric palliative care: a foundation for problem-solving and decision-making. *Pediatric Clinics of North America*, **54**(5), 583–607.

Fierman, A.H. (2010). Voices from the field: controversies in vaccine mandates. *Current Problems in Pediatric and Adolescent Health Care*, **40**(3), 59.

Flanagan-Klygis, E.A., Sharp, L., & Frader, J.E. (2005). Dismissing the family who refuses vaccines: a study of pediatrician attitudes. *Archives of Pediatrics and Adolescent Medicine*, **159**(10), 929–934.

Freed, G.L., Clark, S.J., Butchart, A.T., Singer, D.C., & Davis, M.M. (2010). Parental vaccine safety concerns in 2009. *Pediatrics*, **125**(4), 654–659.

Gust, D.A., Strine, T.W., Maurice, E., et al. (2004). Underimmunization among children: effects of vaccine safety concerns on immunization status. *Pediatrics*, **114**(1), e16–e22.

Gust, D.A., Darling, N., Kennedy, A., & Schwartz, B. (2008). Parents with doubts about vaccines: which vaccines and reasons why. *Pediatrics*, **122**(4), 718–725.

Heininger, U., Klich, K., Stehr, K., & Cherry, J.D. (1997). Clinical findings in *Bordetella pertussis* infections: results of a prospective multicenter surveillance study. *Pediatrics*, **100**(6), E10.

Institute of Medicine, Division of Health Care Services, Division of Health Promotion and Disease Prevention (2000). *Calling the Shots: Immunization Finance Policies and Practices*. Washington, DC: National Academies Press.

Meyer, E.C., Sellers, D.E., Browning, D.M., et al. (2009). Difficult conversations: improving communication skills and relational abilities in health care. *Pediatric Critical Care Medicine*, **10**(3), 352–359.

Moon, M., Taylor, H.A., McDonald, E.L., Hughes, M.T., & Carrese, J.A. (2009). Everyday ethics issues in the outpatient clinical practice of pediatric residents. *Archives of Pediatric and Adolescent Medicine*, **163**(9), 838–843.

Omer, S.B., Pan, W.K., Halsey, N.A., et al. (2006). Nonmedical exemptions to school immunization requirements: secular trends and association of state policies with pertussis incidence. *JAMA*, **296**(14), 1757–1763.

Omer, S.B., Enger, K.S., Moulton, L.H., et al. (2008). Geographic clustering of nonmedical exemptions to school immunization requirements and associations with geographic clustering of pertussis. *American Journal of Epidemiology*, **168**(12), 1389–1396.

Orenstein, W.A., Douglas, R.G., Rodewald, L.E., & Hinman, A.R. (2005). Immunizations in the United States: success, structure, and stress. *Health Affairs (Millwood)*, **24**(3), 599–610.

Plotkin, S.A., Orenstein, W.A., & Offit, P.A. (2008). *Vaccines*, 5th edn. Philadelphia, PA and London: Saunders.

Roush, S.W. & Murphy, T.V. (2007). Historical comparisons of morbidity and mortality for vaccine-preventable diseases in the United States. *JAMA*, **298**(18), 2155–2163.

Smith, P.J., Kennedy, A.M., Wooten, K., Gust, D.A., & Pickering, L.K. (2006). Association between health care providers' influence on parents who have concerns about vaccine safety and vaccination coverage. *Pediatrics*, **118**(5), e1287–e1292.

Stewart, M.A. (1995). Effective physician-patient communication and health outcomes: a review. *Canadian Medical Association Journal*, **152**(9), 1423–1433.

Sturm, L.A., Mays, R.M., & Zimet, G.D. (2005). Parental beliefs and decision making about child and adolescent immunization: from polio to sexually transmitted infections. *Journal of Developmental and Behavioral Pediatrics*, **26**(6), 441–452.

Chapter

36

When institutional, professional, and public health obligations conflict: the controversial case of youth boxing

Stephanya B. Shear, Carolyn Korfiatis, and Douglas S. Diekema

Case narrative

A city police league asked a children's hospital pediatrician to provide ringside medical supervision at a community amateur youth boxing event for at-risk urban boys. Amateur youth boxing is a legal sport performed in a controlled fashion with protective headgear. A licensed provider is required at the ringside in order for all boxing events to occur. The ringside physician provides pre-match assessments of the participants, monitors the boxing bouts, and has the authority to stop matches if they decide that doing so is in the participants' best interests. The ringside physician may also prevent an individual from participating in future matches because of injury, illegal hits, or poor sportsmanship if deemed necessary. Neither professional boxing nor amateur martial arts events give such wide discretion to the ringside physician. Unlike professional boxing, the goal in amateur boxing is to score points rather than to "knock someone out." The police league's at-risk youth program upholds values such as diversity, equal opportunity, and self-confidence.

In the past, this pediatrician has provided assistance at other youth events sponsored by the police league, including football and soccer games. While checking her malpractice coverage to participate, she found herself mired in a larger controversy when several staff in her department expressed vehement opposition to her participation. The pediatrician's colleagues cited the American Academy of Pediatrics (AAP) policy statement "vigorously opposing" youth boxing (Committee on Sports Medicine and Fitness, 1997). The AAP policy does not directly mention ringside assistance; however, the physician's colleagues felt that participating in this program was inconsistent with the hospital's commitment to injury prevention and programs designed to reduce concussions. Some individuals opined that

boxing was nothing more than a "brutal sport" masquerading as "legalized violence," and that the sport did not promote a healthy lifestyle.

Others in the hospital encouraged her to participate, arguing that the boxers' welfare would be best served by the presence of an experienced physician knowledgeable about concussion management rather than an "allied" medical person less familiar with such issues. Supporters also cited insufficient evidence that the risks of amateur boxing exceed those of other potentially dangerous sports for which physicians provide coverage, such as football (Committee on Sports Medicine and Fitness, 1997; Cowie, 2000). The AAP statement concedes that football poses an overall greater risk of injury than amateur boxing but justifies opposition to youth boxing by highlighting its scoring system, which rewards direct blows to the head. The statement notes that the "ultimate victory [in boxing] may be to render the opponent senseless."

The medical arguments against boxing in the AAP statement, such as risk for dementia pugilistica, were extrapolated from professional boxing (Jordan 2000). It is difficult to know whether the injuries sustained from years of professional boxing are risks that apply to amateur boxing, but the evidence suggests the risks of traumatic brain injury in amateur boxing are low (Loosemore et al., 2008). Some differences between the two include different scoring mechanisms, equipment, and time rules (USA Boxing, 2010). Amateur boxing is scored on points without emphasizing the force of a blow whereas the objective in professional boxing is to knock down or knock out the opponent. Professional boxers do not use the protective headgear that amateur boxers are required to wear, and the gloves worn by amateur boxers are designed to absorb shock versus the gloves worn by professional boxers designed to transmit force.

Clinical Ethics in Pediatrics: A Case-Based Textbook, ed. Douglas S. Diekema, Mark R. Mercurio and Mary B. Adam. Published by Cambridge University Press. © Cambridge University Press 2011.

The AAP statement acknowledges these discrepancies but remains firm in its opposition because "the 'safety' of amateur boxing remains unproven."

Finally, the physician was warned that a decision to participate would be perceived as inconsistent with the hospital's mission and values, potentially damaging hospital fundraising efforts given boxing's violent image. Participation in the event might be perceived by some as the equivalent of supporting street fights as a method of anger management.

After considering the controversy surrounding boxing, divergent opinions within her medical group, the AAP statement, and her possible inconsistency in having participated in more harmful sports, the physician contacted her hospital's ethics consult service for assistance in making her decision.

Discussion of ethical issues

This case is complex and includes stakeholders within the medical community and the general community. It addresses not only the medical needs of a vulnerable population, but also the moral responsibility and influence of physicians and hospitals. Public and professional opinion about boxing as a sport strongly influences how people will view this case. The AAP's policy statement, while not directly addressing ringside medical coverage by physicians, specifically condemns youth boxing. The AAP's silence on ringside medical coverage adds to the complexity and controversy by leaving the physician's role open to interpretation. The request to provide medical coverage for a youth boxing event involves ethical issues that extend to youth involved in the sport, the community in which the boxing occurs, the physician who has been asked to provide coverage, the physician's institution and colleagues, and the professional organization to which she belongs. It does not lend itself to clean assessments (Trotter, 2002).

In the case of adult boxing, the basis for tolerating what some perceive as a harmful sport has been the recognition that those who participate have made an autonomous decision to do so. Respect for autonomy would suggest that while we may try to convince adult participants that the sport is harmful and that they might be better off not participating, ultimately it is their decision to make. In general, arguments to ban an activity simply because it is potentially harmful to the autonomous adult who chooses to participate in it are not considered sufficient to justify the infringement on individual liberty. After all, similar arguments can be made for many activities, such as mountain climbing, professional football, motorcycle riding, and around-the-world sailing races, to name but a few. In general, outlawing an activity requires a demonstration that it causes significant harm to those who have not chosen to participate. While many may be offended by the violence in the sport of boxing, it is hard to demonstrate actual harm to individuals other than those who have chosen to participate.

Youth boxing involves minors, however, who may not have developed the full capacity to make truly autonomous decisions about participation in a sport that may impact their future health. The AAP stance opposing youth boxing is partially based in the notion that a person who chooses to participate in boxing is not acting in his own best interest (Committee on Sports Medicine and Fitness, 1997), and while that kind of choice might be tolerated for autonomous adults, it should not be for youth. This would imply that youth boxing should be banned for many of the same reasons other activities (cigarette smoking, drinking alcohol) are restricted to adults – to prevent youth from participating in a harmful activity.

Youth boxing has not been banned, however, and individual physicians must struggle with how to respond to requests for medical coverage of events like this one – a legal police-sponsored youth boxing event. The events will occur whether they are attended by a physician or not, since the league requires medical coverage, which can come from any health care professional, including a paramedic. The sponsors would prefer a physician with expertise in concussion recognition in order to provide the highest level of safety for the youth participating.

Those who oppose physician coverage of youth boxing events argue as a matter of principle. The argument goes as follows: Youth boxing is wrong because it puts youth at risk of injury and glorifies violence. Since it is not in the best interests of youth to be boxing, physician coverage of boxing events tacitly condones an activity that puts youth at risk. Therefore, it is wrong to provide medical coverage of youth boxing because it supports and makes possible an activity that is wrong. Furthermore, since the AAP has argued that youth boxing should be banned because of the risk it poses to youth, then physicians must show their opposition to such events by not providing medical coverage.

It should be noted that this argument from principle is based on several assumptions that may not be true. First, it assumes that youth boxing is actually more harmful than other activities that are not condemned. In fact, this is not the case. Football, rugby, hockey, wrestling, tae kwan do, and a host of other sports put athletes at risk of head injury, and have higher injury rates than youth boxing. However, none of those sports are formally opposed by hospitals or the AAP. Similarly the AAP does not oppose martial arts, where intentional striking or kicking is performed with less controlling oversight from a ringside physician. This would suggest that opposition to boxing is not entirely based on its risk of injury (Cowie, 2000).

What makes boxing different? Some argue that the real harm of boxing is that the intent of the sport is to strike one's opponent, which makes it different than a sport like football, where the goal is to score points. In fact, the goal of youth boxing is to score points. In contrast to adult boxing, where the goal is to knock out one's opponent, the scoring system in youth boxing recognizes only the location of a blow. There are no added points based on the force of the blow, and knockdowns and knockouts are not recognized. It may be true that points are scored by striking one's opponent, but to be fair, every play in football is accompanied by players hitting, tackling, and blocking their opponents, often with great force. While the team's goal may be to score points, the individual defensive back's goal is often to sack the quarterback.

Second, the argument that youth boxing is wrong fails to recognize that participation in youth boxing might actually benefit some youth. The event described in this case is sponsored by the police league, a group whose goals include preventing youth crime and supporting maturity and good citizenship among at-risk teens. The sponsors argue that providing the opportunity to participate in a carefully monitored youth boxing activity provides an option for some kids who might otherwise be drawn toward gang activities, street fights, and drugs. The police department faces the effects of youth violence directly and they feel that by sponsoring this event, the best interests of these youth and the community will be promoted.

Finally, boycotting these events on principle only stands to benefit the youth in question if the boycott successfully ends youth boxing. While the stance "makes a statement," it may not actually represent what is best for the youth participating in these events, which will occur whether the physician agrees to cover the event or not.

Given that youth boxing is legal, it is difficult to argue that it is in the adolescent's best interest not to

have a physician available at a match where injury might occur. In fact, it is surely in the participants' best interest to have the most qualified and experienced medical provider present at ringside, a provider who is given wide discretion and responsibility to stop a match when she feels a participant may be at risk of injury (USA Boxing, 2010). The only valid reason for opposing physician coverage of boxing events has nothing to do with the best interests of those participating, but rather is a principled stance in opposition of the sport. Those who oppose physician coverage of youth boxing events would not object to a physician treating a participant who came to the emergency room to be treated for an injury sustained while boxing.

Even if all physicians agree that boxing should be banned, an argument can still be made that physician participation at the ringside should be allowed and even encouraged. By way of an example, many physicians believe that it is better for adolescents to refrain from sexual activity, and physicians generally do not support or encourage early sexual activity. However, most physicians recognize that if an adolescent chooses to become sexually active, they should do so safely, and they are willing to assist them in getting contraception and learning about safe sexual practices. Likewise, they will offer medical care for the consequences of sexual activity, including pregnancy or sexually transmitted diseases. Although many believe it is in the best interests of adolescents to abstain from sexual activity, it is also in their interests to receive appropriate medical care should they choose to engage in those activities. Further, providing care to these patients affords the physician an opportunity to educate them, thereby decreasing the associated risks.

Why should boxing be different? Even if a physician thinks that boxing is not in a child's best interest, they may feel compelled to provide ringside care in order to make the activity as safe as possible. Ringside physicians are tasked with providing the athletes with pre- and post-bout physicals, they can stop a match to evaluate an athlete, and they have the authority to terminate a bout when they feel it is necessary. Even if the physician has concerns about the sport, it does not follow that they should refrain from providing a medical service that benefits those who choose to participate in the sport.

Could providing ringside medical coverage result in negative consequences for the physician or the physician's institution? Undoubtedly, some adverse publicity can result anytime there is disagreement about a contentious issue. This could result in negative or unflattering publicity towards the hospital. It could even result in the loss of some potential donors. However, ultimately the goal of health care institutions should be focused on the good of the individual patient. If the best interests of youth are served by providing medical coverage at sporting events, including amateur boxing, then institutions should support their physicians in doing so. Opposition to youth boxing is best addressed in the public policy arena, not by denying the best possible medical coverage to youth who choose to participate in a legal activity.

Practical summary

Pediatric sports medicine physicians and programs need to navigate the health imperative to provide medical expertise at youth sporting events, such as boxing, while at the same time recognizing that participation may seem inconsistent with policy recommendations, and that their participation may be perceived negatively. Those who oppose youth boxing for public health or moral reasons should pursue change in the public policy realm. The mere fact that a physician has a personal objection to youth boxing or belongs to a professional medical society that objects to the sport should not preclude the physician from providing ringside medical coverage as a way of maximizing the safety of participants in what remains a legal activity. Certainly physicians should be free to refuse to participate on moral grounds, but we would argue that those who feel an obligation to cover these events do not act wrongly. A physician's presence at the ringside may significantly benefit participants and increase the safety

of the activity. At the same time, the absence of a well-trained physician is unlikely to deter youth from participating in boxing.

Case resolution

The case of physician ringside coverage at a youth boxing event was considered by the ethics committee at the physician's hospital. The ethics committee advised the physician that participation was not inconsistent with her ethical and professional obligations. The hospital administration, however, felt that participation at the ringside was inconsistent with the hospital's goals and image and barred the physician from participating in the event.

References

Committee on Sports Medicine and Fitness, American Academy of Pediatrics (1997). Participation in boxing by children, adolescents, and young adults. *Pediatrics*, **99**(1), 134–135.

Cowie, C. (2000). The ethics of boxing. *British Journal of Sports Medicine*, **34**(3), 230.

Jordan, B.D. (2000). Chronic traumatic brain injury associated with boxing. *Seminars in Neurology*, **20**(2), 179–185.

Loosemore, M., Knowles, C.H., & Whyte G.P. (2008). Amateur boxing and risk of chronic traumatic brain injury. *British Journal of Sports Medicine*, **42**(11), 564–567.

Trotter, G. (2002). Outside outpatient ethics: is it ethical for physicians to serve ringside? *Journal of Clinical Ethics*, **13**(4), 367–374.

USA Boxing (2010). Amateur boxing vs. professional boxing. http://usaboxing.org/about-us/boxing-101/amateur-boxing-vs-professional-boxing. Last accessed December 22, 2010.

Chapter 37

Industry representatives, gift-giving, and conflicts of interest

Ellen L. Blank and D. Micah Hester

Case narrative

During an outpatient rotation in the pediatric gastro-enterology clinic, Dr. Q (a second-year resident) finishes observing a colonoscopy in the operating room and returns to the Doctors' Lounge with the Gastroenterology fellow and attending physician to take a short break before the next procedure. It is lunchtime, and they are hungry. The next procedure will start in 15 minutes, and the cafeteria line will be too long to get lunch and return before the next procedure starts. They all enter the lounge and immediately see a well-dressed man sitting at a table with a 3-foot-long sub sandwich, a plate of brownies, and a display of brand-name skin care dressings commonly used by surgeons, emergency rooms, and in pediatricians' offices. He offers them all lunch. Dr. Q is particularly hungry, having skipped breakfast, and sees the fellow and staff physician accept a sub and a brownie. She pauses only a moment before filling a plate herself. The man at the table only mentions that his company is excited about this new product and hands over a brochure and pen with each plate of food, but demands no more of the physicians' time. At the table, Dr. Q slides the pen into her pocket, briefly opens the brochure, but quickly engages in conversation with the fellow and attending physician, and leaves the brochure on the table as she departs.

A free lunch?

Of course, it is not surprising that in a stressful or busy situation thoughts often go quickly to self-preservation or, in this case, eating lunch. However, the acceptance of the food sets up a particularly powerful impulse to reciprocate in some way. A conflict of interest exists when professional judgment concerning a primary interest is *unduly* influenced by a secondary interest. In this case, the primary interest is good treatment of

patients' wounds to promote the most effective healing, and the secondary interest is satisfaction of personal hunger at lunchtime. Of course, it is not without careful consideration of marketing principles that the sales-person offers food to potential clients. By accepting the food from the salesman, a positive feeling is associated with the salesperson and with the brand-name of the product he represents. Furthermore, the acceptance of the food by the mentors of the resident reinforces that this type of behavior is acceptable even though there are consequences that they may not have carefully considered.

Several ethical concerns arise when physicians participate in these kinds of activities:

- Whose and what interests are and should be served?
- How can a physician be sure that marketing is not *unduly* influential?
- Does the influence of marketing undermine trust in the "social role" of medical professionals? (Erde, 1996; Brody, 2007)

Industry marketing practices and the physician

Scenarios like the one in which Dr. Q finds herself are commonplace (Campbell et al., 2007; Sernyak & Rosenheck, 2007). Even with increasing institutional restrictions regarding interactions of physician-faculty and residents with industry sales representatives (Association of American Medical Colleges [AAMC], 2008), there remain a great many encounters in doctors' offices, hospitals, at medical conferences, and in other settings where physicians and sales representatives from the medical industry discuss drugs or devices approved for patient care, and during those encounters exchange gifts of pens, textbooks, toys, food, and more.

Clinical Ethics in Pediatrics: A Case-Based Textbook, ed. Douglas S. Diekema, Mark R. Mercurio and Mary B. Adam. Published by Cambridge University Press. © Cambridge University Press 2011.

Outside the medical arena, marketing of everyday consumer products includes attracting the attention of a customer, cuing the customer to make mental shortcuts, and then closing the deal. Marketing prescription drugs and medical devices by sales representatives to physicians has the same goal, and one instrument of achieving that goal is gift-giving.

Targeted marketing of pharmaceutical drugs or devices ("detailing") has become ubiquitous since the 1980s and presents a unique marketing situation for the medical industry. While most businesses usually market their goods directly to the consumer who will use those goods, only medical professionals may write prescriptions for controlled drugs and devices, and thus, the medical industry must market to prescribers in the hope that they will choose a particular product to prescribe to the consumer. As such, the medical industry spends tens of billions of dollars per year in detailing to gain access to professionals who write the prescriptions or use specific devices. They do so because it works, and over time the professionals who write the prescriptions become accustomed to attention from the medical industry, expecting more and more of it.

Of course, all this occurs in conjunction with the everyday practice of medicine, a profession governed by certain ethical expectations, aspirations, and obligations. In particular, physicians are expected to act in the best interests of patients, even when this may interfere with their own personal interests. Such expectations arise from the basic trust society, in general, and patients, in particular, have in their medical professionals (Zaner, 1988). However, even small gifts have their effects on behavior, and for physicians this creates a perception that a physician's self-interest may trump the best interests of patients. Accepting these gifts presents a problem for physicians because it creates an urge to reciprocate. Reciprocation is the need to repay in kind what another has given us. But do everyday items like pens and lunch create *disconcerting* influence? In fact, they can. For example, the satisfaction of hunger induces a unique obligation to reciprocate. Strohmetz et al. (2002) demonstrated that as little as the random offering of after-dinner mints at an Italian restaurant resulted in an increase in tipping, which over-compensated for the service given during the meal.

But still we might say that tipping waiters is significantly different behavior than prescribing medications. The former comes in relationship to a service provided, while the latter is in service to others. Tipping, then, can be seen as appropriate reciprocity, but prescribing

medications is an act of intelligent altruism. Further, even if one's prescribing habits could be influenced, physicians think that it would take *significant* personal gain (not trivial trinkets or food) to overcome the intelligent exercise of medical expertise. In fact, physicians commonly express disbelief that their clinical judgment could be influenced by as little as a free meal or a pen (Wazana, 2000). Physicians are well-meaning, intelligent people, after all, and surely can analyze situations well enough to parse legitimate medical considerations from propaganda.

Furthermore, conflicts of interest are simply part-and-parcel of any professional's life. In medicine, one cannot help desiring to act for the benefit of patients, and yet when stressed and fatigued, physicians make mental shortcuts during each working day. The habit of self-serving bias, like any habit, can easily take hold under such conditions. In those moments, it is difficult to evaluate boundaries among our interests. Where is the line between ethically acceptable and unacceptable relationships between physicians and the medical industry? Since physicians consistently underestimate the power of industry, influence of marketing, and the pull of reciprocity to mold their behavior, and since patients need to be able to trust that their physicians will put patients' interests first, it is important to recognize the influential power of marketing and reciprocity in relation to the trust and the fiduciary relationship between health care providers and patients.

To begin, it must be pointed out that multiple studies have shown that the prescribing practices of both residents and veteran practitioners are affected by detailing practices of the medical industry (Wazana, 2000; Schwartz et al., 2001). For example, Chren and Landefeld (1994) found that physicians were 9–21 times more likely to request additions of drugs to hospital formularies after eating a free meal sponsored by a pharmaceutical company. And according to Gibbons and colleagues (1998), patients themselves were able to perceive influences by the medical industry on their physicians that the physicians could not see.

Even more confounding is that physicians do, in fact, perceive industry influence, just not in themselves. For example, a study by Steinman and colleagues (2001) demonstrated that residents perceived their colleagues were *more* influenced by the acceptance of gifts from medical industry than they were. But then, why can physicians see bias in colleagues but not in themselves? For that matter, why can patients see biases that their physicians cannot see? The answer: "self-serving bias," the overestimation of one's objectivity compared with others in the same situation. Such bias becomes a habit – both neuro physiologically and emotive-psychologically. Once self-serving bias occurs, it is very difficult to eradicate (Koriat et al., 1980, Babcock & Loewenstein, 1997).

To put it differently, the thought processes of medical professionals are no different than other humans. Repeated exposure to the same marketing message for a particular drug or device eventually results in mental fatigue, and a mental shortcut from a conscious, controlled to an unconscious, automatic response occurs. As already noted, multiple studies have demonstrated changes in physicians' prescribing practices after repeated exposures to targeted marketing, changes of which the physicians themselves are unaware, and thus without consideration of the moral consequences. So, even though physicians strive to use conscious, controlled responses at all times when caring for patients, as human beings, it would be impossible for all our decisions and behaviors to be so controlled and reflective.

As suggested above, reciprocity is just such a habitual, unconscious response to the actions of others. Research has shown that all human societies, no matter how primitive or advanced, practice some form of reciprocity (Gouldner, 1960), which is centrally important for social rules, ethics, commerce, and social stability (Tiger & Fox, 1998). Why such an impulse exists in humans can be debated, but clearly this impulse to reciprocate is not only a psychological process but has deep moral implications as well.

The moral importance of reciprocity has been considered at least since the time of Aristotle. In a modern framework of reciprocity as a moral concern, ethicist Lawrence Becker (1990) has argued that each agent must operate morally to maintain equilibrium among our exchanges of good (and evils). Each agent should avoid evil because it would result in unhappiness; restitution should be made by the ones who received good or did evil, returns should be fitting and proportional and should be made for the good received – not merely for the good accepted or requested. Retaliation, on Becker's account, is not permitted. Relationships perceived as detrimental should be terminated. The central conclusion that Becker draws in relationship to moral reciprocity is that "right actions" result in a reduction of conflict, and thus, when considering any conflict of interest, one important mark of a "right action" is that it results in reduction of conflict of interest. That is, morally supportable reciprocity requires reflection on what

are the potential consequences of our considerations, with a determined eye towards reducing, not enforcing, conflicts of interest.

Here one important guide is that of "trustworthiness" and maintaining the fiduciary relationship. The patient–physician relationship is an asymmetrical relationship of power, knowledge, and trust (Zaner, 1988). The physician, who comes to the relationship with expertise and authority, is obligated to the patient, who comes with a story of suffering and trust in the physician. This obligation is, in part, one that requires the physician to demonstrate worthiness of that trust both through actions and considerations. Put in more legalistic terms (if one prefers), the physician is the fiduciary (Morreim, 2005), with the obligation of loyalty to the patient (as beneficiary). But whether moral or legal concepts apply, the obligations to patients are clear: in order to maintain the primary interest of patient well-being, conflicts of interests are to be avoided or where unavoidable, intentionally managed and disclosed.

Physicians, industry, and conflicts of interest

Over the past 30 years, the marketing relationships between the medical industry and physicians have intensified – from gift-giving to funded advisory board memberships to sponsored conferences to speakers' bureaus, and more. As a result, some of the ensuing conflicts of interest have resulted in adverse outcomes or the perception of adverse outcomes for patients. Examples of conflicts of interest permeate the medical profession, resulting in a loss of trust by patients in the ability of physicians to act in their best interest. For example, offering free samples of new drugs resulted in brand-name loyalty to medications instead of a preference for the least expensive, effective treatment for patients' ailments. Many residency training programs and continuing medical educational conferences are sustained by contributions from the medical industry. Casting doubt on medical research, the medical literature has been tainted by industry-sponsored clinical trials which produce ghost-written articles, massaged statistics to improve claims of efficacy, suppression of studies demonstrating lack of efficacy, and clinical practice guidelines for best practices whose authors are also paid by pharmaceutical companies (Kassirer, 2005).

It is fair to speculate that almost every physician desires to act in the best interests of patients.

However, doing so can be compromised through any professional relationship with members of medical drug or device companies. While groups like the Accreditation Council for Continuing Medical Education (ACCME), AAMC, and the US Department of Health and Human Services have all produced guidelines/recommendations that define and discuss conflicts of interest, from an ethical point of view, the direct concerns can be characterized simply as both aspirational and confrontational. Conflicts of interest threaten the aspirational attempt always to do what is best for the patient, and confrontationally they could go so far as produce identifiable harm. Either way, ethical peril abounds. When a physician understands how marketing affects thought processes, the physician is in a position to make a controlled decision to limit the context and content of interactions with medical industry. Clearly, voluntary acts of self-interest in light of the known effects of industry detailing would be ethically suspect, at best. However, even involuntary acts must begin to be scrutinized in order to change the habits of self-serving agency that support them. It is not enough, then, simply to say, "I never purposefully change my practices." Instead, we must build new habits of purposeful reflection on our, even unconscious, behavioral motivations. Marketing continues as-is because it works. Because medical industry is beholden to physicians to use their products, physicians are in a strong position to remold their relationships with medical industry in a way that undermines the undue influence of detailing.

After their respective tenures as editors of the *New England Journal of Medicine*, Drs. Marcia Angell (2004) and Jerome Kassirer (2005) each wrote books about conflicts of interest in the relationships between physicians and medical industry that flourished during their tenures. They agreed that the ideal situation for physicians would be to avoid all relationships that posed a conflict of interest, but realized that ideal would be unlikely. They agreed on four strategies to reduce conflicts of interest for physicians, including:

1. no more gifts from medical industry to physicians
2. no more participation in speakers' bureaus
3. no more sales calls by pharmaceutical representatives on academic campuses
4. no more medical industry support of professional medical societies.

In 2006, Brennan et al published a call from the Institute of Medicine to academic institutions to eliminate conflicts of interest with medical industry in their daily practices and to be better role models to their students. In addition to the recommendations made by Angell and Kassirer, the group recommended no more free drug samples, no conflicts of interest related to pharmaceutical companies for physician members of institutional formulary committees, no more direct medical industry support of continuing medical education programs or travel expenses for trainees, no more ghost-written manuscripts, creation of monitoring and enforcement policies at individual institutions, and contracts specifically outlining any financial relationships between physicians and the medical industry. Since the relationships between medical industry, physicians, and medical institutions are complex, the implementation of all of these recommendations remains an unattained goal for many institutions. The ACCME has revised the relationship between medical industry and continuing medical education to separate marketing from education while still allowing interactions of medical industry with medical researchers and practitioners (ACCME, 2007). In response, the pharmaceutical industry has changed some of its marketing practices to comply with the changes made by the ACCME.

Conclusion and suggestions

Since physicians want to (and must) act in the best interests of their patients, there are a few practices that everyone, particularly residents and younger physicians, can adopt to try to avoid/reduce the development of conflicts of interest and self-serving bias. They include (but are not limited to):

1. Accept that conflicts of interest and self-serving bias are going to be a part of the practice of medicine.
2. Avoid interactions with medical industry that involve gifts, food, textbooks, toys or other freely exchanged items from industry. Do not accept trips or honoraria from industry.
3. Discuss new products with sales representatives at an appointed time when patients will not be competing for attention. Then be prepared to listen to the information and ask pertinent questions about efficacy and comparisons to other similar medications, side effects, cost, and

availability to gather more information about the product.

4. Do not participate in speakers' bureaus. Repeating the script written by the company using the company's slides turns the physician into a salesperson for the company's products. The presentations are an advertisement for the company's product.

5. Limit drug sampling, and try to use a variety of similar products by several companies to decrease loyalty to a single brand. Use the samples for people who truly cannot afford to buy medication or as a way to try out the medication to be sure that children in particular can ingest it or sit still for topical applications. Do not use free samples for members of the office staff, family members, or self-medication.

6. When engaging in industry-sponsored research, the agreement should include provisions for doing the research on time so it is useful to the company, use of an independent statistician to assure accuracy of the results, a commitment to reporting negative as well as positive results, listing only the co-authors who contributed meaningfully in writing the paper, disclosure of any conflicts of interest in the consent forms, and recruitment of subjects by people with no conflicts of interest.

7. Read independent evaluations of medical industry drugs and devices for unbiased information. Examples include:

   The Medical Letter (www.medicalletter.com)

   Therapeutics Initiative – Canada (www.ti.ubc.ca)

   Drug and Therapeutics Bulletin – United Kingdom (www.which.net/health/dtb).

References

Accreditation Council for Continuing Medical Education (2007). The ACCME Standards for commercial support: standards to ensure the independence of CME activities. www.accme.org (last accessed November 1, 2010).

Angell, M. (2004). *The Truth About the Drug Companies: How They Deceive Us and What To Do About It*, 2nd edn. New York: Random House.

Association of American Medical Colleges (2008). Industry funding of medical education: Report of an AAMC task force. https://services.aamc.org/publications/showfile.cfm?file=version114.pdf&prd_id=232&prv_id=281&pdf_id=114 (last accessed November 4, 2010).

Babcock, L. & Loewenstein, G. (1997). Explaining bargaining impasse: the role of self-serving biases. *Journal of Economic Perspectives*, **11**(1), 109–126.

Becker, L.C. (1990). *Reciprocity*, 2nd edn. Chicago: University of Chicago Press.

Brennan, T.A., Rothman, D.J., Blank, L., et al. (2006). Health industry practices that create conflicts of interest; a policy proposal for academic medical centers. *JAMA*, **295**(4), 429–433.

Brody, H. (2007). *Hooked: Ethics, the Medical Profession and the Pharmaceutical Industry*. Lanham, MD: Rowman & Littlefield.

Campbell, E.G., Gruen, R.L., Mountford, J., et al. (2007). A national survey of physician-industry relationships. *New England Journal of Medicine*, **356**(17), 1742–1750.

Chren, M.-M. & Landefeld, C.S. (1994). Physicians' behavior and their interactions with drug companies: a controlled study of physicians who requested additions to a hospital drug formulary. *JAMA*, **271**(9), 684–689.

Erde, E.J. (1996). Conflicts of interest in medicine: a philosophical and ethical morphology, In *Conflicts of Interest in Clinical Practice and Research*, ed. R.G. Speece, D.S. Shimm, & A.E. Buchanan. New York: Oxford University Press, 12–41.

Gibbons, R.V., Landry, F.J., Blouch, D.L., et al. (1998). A comparison of physicians' and patients' attitudes toward pharmaceutical industry gifts. *Journal of General Internal Medicine*, **33**(March), 151–154.

Gouldner, A.W. (1960). The norm of reciprocity: a preliminary statement. *American Sociological Review*, **25**(2), 161–178.

Kassirer, J.P. (2005). *On the Take: How Medicine's Complicity with Big Business Can Endanger Your Health*. New York: Oxford University Press.

Koriat, A., Lichtenstein, S., & Fischhoff, B. (1980). Reasons for confidence. *Journal of Experimental Psychology: Human Learning and Memory*, **6**(2), 194–198.

Morreim, E.H. (2005). The clinical investigator as fiduciary: discarding a misguided idea. *Journal of Law, Medicine, and Ethics*, **3**(3), 586–598.

Schwartz, T.L., Kuhles, D.J., Wade, M., & Masand, P.S. (2001). Newly admitted psychiatric patient prescriptions and pharmaceutical sales visits. *Annals of Clinical Psychiatry*, **13**(3), 159–162.

Sernyak, M. & Rosenheck, R. (2007). Experience of VA psychiatrists with pharmaceutical detailing of antipsychotic medications. *Psychiatric Services*, **58**(10), 1292–1296.

Steinman, M.A., Shlipak, M.G., & McPhee, S.J. (2001). Of principles and pens: attitudes and practices of medicine house staff toward pharmaceutical industry promotions. *American Journal of Medicine*, **110**, 551–557.

Strohmetz, D.B., Rind, B., Fisher, R., & Lynn, M. (2002). Sweetening the till: the use of candy to increase restaurant tipping. *Journal of Applied Social Psychology*, **32**(2), 300–309.

Tiger, L. & Fox. R. (1998). *The Imperial Animal.* New Brunswick, NJ: Transaction Publishers.

Wazana, A. (2000). Physicians and the pharmaceutical industry. Is a gift ever just a gift? *JAMA*, **283**(3), 373–380.

Zaner, R.M. (1988). *Ethics and the Clinical Encounter.* Englewood Cliffs, NJ: Prentice Hall.

38

Patient participation in medical training

Armand H. Matheny Antommaria

Case narrative

Tracy, a new intern, is on her first rotation in the busy emergency department. Her third patient is an otherwise healthy 23-day-old female infant with a temperature of 101.3°F. After presenting her history and physical examination findings to her attending physician, she recommends performing a venepuncture, a bladder catheterization, and a lumbar puncture (LP) to obtain specimens for analysis and culture. The attending physician agrees with the plan and asks Tracy whether she is comfortable performing the LP by herself. Tracy observed a number of LPs as a third year medical student, attempted several as a fourth year medical student but does not yet feel proficient. She, however, does not want to seem incapable or to slow her attending physician down. She hesitantly says yes.

After describing the risks, benefits, and alternatives, she obtains consent from the patient's parents who want to stay in the room. Once the technician has drawn the blood and collected the urine, he helps Tracy set up for the procedure. The gown and mask are hot, and combined with her anxiety, make her begin to sweat. The patient is more vigorous than Tracy had anticipated and the technician is having trouble holding her still to Tracy's satisfaction. Her first attempt is unsuccessful and, as she asks for a second LP needle, the patient's father asks Tracy if she has ever done this before. He is concerned that his daughter is experiencing unnecessary pain. Tracy considers how to answer this question, concerned she may lose the opportunity to learn this essential skill.

Patient participation in medical education

Patients participate extensively in the various phases of medical education. Undergraduate premedical students shadow patients' primary care providers observing their clinical encounters. During their physical diagnosis classes, medical students practice taking histories and/or performing physical examinations on hospitalized patients. Medical students, residents, and fellows provide direct patient care as part of larger teams. This may include practicing intimate examinations, invasive procedures, or surgical skills on patients.

It is important to note that, while this discussion will focus on trainees, these issues are not unique to them. Learning is not confined to a particular time at the beginning of one's medical career. Established providers need to learn new techniques. For example, practicing surgeons needed to learn laparoscopic techniques as they were developed. In addition, there may be sufficient variation in providers' performance to raise similar issues about the disclosure of risks and consent (Burger et al., 2007).

Trainees have the opportunity to learn through these practices. Participation in medical education, however, entails potential risks for patients (Gawande, 2002). Observation poses the potential risks of violating patients' privacy and confidentiality. While more experienced medical students and residents contribute to patients' care, they may impose on patients' time. In the middle of the night, parents may object to three separate individuals asking similar questions and performing the same examination on their child who has already waited 6 hours in the emergency department and needs to sleep. Learning procedures may also cause pain or broader harm. If Tracy's patient was pretreated with antibiotics, the cerebral spinal fluid cell count would be particularly important to exclude meningitis because the culture may be uninformative. Tracy may not only be more likely to need several attempts causing additional pain but also be more likely to obtain a

Clinical Ethics in Pediatrics: A Case-Based Textbook, ed. Douglas S. Diekema, Mark R. Mercurio and Mary B. Adam. Published by Cambridge University Press. © Cambridge University Press 2011.

traumatic "tap" making the cell count difficult to interpret. This outcome could potentially necessitate treatment for meningitis because it cannot be excluded. These potential risks vary in both type and magnitude.

Potential conflict of interests

The tension between the duty to care for patients and the need to learn but potentially cause harm creates a conflict of interests. A conflict of interests exists when an individual has a professional duty which may be unduly influenced by a significant personal interest (Beauchamp & Childress, 2009, p. 314). In addition to actual conflicts of interests, there are potential and perceived conflicts of interests. Health care providers have a fiduciary obligation to their patients, meaning they have an obligation to place their patients' interests before their own. Conflicts of interest arise in a variety of circumstances in health care, including when reimbursement systems create personal financial interests or clinical research creates personal financial or intellectual interests.

Conflicts of interest are addressed through disclosure and management. For example, in clinical research, the purposes of the study, its potential benefits and risks, and compensation are disclosed to potential participants. Disclosure reinforces potential participants' autonomy or self-determination by enabling them to decide whether or not to participate. Individuals are not, however, always able to evaluate or compensate for the potential conflict. In some cases, therefore, additional strategies are utilized to manage, mitigate, or eliminate them (Beauchamp & Childress, 2009, p. 316). For example, the health care institutions and the pharmaceutical industry have prohibited certain types of interactions between clinicians and pharmaceutical representatives such as entertaining at sporting events.

Informed consent

One means for managing the potential conflict of interests entailed by patient participation in medical education is disclosure and permitting the patient to decide whether or not to participate as part of the informed consent process. In the informed consent process, providers are generally obligated to disclose the patient's condition, the proposed intervention, its risk and benefits, and the alternatives. There are three major standards for disclosure (Beauchamp & Childress, 2009, pp. 122–124). The professional practice standard requires

providers to disclose what their colleagues would. Current professional practice does not necessarily involve disclosing trainees' participation. This standard is problematic in part because it may be difficult to identify the relevant professional community or its shared practice. More importantly, the simple fact that the practice is shared does not provide an ethical justification for it.

The two alternative standards are the reasonable person and the subjective standards. The reasonable person standard requires one to disclose information that would be relevant to a reasonable person and the subjective standard to disclose information relevant to the particular patient. Individual patients may have particular needs or interests that make certain information relevant to them. A professional pianist with a hand injury, for example, may have greater concerns about the implications of the proposed treatment on his/her dexterity or sensation. While it represents an ideal, the subjective standard is problematic in clinical practice because it may be difficult for providers to anticipate the specific information needs of individual patients. The reasonable person standard is, therefore, preferable.

Analogous to describing the patient's condition, the reasonable person standard would require providers to introduce themselves and explain their level of training and role in the patient's care in addition to the risks and benefits of their participation. The literature suggests that providers often neglect to explain their role in patient care and, even if they do, patients may be unfamiliar with the terminology they use. In an observational study of patient–physician interactions in an emergency department, Santen et al. (2008) found that residents identified themselves as residents only 7% of the time and attending physicians introduced themselves as the supervising physician only 6% of the time. They also found that patients had limited knowledge of the terms the medical profession uses to describe physicians' level of training. For example, only 58% of patients agreed with the statement "A resident has completed medical school." Such introductions, therefore, must rely on simpler language.

Risks

As previously described, the potential risks of participating in medical education include imposition on patients' time, increased discomfort or pain, unsuccessful or inadequate procedures, and iatrogenic injury. Performing pelvic examinations on anesthetized women (Coldicott et al., 2003) and practicing procedures on the newly dead (Berger et al., 2002) are specific topics within this debate that highlight the wide scope of harm that should be considered. At its worst, anesthesia was seen by some as an opportunity to have multiple trainees, including those not directly involved in a patient's care, practice their pelvic examination skills without the woman's knowledge or consent. It was argued that anesthesia made it easier to perform the examination and decreased discomfort to the patient. The primary harms in this case are the affront to the patient's dignity and the potential loss of trust in the medical profession should the patient inadvertently find out after the fact.

The newly dead were seen as an opportunity to practice techniques, such as intubation or cricothyroidotomy, without the risk of harming the patient. Dead bodies, it may be argued, are beyond harm and without rights, and next of kin have limited authority over them. Practicing procedures on the newly dead without consent may also be perceived as demonstrating a lack of respect for the dead and cause a loss of faith in the profession should it be discovered. In addition, it delays allowing the family to view the body and say their goodbyes. While different than physical injury, such affronts to patients' dignity and risks to professional status are nonetheless significant.

Alternatives

Requiring that the participation of trainees be addressed as part of informed consent necessitates that there are true alternatives available. In some cases it may be feasible to have a more senior or experienced team member perform the intervention or procedure him/herself. In others, patients may be admitted to hospitalist teams without housestaff involvement. Identifying alternatives becomes more complex in systems of care that are dependent on trainees. While one might have the attending surgeon perform rather than supervise the surgery, the system may rely on trainees to assist and/or to provide follow-up care. Is an attending surgeon morally obligated to return to the hospital to evaluate a postoperative fever in a patient who refused the participation of residents if the system is designed to rely on residents for in-house call coverage? The alternative in some cases may be the transfer to a nonteaching facility.

In addition to disclosure and informed consent, there are other ways to manage these potential conflicts

of interest. One is to reduce the risks to patients by using other training methods, such as peer teaching, simulated patients, simulation, animal models, and cadavers to prepare students prior to patient contact (Ziv et al., 2003). (It should be noted that these methods, particularly peer teaching and animal models, raise their own ethical concerns.) Another is for training programs to develop formal competence standards for when direct supervision is no longer required. Reliance on time- or volume-based standards is insufficient, as evidence demonstrates that individuals develop competency at varying rates. There are a variety of proposals regarding how competence should be measured, but all require increased data collection (Kestin, 1995).

Objections and replies

There have been a variety of objections to proposals that informed consent be required for patient participation in medical education. The major themes are that patients provide implied or actual consent, patients may already opt out, and that consent is unnecessary. Reasons offered why consent should not be required include that the benefits outweigh the burdens, patients have an obligation to participate in medical education, and requiring consent will undermine medical education. Each of these objections, however, is insufficient (Mercurio, 2008).

Actual or implied consent

Some contend that patients provide implied or actual consent to participation. One version of this claim is that patients, in seeking care at a teaching hospital, have given implied consent. This assertion is unsuccessful because patients lack both the requisite knowledge and choice. Empirical data suggest that patients are unable to differentiate between teaching and nonteaching hospitals and are unfamiliar with the medical education process, including the roles of individuals at different levels of training. In addition, patients may not have control over where they receive treatment. If they require Emergency Medical Services, protocol may require them to be taken to the nearest hospital. More importantly, many patients do not choose their health care insurance, it is provided by their employers. The policies frequently provide strong financial incentives to receive care within specific health care systems. These considerations undermine the contention that patients have adequate information or control to provide implied consent.

Others argue that by signing the general terms of admission, patients provide their actual consent. This "consent" is also not informed. The documents do not specify the potential risk and benefits of participation. In addition, patients are asked to consent to a bundle of requirements at one time rather than individual components. This is coercive.

Opt-out

Informal opt-out systems, where patients are permitted to refuse to participate rather than required to consent, are currently unjust. Historically, participation in medical education was largely determined by the patients' ability to pay. Training occurred primarily at public hospitals. Allocating involvement according to ability to pay is unjust because ability to pay is an ethically irrelevant consideration. Changes in the delivery of health care have changed this practice to some degree. It may, however, persist in informal opt-out systems in which some patients are permitted to refuse the involvement of trainees. This ability is generally reserved for VIP patients or health care providers. For an opt-out system to be fair, all patients would need to be made aware of their ability to refuse.

Consent unnecessary

While the discussion has principally focused on the harms, patients may benefit by participating in medical education. Patients may receive more attention from trainees or be gratified by helping them learn. While the data are equivocal, some argue that patients receive a higher level of care in teaching hospitals. Neither of these arguments is, however, sufficient. The subjective benefit of helping a trainee learn is contingent on consent. Even if there was a preponderance of benefit over burden, arguing that consent is not required is inappropriately paternalistic.

Others contend that consent is unnecessary because patients have an obligation to participate in medical education. This argument takes a variety of forms. (Some parallels can be drawn to the literature on patients' obligation to participate in research [Shapshay & Pimple, 2007]. The major disanalogy is that educational activities are frequently more directly related to patients' treatment.) The first form of the argument focuses on benefits the patients have previously received. Because patients received benefits from medical education in the past, it would be unjust for them not to participate in the present. A second form of the argument focuses on the future benefit to patients. Patients will be dependent on the supply of trained clinicians in the future and, therefore, are obligated to participate in their training now. The third form of the argument focuses on the benefits not to the individual patient him/herself but to other patients. Patients have a duty to help others by helping to maintain the supply of trained physicians. While these arguments may demonstrate that patients have a general duty to participate in medical education, they do not demonstrate that patients have a duty to participate in any or all specific instances of medical education or that this duty should be unilaterally enforced.

Finally, some contend that the requirement to consent is impractical. If consent was required, this argument contends, the number of patients who would refuse would be sufficient to undermine the education process and there would not be an adequate supply of trained physicians. Interpreting data regarding patients' willingness to participate in medical education is complex. Many studies rely on hypothetical situations and patients' responses may not reflect their actual behavior. Better studies seek the informed consent from patients for trainee participation in their actual health care. These include studies of the willingness of patients in emergency departments to have students perform procedures, such as suturing, obtaining intravenous access, and splinting, on them. Santen et al. (2005), for example, found that 90% of patients consented. Such studies suggest that a sufficient number of patients would consent that the system would not be significantly impaired.

Case resolution

Returning to the case, one can imagine the attending physician knowing, based on the residency program records, that Tracy had not yet demonstrated competency in performing lumbar punctures on infants. After agreeing with Tracy's plan, the attending physician might go into the patient's room with Tracy while she sought informed consent from the patient's parents. The conversation would include a discussion of the additional risks and benefits of her performing the procedure such as multiple attempts and greater discomfort. The attending physician might support Tracy by affirming her confidence in Tracy and reinforcing that she will be present during the procedure and will complete it if Tracy is unsuccessful. There is good reason to believe that the parents will agree to let Tracy attempt the lumbar puncture. In another circumstance, such as when the cerebral spinal fluid culture will be pretreated, the attending physician might decide that Tracy's lack of competence precludes her from attempting the procedure.

Conclusion and key points

- Students and other trainees should be adequately prepared before interacting with actual patients. Methods include simulated patients and simulation.
- Attending physicians and training programs should assess trainees' competencies, provide graduated responsibilities, and ensure adequate supervision.
- All providers should introduce themselves to patients and their families. Their introduction should include a description of their level of training and role in patient care.
- Consent should be sought for trainee participation in patient care if it alters the risk–benefit ratio in a way that would be relevant to a reasonable person.
- Systems should provide alternatives to patients who decline to participate in medical education.

References

Beauchamp, T.L. & Childress, J.F. (2009). *Principles of Biomedical Ethics*, 6th edn. New York: Oxford University Press.

Berger, J.T., Rosner, F., & Cassell, E.J. (2002). Ethics of practicing medical procedures on newly dead and nearly dead patients. *Journal of General Internal Medicine*, **17**, 774–778.

Burger, I., Schill, K., & Goodman, S. (2007). Disclosure of individual surgeon's performance rates during informed consent: ethical and epistemological considerations. *Annals of Surgery*, **245**, 507–513.

Coldicott, Y., Pope, C., & Roberts, C. (2003). The ethics of intimate examinations – teaching tomorrow's doctors. *British Medical Journal*, **326**, 97–101.

Gawande, A. (2002). The learning curve. *The New Yorker*, January 28, 52–61. Available at: http://archives.newyorker.com/?i=2002-01-28#folio=060 (last accessed December 3, 2010).

Kestin, I.G. (1995). A statistical approach to measuring the competence of anaesthetic trainees at practical procedures. *British Journal of Anaesthesia*, **75**, 805–809.

Mercurio, M.R. (2008). An analysis of candidate ethical justifications for allowing inexperienced physicians-in-training to perform invasive procedures. *Journal of Medicine and Philosophy*, **33**, 44–57.

Santen, S.A., Hemphill, R.R., Spanier, C.M., et al. (2005). "Sorry, it's my first time!" Will patients consent to medical students learning procedures? *Medical Education*, **39**, 365–369.

Santen, S.A., Rotter, T.S., & Hemphill, R.R. (2008). Patients do not know the level of training of their doctors because doctors do not tell them. *Journal of General Internal Medicine*, **23**, 607–610.

Shapshay, S. & Pimple K.D. (2007). Participation in biomedical research is an imperfect moral duty: a response to John Harris. *Journal of Medical Ethics*, **33**, 414–417.

Ziv, A., Wolpe, P.R., Small, S.D., et al. (2003). Simulation-based medical education: an ethical imperative. *Academic Medicine*, **78**, 783–788.

Chapter 39

Boundary issues in pediatrics

Ian R. Holzman

Case narrative

Sally will be completing her pediatric residency in 2 months and will be starting a fellowship in pediatric infectious diseases at the same medical center. Her husband, Ben, is a violinist with the local symphony orchestra. They have a 23-month-old daughter, Eve. Eve receives her medical care from a pediatric solo practitioner, Dr. Kaplan, who Sally met during her first rotation in the well baby nursery where he was her teaching attending physician.

One Friday evening, after a particularly long and difficult day at the hospital, Sally comes home and finds that her daughter seems irritable, doesn't want to eat and might have a fever (she opts not to take Eve's temperature since Eve usually has a temper tantrum around having her temperature taken and Sally doesn't have the energy for a fight). Ben hasn't noticed anything unusual and is getting ready to go off to a performance where he has a solo part. Sally decides to perform a quick exam rather than bothering Dr. Kaplan who would likely send them to the emergency room. Although Eve is not very cooperative, Sally thinks she might have a red throat and some swollen lymph nodes (although her exam was less than optimal) and decides to start an antibiotic that she happens to have sitting in the medicine cabinet.

Eve eventually goes to sleep but awakes a few times and still seems warm. The next morning Eve isn't really better but Sally decides to give the antibiotics some time to work. Although Ben suggests they call Dr. Kaplan, Sally is reluctant to bother him, especially now that she has begun antibiotic treatment and feels confident in her ability to diagnose strep throat. On Sunday, Eve seems more lethargic and Ben decides to call Dr. Kaplan, just to "make sure" everything is being done correctly. Dr. Kaplan seems very concerned and

suggests he meet them at the emergency department. Sally bristles at the suggestion but finally agrees to go to the emergency room. Eve is diagnosed with bacterial meningitis and admitted to the hospital.

Introduction

All physicians are held to a variety of professional standards both for their medical competence and for their behavior. Some standards are directed specifically to one or another specialty while others can be generalized to anyone caring for patients. Pediatricians (and the pediatric surgical subspecialties) routinely interact with a patient and members of the patient's family, adding another dimension to their practices. The complex web of relationships connecting the pediatrician with her patient, the patient's family, and others in the community plays an important role in the consideration of issues requiring limits or boundaries to be set. It is part of a pediatrician's role as a professional to recognize important responsibilities to patients and families that include a collaborative relationship with the patient and family (Fallat et al., 2007). In this chapter, we will examine a number of "boundary issues" including the provision of care to one's own children, other family members, and the children of close friends; romantic relationships with family members of patients; the acceptance of gifts from patients and families; and political petitions in the office setting.

Providing medical care to one's children and the children of close relatives and friends

The case of Sally, Ben, and Eve captures some of the important problems with providing medical care for family members and the children of close friends. Sally

Clinical Ethics in Pediatrics: A Case-Based Textbook, ed. Douglas S. Diekema, Mark R. Mercurio and Mary B. Adam. Published by Cambridge University Press. © Cambridge University Press 2011.

is a dedicated and good physician who wants to do the right thing. She has a particular interest in infectious diseases and is likely to be knowledgeable in the management of streptococcal pharyngitis. Her husband, Ben, knows little about medicine and appropriately trusts his wife's judgment. Eve's pediatrician is someone Sally trusts but Sally's relationship with Dr. Kaplan leads her to want to be protective of his time. So what went awry?

Providing medical care for one's own children, relatives, and close friends is an issue that confronts most physicians (La Puma et al., 1991; La Puma & Priest, 1992; Dusdieker et al., 1993; Reagan et al., 1994). Survey studies (Walter et al., 2009, 2010) of physicians indicate that physicians often do provide such care. Why, then, is this a potential problem? The feelings a pediatrician has for their patients are described as caring and empathetic, but this is not the same as the more complex feelings we have for our own children and loved ones (Mailhot, 2002). The personal emotional impact of diagnosing a serious illness is far greater in the case of a loved one than a patient, no matter how much concern we have for our patients. Pediatricians are very unlikely to remain totally objective when dealing with family members and close friends. Depending on the specific circumstances, it is possible that the pediatrician/parent will function with incomplete information (a complete history and physical examination will not be done). When dealing with an adolescent (either one's own child or the child of a close friend or relative) it is likely that patient will withhold relevant but sensitive information. While the good pediatrician strives to obtain information on "drugs, sex, and rock and roll" when they have a trusting and confidential relationship with their adolescent patients, obtaining the same information from an adolescent patient with whom the physician has a close personal relationship may prove more challenging.

If there are fundamental problems with providing such care, why does this occur so commonly? The leading explanation given by pediatricians is convenience (Walter et al., 2009). For Sally, her husband was leaving for work and she was exceedingly tired after a busy day. Furthermore, Dr. Kaplan's office was closed (the second most common reason for treating one's own child is symptoms occurring after hours) and a trip to the emergency room seemed daunting. Sally certainly felt that she could identify strep throat and knew the treatment. Confidence in one's own diagnostic and treatment skills is a third commonly cited reason that

physicians treat a family member (Walter et al., 2009). While it is commonly acknowledged that the physician who self-treats has a fool for a patient, many physicians fail to recognize that the same rule may extend to treating family members and, in this case, one's child.

Sally's good judgment was clouded by fatigue as well as the teacher–student relationship that Sally had with Dr. Kaplan. While the literature clearly demonstrates how commonly physicians provide care to family members, the pediatrician must be aware of this boundary issue and, as such, should remain alert to the dangers it presents. Given the high prevalence of physicians treating family members and children of friends and family, the most practical solution is to limit such treatment to minor conditions (and emergencies). Diagnosis and treatment that falls under the general rubric of "first aid" and/or common knowledge is less concerning than the kind of diagnosis and intervention normally performed only by a licensed physician. Sally "thought" her daughter might have had streptococcal pharyngitis but she really wasn't sure. Starting antibiotics was something she would not have done or recommended for a patient in her office. The next morning she should have called Dr. Kaplan and let him take over the care of Eve. Had she told him her diagnosis wasn't "firm," that she knew the use of antibiotics in that particular setting might not be appropriate, and that Eve still seemed less active, he certainly would have suggested she bring Eve into the office for a quick exam and confirmation of the diagnosis and appropriate treatment. Even in a situation where an appropriate physician is either far away or not available, the responsibility to contact the child's primary care physician and inform that person of what you have diagnosed and how you are treating it rests with the parent/pediatrician. While such contact might not easily prevent the rare case of misdiagnosis and/or mistreatment, it will improve continuity of care and assure that the child's medical record is complete. If the pediatrician does not have a record of illnesses and/or treatments provided by the parent/physician, the pediatrician will be less able to make appropriate medical decisions in the future.

Intimate relationships with patients and family members of patients

The obvious prohibition of any romantic or sexual relationship between a pediatrician and the child in the care of the pediatrician requires little discussion. Such a relationship prevents the pediatrician from providing rational and impartial care to the child/patient, is likely to be illegal in the vast majority of cases, and would almost certainly represent an abuse of power in the physician–patient relationship that would ultimately cause harm to the patient. It is hard to imagine a scenario where it would be acceptable in pediatric practice. The use of an appropriate chaperone (Feldman et al., 2009) when indicated and a heightened sensitivity to this issue when performing sensitive portions of the exam are crucial. Although less common, there is also an issue as to whether a physician should have a romantic or sexual relationship with a former pediatric patient who has reached adulthood. The American College of Obstetricians and Gynecologists (2007) has stated that such a relationship may also be unethical because of "the former patient's feeling of dependency, obligation or gratitude (as well as) the former patient's vulnerability." Similar issues likely exist for pediatricians.

A relationship with a parent or guardian of a child who resides in the pediatrician's practice presents an even more complex situation. The pediatrician is expected to provide unbiased and unemotional care for the young patient. We have already seen how difficult this may be for a pediatrician when caring for one's own children. The same lack of objectivity can easily arise in a setting in which the pediatrician is having a relationship with the patient's parent or guardian. Families expect the pediatrician's office to provide a safe environment dedicated to the care of their child. From that perspective it is easy to see that any romantic or sexual advance by a pediatrician to a parent or guardian irrevocably changes the dynamic of a patient visit. This is often the case even when a parent or guardian makes personal advances toward the pediatrician. If a pediatrician believes that the "agenda" of an office visit or repeated visits is other than the care of the child, it is imperative that the pediatrician bring this concern to the parent or guardian privately. If there is an admission of romantic feelings on either side, it is probably best to insist that the child receive medical care from a different provider and arrangements for such a transfer of care should be undertaken. Separate documentation of this plan should be kept by the pediatrician, and every attempt to prevent the child from becoming harmed in these interactions is mandatory.

Changing providers may eliminate any potential problem; however, such a solution may be impractical in an area with limited pediatrician availability. Rural providers in particular may raise the valid concern that strictly prohibiting any personal relationship with the parent of a patient may represent an unfair impingement upon the personal life of the pediatrician. A pediatrician in a sparsely populated rural area who is interested in finding a partner is likely to have a limited number of possible people with whom to interact. While there may not be a simple answer to this very complex boundary issue, openness and transparency may possibly prevent inappropriate medical decisions that could impact a child's care. The older the pediatric patient is, the more likely that a relationship with a parent or guardian will result in unintended consequences for the patient. Providing medical care for an adolescent is often a complex process. Caring for an adolescent who believes their pediatrician is romantically involved with a parent or guardian may create an uncomfortable situation for the adolescent patient. Regardless of whether there is any justification for such a relationship to continue, it is imperative that the issues be brought into the open in order to assure the patient receives optimal medical care. In most cases, transfer of the child's care to another doctor would be the best solution. When confronted with this complex boundary issue, it is important for the pediatrician to be aware of the potential impact on the child as well as the possible need for independent counseling services.

Gifts from patients and their families

The majority of pediatricians are likely to have received gifts at some time from patients' families (Nadelson & Notman, 2002; Gaufberg, 2007). In most cases, such gifts are small, socially acceptable, and very consistent with local custom. They are viewed by all concerned as personal thank-you gestures that are intended to convey no more than gratitude. Accepting such gifts is not a violation of professional boundaries. Nevertheless, there are gifts that do present significant problems for the pediatrician. From the outset, it is clear that there is not a single bright line indicating whether a gift is small, inconsequential, and appropriate to accept as opposed to when a gift should be rejected because of its value. Between cookies and a car there is a vast middle ground. Geographic location, the social strata and means of employment of families in the practice, and local custom all play a role in evaluating the appropriateness of a gift. If a gift seems inappropriate or if the physician would not want others to know about it, the physician should be wary of accepting it. It is worth considering the option of asking the person to consider donating an equivalent monetary amount to charity as an acknowledgment of their appreciation.

The fundamental ethical concern that accompanies the acceptance of gifts by a physician relates to the influence the gift may have on the care the child/patient receives. Every patient deserves the best medical care the pediatrician can provide, and no gift should be required to obtain that care. From the pediatrician's perspective, does offer of a "large" gift seem intended to obligate the pediatrician to do something above and beyond regular care? What if the gift giver requested a home visit the next time their child was ill? While more convenient for the family, does it represent "better" care, especially since neither normal office equipment nor the complete medical record will be available? But that really isn't the major problem. When accepting a valuable gift leaves the physician feeling obligated to accede to special requests in the future, the situation, as in many boundary issues, can cloud one's judgment. The physician may feel obliged to prescribe antibiotics when they are not indicated, forgo an uncomfortable diagnostic procedure, or overlook issues of neglect or abuse. Gifts naturally invoke a sense of obligation on the part of the person receiving the gift. It takes a keen awareness of these issues, at the outset, to prevent the pediatrician from being placed in an untenable position.

A secondary issue raised by gift-giving is the possibility that the gift is not being given out of gratitude or the wish to "buy" better care, but is part of a desire for a potentially inappropriate relationship. As discussed earlier, this is clearly a significant boundary issue that the pediatrician must confront. The pediatrician should always ask whether her own behavior is in any way responsible for eliciting the gift. If the pediatrician believes she might have done something that the parent is misinterpreting, it is important to discuss this with the parent so that no further misinterpretation is possible. Defining and clarifying boundary issues is essential if they are to be well managed.

Political and policy issues in the office

A final boundary issue worth examining is one that has not received much attention, but may be increasingly important in a politically divided environment. Is a pediatrician's office an appropriate place for political (loosely defined to include a number of polarizing issues such as gun control, abortion, and immunizations) petitions? We have already seen how complex the interactions among physicians, families, and patients can be. Is there a problem with the pediatrician making her political leanings known? Clearly pediatricians have every right to have political and societal views, belong to one or another party, campaign for candidates, run for office, and attend rallies (Gruen et al., 2006). There is nothing about being a professional that restricts political activism. If a physician chooses an unpopular stance or candidate, his patients (or their families) can choose to continue using his services or pick a different pediatrician. If there is no other accessible pediatrician they can avoid starting political discussions with the physician and limit office visits to medical issues and pleasantries about family or the weather (the norm for a visit anyway).

Physicians should in general avoid initiating discussions of politics with their patients and families. Asking a patient or parent to reveal their political opinions in the office setting can make the members of the family feel very uncomfortable and should be avoided. Patients choose to receive medical care from a professional whom they trust and with whom they want to be in a trusting and caring relationship. If this physician's political opinions are similar to the parent's, that may have contributed to a parent's or patient's decision to seek care from him. Nevertheless, it is appropriate that medical care and politics remain separate endeavors. Physicians appropriately advocate for political issues and candidates, but these activities should be kept separate from the office and the patient care visit.

A clear boundary issue occurs when there is an expectation that a patient or family will support, in writing, a particular position that the pediatrician supports (gun control, abortion, legalizing drugs, banning required immunizations, etc.). A petition clearly displayed in the waiting room or given to a patient by the receptionist oversteps the boundary of professionalism. It places the patient or family member in the position of being concerned about how the doctor will respond to them if they refuse to sign the petition and clearly indicates a lack of respect for the autonomy of the patient or family member. Whether or not a patient's concerns about how the doctor will treat them are real, the mere possibility of a negative outcome raises this to the level of a serious boundary issue. A prominently displayed sign as one walks into the office that announces that Dr. Q would prefer only to care for patients or families who believe in X, Y, or Z would also be blatantly unprofessional. Such a notice posted at a physician's office would raise a valid concern on the part of patients and families as to whether the pediatrician can provide unbiased care to those who disagree politically.

Conclusion

We have examined four separate boundary issues that may confront pediatricians in their practice of medicine. While each has unique aspects, they share the common theme of requiring pediatricians to be constantly aware of the personal boundaries that might affect the practice of pediatrics. Caring for family members and children of close friends is a very common occurrence that requires a fair amount of self-reflection and understanding to prevent mishaps that can cause serious medical harm. Romantic or sexual relationships with family members of patients and former patients could well be more common than realized. While these relationships may not be totally preventable, an awareness of the possible adverse effects they might have on the medical care of patients is critical. Accepting gifts is likely a universal occurrence. Inappropriately large gifts present unique challenges that require careful scrutiny of the possible future consequences and should almost always be refused. The last boundary issue, political pressure in the office setting, is, remarkably, an unexplored issue that could have a negative impact on the health care of patients and represents on unprofessional lack of awareness of the importance of respect for individuals in the practice of medicine.

References

American College of Obstetricians and Gynecologists (2007). Sexual misconduct. *Obstetrics and Gynecology*, 110, 441–443.

Dusdieker, L.B., Murph, J.R., Murph, W.E., & Dungy, C.I. (1993). Physicians treating their own children. *American Journal of Diseases of Childhood*, 147, 146–149.

Fallat, M. E., Glover, J., & The Committee on Bioethics, American Academy of Pediatrics (2007). Professionalism in pediatrics. *Pediatrics*, 120(4), e1123–e1133.

Feldman, K.W., Jenkins, C., Laney, T., & Seidel, K. (2009). Towards instituting a chaperone policy in outpatient pediatric clinics. *Child Abuse and Neglect*, 33, 709–716.

Gaufberg, E. (2007). Should physicians accept gifts from patients? *American Family Physician*, 76, 437–438.

Gruen, R.L., Campbell, E.G., & Blumenthal, D. (2006). Public roles of US physicians: community participation, political involvement and collective advocacy. *Journal of the American Medical Association*, 296, 2467–2475.

La Puma, J. & Priest, E.R. (1992). Is there a doctor in the house: an analysis of the practice of physicians treating their own families. *Journal of the American Medical Association*, 267, 1810–1812.

La Puma, J., Stocking, C.B., LaVoie, D., & Darling, C.A. (1991). When physicians treat members of their own families. Practices in a community hospital. *New England Journal of Medicine*, 325, 1290–1294.

Mailhot, M. (2002). Caring for our own families. *Canadian Family Physician*, 48, 546–547.

Nadelson, C. & Notman, M.T. (2002). Boundaries in the doctor-patient relationship. *Theoretical Medicine*, 23, 191–201.

Reagan, B., Reagan, P., & Sinclair, A. (1994). Common sense and thick hide. Physicians providing care to their own family members. *Archives of Family Medicine*, 3, 599–614.

Walter, J.K., Pappano, E., & Ross, L.F. (2009). A descriptive and moral evaluation of providing informal medical care to one's own children. *Journal of Clinical Ethics*, 20, 353–361.

Walter, J.K., Lang, C.W., & Ross, L.F. (2010). When physicians forego the doctor-patient relationship, should they elect to self-prescribe or curbside? An empirical and ethical analysis. *Journal of Medical Ethics*, 36, 19–23.

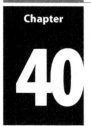

40

The impaired, incompetent, or unethical provider

Jennifer Guon and Douglas S. Diekema

Case narrative

A pediatric resident is seeing a 4-month-old female who is post-op from pyloric stenosis repair. The child presents with a high fever and no obvious signs of infection. Because of her post-op status, the general surgery resident is seeing the patient along with the pediatric resident in the emergency department. Both of the residents believe the child needs to have a catheterized urine specimen collected, but have been unsuccessful at performing the procedure because the child has labial adhesions. As both residents stand over the child, the surgical resident looks at the pediatric resident and says, "We need the urine sample, and there is an easy way to fix this." He grasps the labia and pulls them apart, leaving a raw, bleeding labial surface. He then walks out of the room. When the pediatric resident asks her attending physician for advice, she is told to make no mention of the event in the chart and to say nothing to the family.

Introduction

Responding to other physicians whose behavior or clinical practice appears incompetent or unethical presents many difficult challenges. Many physicians feel some duty of loyalty to their peers. Minimally, this duty requires that physicians not take action that may harm a colleague's career unless there is sufficient evidence to justify that action. At the same time, clinicians have an independent obligation to protect patients who may be receiving substandard care.

The medical field is, in theory, intended to be a self-regulating profession. The idea of self-regulation originates from the idea that medical professionals are best suited to both establish and to monitor each other's compliance with a specific set of professional values (Wynia, 2010). Despite this belief in self-regulation,

a recent study in *The Journal of the American Medical Association* discovered that out of 1120 physicians surveyed, only 64% agreed that there is a professional commitment to report significantly impaired or otherwise incompetent physicians. Only 69% of physicians reported feeling prepared to adequately deal with incompetent colleagues. Furthermore, of those reporting personal and direct knowledge of an incompetent colleague in their hospital, group, or practice, one third failed to report this colleague to the relevant authorities (DesRoches et al., 2010).

This chapter explores the ethical issues that arise when a physician becomes aware of a colleague who has delivered substandard care or behaved in a way that appears to be unethical. Three main issues to be considered include: (1) how to determine when intervention is necessary; (2) how to balance the ethical obligations owed to colleagues against the ethical obligations owed to patients; and (3) identifying actionable strategies available to providers when it appears that a colleague has delivered substandard care.

Identifying incompetent or unethical behavior

Before considering the ethical challenges that arise after witnessing a physician's incompetent or unethical behavior, it is first necessary to determine whether the physician's actions may properly be categorized as incompetent or unethical. A proper assessment of the surrounding facts should precede any decision to intervene in another physician's practice. Several questions might be helpful:

1. Do you know for certain who is responsible for the behavior in question?

2. Are you certain that the decisions made constitute a violation of well-accepted standards of practice?

3. Is there a genuine impropriety and to what degree?

4. Are there data that support any contention that the behavior or approach in question violates good medical practice or causes harm to patients?

It is important to remember that not all adverse outcomes are due to physician incompetence. A witnessing physician must first distinguish between disagreements over reasonable medical alternatives and actions that other reasonable physicians would not be willing to defend, such as those that fall below the standard of care.

Judgments about competence can be difficult in medicine because in many cases there is not a clear consensus on a single best approach to a given problem. In determining whether unethical or incompetent behavior has occurred, Haavi Morreim (1993) suggests five categories of medical decision-making that might result in an adverse patient outcome. These range from events completely outside the physician's control, to gross violations in medical decision-making and the standard of care:

1. Adverse events that occur completely independent of the actions of the provider. An example would be a parent giving their child an overdose of medicine at home despite thorough instructions and proper dosing by the physician.

2. Adverse events that occur despite the physician following standard practice, such as side effects resulting from medication administered in the usual manner.

3. Situations where good physicians disagree about the proper course of action. In these situations, one physician may not manage a patient the same way as a colleague, but most would recognize that each physician is nonetheless practicing in an acceptable fashion.

4. Situations in which a physician exercises poor, but not horrible, judgment or skill. All physicians do this from time to time. These are cases where an isolated mistake has occurred, but absent a pattern, we do not identify this physician as being incompetent.

5. Egregious violations of the accepted standard of care. Here, nearly all physicians would agree that the physician acted below the accepted standard of care.

If the observed medical care fits into one of the first three categories, the provider has acted reasonably.

Even if there is a bad outcome, we should not consider the physician to have acted incompetently. The last two categories represent situations in which lapses in judgment occurred and education or correction may be appropriate. In the case we have presented, the surgeon's behavior falls into one of these latter two categories. It is generally not recommended that fused labia be pulled apart because it is painful, it leaves the formerly fused surfaces raw and bleeding, and the labia frequently fuse together again. Was his behavior simply misguided? Did the provider simply not know better? If that is the case, education may be sufficient. If it was a case of simply not knowing better, is there a pattern of behavior suggesting that he may not be capable of practicing safely? On the other hand, if this represents willful disregard of standard of care, punishment or discipline may be appropriate.

Ethical considerations

Over time, the physician's role has morphed into that of both healer and professional. The healer acts to treat the sick whereas the professional is expected to take part in maintaining the standards of those who practice medicine (Cruess & Cruess, 1997). Physicians have duties to their patients, to the public, and to their colleagues. While there is a duty not to harm the reputation or career of other physicians without sufficient justification, the physician's duty is first and foremost to his or her patient and the public. This duty requires taking action when confronted with another physician who shows a pattern of incompetent or unethical behavior. This is for good reason: viewed as both the healer and professional, physicians are entrusted to assess and report their colleagues because, as is the case in most professions, those outside of the profession such as patients often have insufficient knowledge to know when a physician's actions fall short (Dwyer, 1994). One could also argue that a physician's duty to his or her colleagues includes making sure that they practice medicine according to accepted standards.

The duty of care and duty to report exists not just among colleagues of equal standing, but may extend to residents and medical students when faced with senior physicians who are observed practicing clearly incompetent or unethical medicine. Occasionally, residents will disagree with an attending physician. In one survey, 89% of housestaff reported one or more ethical disagreements in the preceding year with attending physicians. In contrast, only 20% of faculty surveyed could recall a situation in the previous year in which a house officer had been troubled by an ethical disagreement with them regarding patient care. Only one-third of residents had discussed their disagreement with the attending physician (Shreves & Moss, 1996).

James Dwyer (1994) discusses the ethical principle *"primum non tacere"* ("do not be silent") – the obligation to speak up when something wrong has been done. The danger of a resident or medical student speaking up is, of course, that doing so may not be well received by a superior and could place the resident or student at risk of repercussions. The increased vulnerability to adverse consequences does not remove a trainee's ethical duty to report. Failure to speak up about a superior may, in fact, create practical problems for the trainee if it is later determined that the trainee was aware of a problem and covered it up. Maintaining silence (or failing to document anything on the chart as the pediatric resident was advised in this case) may not only represent a failure to care, but may result in legal liability for medical negligence or fraudulent concealment. Confronting a superior requires the virtues of courage and discernment. While trivial or reasonable disagreements do not merit further action, if the patient has been or may be caused substantial harm, a duty exists to advocate on his or her behalf.

How to intervene: suggestions for process and procedure

Once it has been determined that the physician has not adhered to a reasonable standard of care, the correct treatment and steps may differ depending on whether the physician is impaired, incompetent, or acted unethically. The American Medical Association (AMA) (2004) clearly outlines the reporting obligations of a physician witnessing an impaired, incompetent, or unethical colleague based on the duty to protect patients from harm.

An impaired physician is one who is unable to practice medicine with reasonable skill and safety because of physical or mental illness such as addiction or depression. In the case of mental illness or addiction, a proper evaluation and formal treatment program may allow recovery of skills. A colleague may have both an ethical and legal duty to report an impaired physician if that physician continues to practice despite offers of assistance and referral to a physician state health program (American Medical Association, 2004).

Incompetent behavior occurs when a physician provides substandard medical care out of ignorance or lack of skill that is not the result of physical or mental illness. Many physicians occasionally make a mistake out of ignorance or lack of skill and can be readily corrected through education. This education can often occur on the spot or at a later time. As discussed above, more global incompetence occurs when a physician demonstrates a pattern of ignorant or unskillful practice, and may not be as easily correctable by simply providing education at the time (Morreim, 1993). According to the AMA, incompetence that poses an "immediate threat to the health and safety of patients should be reported directly to the state licensing board" (American Medical Association, 2004).

Unethical behavior occurs when a physician knowingly and willfully violates fundamental and well-accepted norms of conduct toward others, especially his or her patients (Morreim, 1993). Unethical conduct should be reported to the proper clinical authority and if such conduct violates state licensing or criminal statutes, the physician should be reported to the proper state licensing board or law enforcement authorities (American Medical Association, 2004).

It is important to recognize that most states have programs for impaired physicians in need of assistance. The Federation of State Physician Health Programs website (2010) is a useful tool for locating each state's resources. The types of programs offered will vary in each state. Some state resources are limited to chemical dependency programs whereas other states cover a variety of programs ranging from chemical dependency to mental and behavioral health assistance.

Case resolution and discussion

Although a physician's first duty is always to the patient and her family, there is a corresponding duty to establish whether or not the surgical resident's actions did in fact breach some well-established standard of care or ethics before reporting his behavior or discussing it with the family. It is generally recommended that fused labia not be pulled apart because it is painful, and the labia are likely to fuse again. If any treatment is recommended for labial adhesions, it is the application of small amounts of estrogen cream. The surgical resident in this situation caused pain to the baby by pulling the labia apart that will persist until the raw surfaces have healed. Furthermore, except in emergency situations where a child's life is imminently threatened, or a delay would result in significant suffering or risk to the child, the physician cannot do something to a child without the permission of the child's parent or guardian. Touching without consent is considered a battery under the law. Therefore in this case, the surgical resident did something that is not accepted as good medical care, caused pain to the baby, and did so without permission of the parents.

Once it has been established that the surgical resident's actions fell below the standard of care, a proper evaluation of his behavior is necessary to determine whether he was simply ignorant of the proper standard of care or whether these actions constitute unethical behavior. If the surgical resident's behavior can be readily corrected through education, your duty may not require reporting to anyone else. If, however, your attempt to address this directly with the surgical resident has been unsuccessful, you should now report his actions to a higher level. Residents should first report to their attending or supervising physician, or may also contact the Chief Resident, the Housestaff Director, or an ethics consultant. Attending physicians might contact a division head, department head, ethics consultant, or Medical Director.

Finally, the parents should be informed of the error. Their child now has raw, bleeding labial surfaces that require explanation and some instruction for how to care for them. Although the parents may think that this was standard practice, it would be improper not to inform them otherwise. The parents may be informed of the resident's actions in a way that does not place blame. For example, one might say, "I think it's important for you to know that I would have done this differently. I don't generally recommend that anyone pull apart labia that are fused, because it hurts and it is not necessary. The other doctor apparently felt differently, and I've expressed my concerns to him." The proper course of action requires the colleague to first assess whether the resident's actions conformed to a proper standard of care, educating the resident if his actions constituted incompetence, and finally reporting him to a higher authority if education is deemed insufficient.

References

American Medical Association (2004). Opinion 9.031: Reporting Impaired, Incompetent, or Unethical Colleagues. Available at www.ama-assn.org/ama/pub/physician-resources/medical-ethics/code-medical-ethics/opinion9031.shtml (last accessed September 21, 2010).

Cruess, R. & Cruess, S. (1997). Teaching medicine as a profession in the service of healing. *Academic Medicine*, **72**, 941–952.

DesRoches, C.M., Rao, S.R., Fromson, J.A., et. al. (2010). Physicians' perceptions, preparedness for reporting, and experiences related to impaired and incompetent colleagues. *JAMA*, **304**, 187–193.

Dwyer, J. (1994). Primum non tacere: an ethics of speaking up. *Hastings Center Report*, **24**(1), 13–18.

Federation of State Physician Health Programs (2010). State programs. Available at www.fsphp.org/State_Programs.html.

Morreim, E.H. (1993). Am I my brother's warden? Responding to the unethical or incompetent colleague. *Hastings Center Report*, **23**, 19–27.

Shreves, J.G. & Moss, A.H. (1996). Residents' ethical disagreements with attending physicians: an unrecognized problem. *Academic Medicine*, **10**, 1103–1105.

Wynia, M.K. (2010). The role of professionalism and self-regulation in detecting impaired or incompetent physicians. *JAMA*, **304**, 210–212.

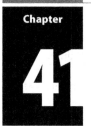

Ethics committees and consultation services

41

Denise M. Dudzinski

Case narrative

Baby Zelda's 18-year-old mother had complications during pregnancy that included a urinary tract infection, prolonged ruptured amniotic membranes, fetal distress, and amnionitis. Baby Zelda was born prematurely at 25 weeks gestational age and was resuscitated and ventilated at birth. She needed antibiotics, transfusions, vasopressors, and analgesia. About a week after birth she developed necrotizing enterocolitis. Surgeons found an irreversibly non-functioning bowel with such extensive intestinal involvement that surgical resection could neither extend nor improve the quality of her life. Her pain, manifested in grimaces and writhing movements, was escalating despite aggressive pain management, and peritonitis developed. All members of her care team favored shifting to comfort care. They recommended that invasive and uncomfortable medical interventions be forgone and all therapies serve a single purpose – to keep Baby Zelda as comfortable as possible for the duration of her short life. Baby Zelda's bedside nurses agreed that her pain was "as bad as anyone can remember for a patient in this NICU" (McCormick & Woodrum, 2008, p. 22). Baby Zelda's young parents, self-described as "poor and used to living a simple rural life," were stunned and believed Zelda would improve if aggressive medical treatment continued. As often happens, the providers continued life-sustaining treatment for several days to give Zelda's grieving, devastated parents time to come to terms with the tragedy. When Zelda's parents were unwavering in their insistence on continuing aggressive treatment indefinitely, the care team requested an ethics consultation (case, described above, comes from McCormick & Woodrum, 2008, p. 26).

What is an ethics consultation?

An ethics consultation is a service provided to patients, surrogates, parents, health care providers, and others involved in patient care to address "uncertainty or conflict regarding value-laden issues that emerge in health care" (Task Force on The Core Competencies for Healthcare Ethics Consultation, 2011). The goals of ethics consultation are to: (1) identify and analyze the ethical issues in clinical cases, policies, or practices; (2) facilitate conflict resolution in the interest of achieving ethically sound consensus; and (3) give those involved tools and information to assist them in addressing ethical issues in health care (Task Force on The Core Competencies for Healthcare Ethics Consultation, 2011).

In Zelda's case, parents and providers held different opinions about the best course of treatment. Both Zelda's parents and the members of her care team were moral agents – responsible for decisions that affect the baby. Therefore all parties wanted to make the best decisions they could. Ethics consultants can help them identify ethical issues, areas of agreement, points of disagreement, and potential compromises and resolutions.

Requesting an ethics consultation

Ethics consultations are typically available in acute care facilities, hospices, and some clinics. The consultant is either paged or a contact number is provided. Some services are available 24 hours a day/7 days a week, while others may only be available during normal business hours.

When an ethics consultant is paged, s/he will return the page in a matter of minutes or hours. Institutions' policies may specify how quickly an ethics page will be returned, but usually a response can be expected

---

Clinical Ethics in Pediatrics: A Case-Based Textbook, ed. Douglas S. Diekema, Mark R. Mercurio and Mary B. Adam. Published by Cambridge University Press. © Cambridge University Press 2011.

within the day. Ethics consultations can take hours or days to complete, since consultants need to speak with many individuals and schedule a meeting with busy providers. An ethics consultant will talk with the caller to ascertain the reason for the call and the patient it pertains to, the ethical issue the caller would like to address, the other providers and family members who should be included, and the caller's perspective on the issues. The consultant will also determine whether the parents have been informed of the consultation and whether a referral to another service, such as palliative care, is in order.

Patients, parents, family, and surrogates should be (and usually are) permitted to request an ethics consultation (Fox et al., 2007); however, this is less common than requests from health care providers. Information about how to request a consultation is often included in patient and staff information. Parents can also ask a nurse or social worker to page the ethics consultant for them.

Models for ethics consultation

There are three common models for ethics consultation services: individual consultant, full ethics committee, and subcommittee models. Consultation is often provided by individuals employed or contracted by the health care institution. Doctors, nurses, social workers, chaplains, philosophers, theologians, and bioethicists serve as ethics consultants. Most volunteer or are paid modestly to provide part-time consultation; however, some institutions, academic medical centers, and health systems employ full-time ethicists. In responding to a call, consultants review the medical record and usually write a note. In the pediatric setting, the consultant works with parents and providers to determine whether and how to include the patient in the consultation.

According to a 2000 survey of ethics committees, 5% of consultants had completed a fellowship or graduate degree program in bioethics, 41% were trained through formal mentoring from an experienced committee member, and 45% learned independently (which may include self-study, continuing education, and certificate programs) (Fox et al., 2007). Ideally, consultants should have some formal bioethics training as well as mentoring; however, lack of funding and the volunteer nature of ethics consultation impacts the educational preparation of consultants. The increasing availability of continuing education and certificate programs,

online training, and the movement toward privileging or credentialing consultants will likely lead to improved educational standards (Dubler et al., 2009).

In some institutions the entire committee convenes to discuss the case with providers, patients, and surrogates. Other institutions enlist a small group of committee members or consultants. The committee models allow collective expertise of consultants to improve the quality of the consultation; however, they also tend to be less nimble than the individual model.

Sometimes multiple models are employed depending on the type of consultation. For example, an individual consultant may call a committee meeting when one party (usually the care providers) strongly recommends withholding or withdrawing treatments it believes are medically futile, but the other party (usually the family) strongly believes that treatments are beneficial and should continue.

The process of ethics consultation

In cases like Zelda's, where all options entail suffering and no option seems "good," parents and providers still have to make choices. Ethics consultations are often called when trust between parents and providers is in jeopardy. Ethics consultants try to foster honesty, candor, sympathy, respectful communication, and a spirit of collaboration rather than confrontation. The consultation offers a fair process and fresh perspective to explore value differences. Hence the oppositional stance of both parties may ease, shared values can be embraced, and a commitment to resolution can be refreshed. Ethics consultants *collaborate* with providers and parents to forge ethically sound compromise and discover new strategies and options. We help everyone understand the ethical rationale for various options so that primary decision-makers can make more informed and ethically sound decisions.

To ensure fairness, and in keeping with guidelines from *The Core Competencies for Healthcare Ethics Consultation*, all involved in making treatment decisions for a child, particularly parents, should be informed of and included in the consultation (Fletcher & Moseley, 2003). However, a recent survey of pediatric ethics consultation services found that only 73% "usually or always" meet with the patient and family (Kesselheim et al., 2010). There are a variety of ways that parents can be included in the consultation: one-on-one discussions with the consultant, by including the consultants in patient care conferences with parents, and/or by inviting parents to the consultation meeting with providers. With the guidance and collaboration of parents and providers, the perspectives of older and more mature children should be sought when the ethics consultation pertains to their care.

The ethics consultation process itself sometimes reduces the moral distress that providers and parents feel by naming and explaining the issues that have given rise to the distress (Tiedje, 2000). Ethics consultants begin by trying to sympathetically understand all points of view. Only after listening to first hand perspectives do we scrutinize and analyze the various points of view, guided by ethical norms, the bioethics literature, and our professional experience.

The consultants in Zelda's case quickly recognized the moral distress providers, especially the primary nurses, were feeling. "(We) empathized with the immediate caregivers' suffering as they attended to a baby they could not heal but could only attend to through a protracted and painful process of dying" (McCormick & Woodrum, 2008, p. 23) Treatment in the neonatal intensive care unit often entails suffering for the baby – less human touch and parental bonding as well as pain and discomfort from invasive treatments and underlying diseases. It is not inflicting pain per se that causes moral distress, provided providers are doing their best to minimize it, but rather the realization that there was no positive trade-off for the suffering – no promise to ameliorate symptoms or cure Zelda. Proportionality is the ethical requirement to balance a "reasonable prospect" of benefit with tolerable, unduly excessive harms (Beauchamp & Childress, 2001). To the providers and the ethics consultants, continuation of ICU-level support did not meet the requirements of proportionality.

Likewise the consultants sympathized with the parents, recognizing their inclination to advocate for anything that might prolong their child's survival. Through the course of the consultation, it appeared that the parents erroneously believed that continued treatment might improve outcome or allow time to improve prognosis. Or perhaps they just could not bear to stop the only measures that were keeping their baby alive. As anguishing as shifting to comfort care might be for parents, Zelda was dying inevitably and imminently. None of the treatments could stop that, but one treatment plan could bring some measure of peace through her final hours or days – a shift to comfort care. The unanimity with which treating providers shared this perspective is compelling for the ethics consultants

because it suggests that prognosis was quite certain. Very often the clinical picture is more ambiguous, leading to multiple ethically defensible courses of action. But that was not the case here. The conclusion that the best treatment option is palliative care is well supported as reflecting the best interest of the child, even in the face of the parents' legitimate claim that they are the legal decision-makers.

Standards for ethics consultation

Many providers have little or no experience with ethics consultations and they may have expectations that are best clarified or dispelled early. I often advise callers that the purpose of the consultation is to understand the rationale for various values and perspectives, give everyone involved a chance to voice their opinions and concerns, and to collectively imagine courses of action and compromises that might lead to resolution of the conflict. The ethics consultant *facilitates* this collaborative process, helps to clarify values that inform various perspectives, identifies areas of agreement and disagreement, and provides an ethical analysis with reference to bioethics and medical literature as well as relevant policies. He or she makes recommendations designed to inform and improve the *decision-making* of parents and providers. I emphasize that we are not judges and we never usurp the authority of the attending physician and the parents to make final decisions. We play an advisory role.

Because ethics consultations are designed to clarify values – which takes time – ethics consultations are not usually efficient in medical emergencies. Occasionally the consultant may be able to promptly provide general education, but in a clinical emergency, providers should address the ethical conflict as best they can and then enlist the consultation service in a debriefing/educational session after the fact.

Steps to resolution of Zelda's case

In the ethical analysis of Zelda's case, McCormick and Woodrum likely investigated and placed a note in the chart documenting the answers to the questions below. Ethics consultants should be mindful of the distinction between *clinical* and *ethics* recommendations. The ethics consultant's recommendations should not *direct* clinical care, although they might certainly *influence* it. For example, a recommendation to remove the ventilator directs clinical care, and suggests that the ethics consultant has usurped the legitimate authority of the attending physician to make clinical decisions. In contrast, statements such as those below frame the recommendations in terms of the ethical analysis and impact patient care indirectly by influencing the judgments of the primary decision-makers.

Do the parents misunderstand the diagnosis and prognosis? Sometimes teams or providers inadvertently convey optimism that may be misconstrued by parents. A doctor might be encouraged that Zelda was more comfortable one day, but the parents interpret her optimism as a sign of recovery. The consultant might suggest designating one provider to communicate with family. In addition, the parents' perspective may be grounded in misinformation (which can be corrected) or in deeply held values about the meaning of suffering that can be explored in depth (as in Zelda's case).

Can the baby's pain be better managed while on the ventilator? The moral distress of providers is primarily generated from their part in inflicting and witnessing Zelda's pain (a violation of the duty of nonmaleficence) without prospect of benefit (in keeping with their duty of beneficence). If pain could be better managed, this could allow parents more time to come to terms with Zelda's terminal illness and for them to say goodbye. This might also be achieved with time trials, where clinical interventions are continued for short periods of time and parents and providers come together to determine whether the benefits each hoped for were achieved during the trial period.

Are there other ways to reach agreement? If the parents do not change their minds, whose decision should prevail? The courts are likely to focus on the procedural question of "who should decide" rather than "what should be done," thereby favoring parental decisions and not directly addressing the best interest concerns raised by providers (McCormick & Woodrum, 2008). If the underlying reason for the parents' position is that a choice for comfort care is tantamount to abandoning their child, they may be persuaded if an experienced doctor with good communication skills compassionately *tells* the parents *why* they plan to shift to comfort care and *how* they will honor some of the parents' values in doing so, rather than burdening parents with a false choice between a treatment no provider finds therapeutic (and therefore need never be offered) and the sole therapeutic option. Parents should have a say in *how* the comfort care plan will be implemented. If these strategies fail, then legally the parents' decision prevails.

Ethics committees

McCormick and Woodrum brought Zelda's case to the ethics committee. The ethics committee concurred with the consultants' recommendation to shift to comfort care. This demonstrates a primary function of ethics committees to peer-review ethics consultations. Ethics committees also serve to review and/or draft institutional policies, educate hospital employees and the public, and contribute to the quality improvement of the institution as a whole (Hackler & Hester, 2008). Hospitals, hospices, long-term care facilities, health systems, and some community clinics have ethics committees. The Joint Commission on Accreditation for Health Care mandates that health care institutions have a mechanism for staff and patients to seek guidance on ethical issues (Caulfield, 2007). In most hospitals, the ethics committee fulfills this function. In this capacity, the ethics consultation service may be under the guise of the ethics committee.

The ethics committee is made up of a multidisciplinary group of professionals employed or affiliated with the institution, which may include physicians, nurses, social workers, administrators, bioethicists, chaplains, lawyers, and community members. Service on the committee is usually voluntary or by appointment. Those interested in bioethics may volunteer to serve, or representatives from key constituencies may be appointed or invited. The chair of the ethics committee is often a member of the professional staff with reporting responsibilities to hospital leadership. Policies vary as to who can serve as the chair and to whom s/he reports.

By culture and policy, ethics committees typically play an advisory role, providing guidance to clinicians, surrogates, and hospital leadership designed to inform clinical and institutional decision-making. Because ethics committees and consultation services are enlisted when ethical conflicts emerge, they need sufficient freedom to make recommendations that may be unpopular. Members of the committee should honestly and openly address the conflict of interest posed by trying to provide a fair process inclusive of vulnerable families while still functioning as a hospital committee, whose health and success is partially dependent on the good graces of hospital leadership.

Ethics committees are often charged with drafting or reviewing hospital policies such as do-not-resuscitate orders, "Baby Doe" guidelines, withdrawing and withholding treatment (including medical futility policies), informed consent, confidentiality, surrogate decision-making, organ donation, and charity care policies. It is also imperative that ethics committees draft policies and/or bylaws governing the committee itself, which address the committee's mission, scope, and responsibilities. Policies should address how the consultant is contacted, the timeframe for a response or initiation of the consultation, the consultant's role and responsibility, and the limits of the ethics consultation (e.g., it will not be a mechanism to address patient or professional complaints).

Finally ethics committees educate health care professionals and the public. First, committees educate themselves. New members may be asked to read selected articles and books or attend continuing education programs to prepare them for their work on the committee. Likewise ethics committees often engage in ongoing professional education by setting aside time at meetings to review pertinent literature or by having annual retreats or workshops.

Second, committees educate hospital staff through employee orientation, bioethics grand rounds, and other educational activities. Committee members also educate during the normal course of their clinical activities and they debrief/consult with health care professionals when ethically challenging cases arise.

Third, the committee may educate patients, families, and the public. Admission packets may describe the nature of the consultation service. Patients are educated during the course of a consultation and in educational sessions on advance directives, for example.

Ethics committees also contribute to the quality improvement of the institution. Some ethics committees, notably those involved in larger health systems or academic medical centers, provide expertise on organizational ethics issues and assess the efficacy of informal and formal educational and consultation work.

Resolution of the case

Although the ethics committee concurred with McCormick and Woodrum's recommendation to discontinue life-sustaining therapies and shift to comfort care, Zelda's parents chose not to heed that advice. The ethics committee enlisted the hospital administration to consider whether a *parens patriae* legal appeal was warranted. This approach allows the court to take over medical decision-making from parents if the court believes that the parents are not acting in the best interest of Baby Zelda. After reviewing case law, hospital counsel determined that the courts would be unlikely to intervene, therefore supportive care continued along with more aggressive pain management, and Baby Zelda died several days later on life-support systems. McCormick and Woodrum (2008) conclude that court action fosters adversarial relationships and is almost never appropriate, because it undermines opportunities to come to a consensus that honors the best interest of the child.

References

Aulisio, M.P., Arnold, R.M., & Youngner, S.J. (eds.) (2003). *Ethics Consultation: From Theory to Practice*. Baltimore: The Johns Hopkins University Press.

Beauchamp, T. & Childress, J. (2001). *Principles of Biomedical Ethics*. Oxford: Oxford University Press.

Caulfield, S.E. (2007). Health care facility ethics committees: new issues in the age of transparency. *American Bar Association, Human Rights*, **34**(4).

Dubler, N.N., Webber, M.P., Swiderski, D.M. & Faculty and The National Working Group For The Clinical Ethics Credentialing Project (2009). Charting the future: credentialing, privileging, quality, and education in clinical ethics consultation. *Hastings Center Report*, **6**, 23–33.

Fletcher, J.C. & Moseley, K.L. (2003). The structure and process of ethics consultation services. In *Ethics Consultation: From Theory to Practice*, ed. M.P. Aulisio, R.M. Arnold, & S.J. Youngner. Baltimore, MD: Johns Hopkins University Press.

Fox, E., Myers, S., & Pearlman, R.A. (2007). Ethics consultation in United States hospitals: a national survey. *American Journal of Bioethics*, **7**, 13–25.

Hackler, C. & Hester, D.M. (2008). Introduction: What should an HEC look and act like? *Ethics by Committee: a Textbook on Consultation, Organization, and Education for Hospital Ethics Committees*. Plymouth, UK: Rowman & Littlefield Publishers.

Kesselheim, J.C., Johnson, J., & Joffe, S. (2010). Ethics consultation in children's hospitals: results from a survey of pediatric clinical ethicists. *Pediatrics*, **125**, 742–746.

McCormick, T.R. & Woodrum, D. (2008). When a baby dies in pain. In *Complex Ethics Consultations: Cases that Haunt Us*, ed. P.J. Ford & D.M. Dudzinski. New York: Cambridge University Press.

Task Force on The Core Competencies for Healthcare Ethics Consultation (2011). *Core Competencies for Healthcare Ethics Consultation*, 2nd edn. Glenview, IL: American Society for Bioethics and Humanities.

Tiedje, L. B. (2000). Moral distress in perinatal nursing. *Journal of Perinatal and Neonatal Nursing*, **14**, 36–43.

Index

Printed in the United States
By Bookmasters